ESSENTIALS OF

CLINICAL LABORATORY SCIENCE

ESSENTIALS OF
CLINICAL LABORATORY SCIENCE

John W. Ridley, Ph.D., RN, MT (ASCP)

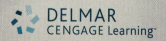

DELMAR
CENGAGE Learning™

Australia • Brazil • Japan • Korea • Mexico • Singapore • Spain • United Kingdom • United States

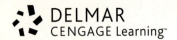

Essentials of Clinical Laboratory Science
John W. Ridley

Vice President, Career and Professional
  Editorial: Dave Garza

Director of Learning Solutions:
  Matthew Kane

Senior Acquisitions Editor:
  Sherry Dickinson

Managing Editor: Marah Bellegarde

Product Manager: Natalie Pashoukos

Editorial Assistant: Anthony Souza

Vice President, Career and Professional
  Marketing: Jennifer Ann Baker

Marketing Director: Wendy Mapstone

Senior Marketing Manager:
  Kristin McNary

Marketing Coordinator: Erica Ropitzky

Production Director: Carolyn Miller

Production Manager: Andrew Crouth

Content Project Manager:
  Anne Sherman

Senior Art Director: David Arsenault

For product information and technology assistance, contact us at
Professional & Career Group Customer Support, 1-800-648-7450
For permission to use material from this text or product,
submit all requests online at **cengage.com/permissions.**
Further permissions questions can be e-mailed to
permissionrequest@cengage.com.

Library of Congress Control Number: 2009934176
ISBN-13: 978-1-4354-4814-8
ISBN-10: 1-4354-4814-6

Delmar
5 Maxwell Drive
Clifton Park, NY 12065-2919
USA

Cengage Learning products are represented in Canada by Nelson Education, Ltd.

For your lifelong learning solutions, visit **delmar.cengage.com**
Visit our corporate website at **cengage.com**.

Notice to the Reader

Printed in the United States
1 2 3 4 5 6 7 12 11 10

CONTENTS

CHAPTER 2   LABORATORY PERSONNEL CREDENTIALING AND FACILITY ACCREDITATION   27

CHAPTER 3 MEDICAL LAW, ETHICS, AND MORAL
ISSUES OF HEALTH CARE   61

CHAPTER 7 | MEDICAL ECONOMICS AND LABORATORY EQUIPMENT 155

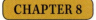 **CHAPTER 8**   PIPETTING AND USE OF GLASSWARE   185

LEARNING OBJECTIVES 185

KEY TERMS 185

CHAPTER 9   LABORATORY MATHEMATICS   207

CHAPTER 12 PROCEDURES FOR URINALYSIS AND BODY FLUIDS   287

PREFACE

Essentials of Clinical Laboratory Science is written in part to reflect the changing scope of duties and to enhance the professional image of the medical laboratory, but is intended primarily to improve the understanding of those entering the laboratory professions. Most ordinary citizens and even some health care professionals do not know what the terms *medical technician* or *medical technologist* even mean. Although these terms are still widely employed, they are changing. At least one professional certification agency, some state-sponsored programs, and various publications now use the terms *clinical laboratory technician* (CLT) or *clinical laboratory scientist*, respectively, as more reflective of a new image for these two basic levels of laboratory professionals. Perhaps the new names for laboratory workers will bolster the public's perception of what laboratorians do and the educational and training qualifications required. All professional agencies may soon use similarly descriptive names in the laboratory arena. For instance, the ASCP Board of Registry (BOR), formed from the 2009 merger of the National Credentialing Agency (NCA) with the American Society for Clinical Pathology (ASCP), now calls the technician level by the term *medical laboratory technician* (MLT) and the technologist level by the term *medical laboratory scientist*.

This textbook provides the background and rationale for the elements involved in teaching laboratory science and its associated skills. It focuses on providing a foundation for all aspects of laboratory medicine and should be taught early in the program schedule. Many who enter laboratory professions have no understanding of the necessity for accurate test values and the care that must go into developing and performing laboratory procedures. The values of efficiency, accuracy, and professionalism are adressed in this publication. Regulations, laws, and scope of practice issues are covered as well.

WHY THIS BOOK WAS WRITTEN

Essentials of Clinical Laboratory Science is designed to provide the primary knowledge and skills necessary to enable a smooth transition into the clinical laboratory profession for the medical laboratory scientist or technician.

Most introductory texts for clinical laboratory students seem to focus on the "how to" without laying the foundation on which all technical skills are built.

Teaching the basics of human anatomy and physiology, and how laboratory procedures correlate with abnormal conditions of the body, is a Herculean challenge. In addition, many laboratory technical students have little concept of the role of the laboratory within the context of the entire scope of a medical facility. As a compilation of information and experience gathered over 30 years, this textbook not only pulls together key physiological and interpretive knowledge, but also describes the basic operations of the medical laboratory and the health care facility in which it is an important and indispensable unit.

Through study of this material, both the medical laboratory scientist and technician will understand their respective roles and scope of functions as well as professional responsibilities when embracing a career in laboratory medicine. Even though primarily intended to train students to function proficiently in today's clinical laboratory, this book has other uses. It provides the kind of comprehensive knowledge valuable to the phlebotomist as well as other health professionals and students in a variety of occupational areas related to medicine. It could also be used as a resource for orienting health care professionals to the role that laboratory personnel play in overall health care. This book is an excellent primer on infection control and the organization of the health care industry. In addition, it covers the impact of morals and ethics on the legal system that governs health care services.

Medical personnel who perform basic tests in a physician's office laboratory or who perform regulated procedures included in point-of-care testing will also benefit from this book. Training in the basic principles of laboratory testing may soon be necessary even for those outside the traditional medical professions, as new and simpler instruments already available today will most assuredly enable a host of others, including patients, their families, and laypersons, to operate the equipment in sites other than a hospital laboratory.

As much as any other health care profession, clinical laboratory technology requires advanced scientific background and the ability to synthesize information and use critical thinking. Although no official statistics are available, it has been said that 80% of medical diagnoses are made or confirmed by laboratory values. The laboratory is the sleuth of the medical arena as a whole, and it is not unusual that a disease process initially suspected turns out to be totally different when laboratory values are weighed.

Standards for various states and educational institutions require differing competencies and objectives for preparing health care professionals for a career in laboratory medicine. In addition to certain shared duties and job requirements, certain requirements such as maintaining professional status and adhering to current safety practices in the laboratory apply equally to both the medical laboratory technician and the medical laboratory scientist. For instance, some sections of this book, such as the economics of health care and the laboratory in particular, might be more appropriate for the scientist-level student. The author has made every effort to prepare a book that will provide for any and all of these wide-ranging sets of duties for both the medical laboratory technician and medical laboratory scientist. Individual instructors will be able to easily gauge the appropriate level for their students due to the organization of the book.

ORGANIZATION OF THE TEXTBOOK

A topical overview in the early portions of this book acquaints the student of laboratory medicine to the beginnings of laboratory practice, how it has changed, and the requirements for entering into and being effective in providing valuable clinical services. Discussion of issues affecting laboratory workers and the role they may play in improving the profession and being flexible in accepting the changes that will invariably occur lay the groundwork for the latter part of the book. The book concludes with a presentation of basic manual procedures for all major departments of the clinical laboratory.

History of the Laboratory

The history of the development of medical laboratory technology is important; the new student should know some of the pioneers who were the first to discover or develop theories and procedures. *As Solomon's asserted [Ecclesiastes 1:9 (NIV):9]*, "What has been will be again, what has been done will be done again; there is nothing new under the sun." The birth of laboratory technology occurred thousands of years ago with the ancient Egyptian physicians and with medical practitioners in the Middle Ages who developed systematic procedures, although misguided in some respects, to diagnose various ailments.

Accreditation of Facilities and Personnel Certification

The competency of facilities as well as the personnel who are employed there must be documented. Licensure, mandatory accreditation, and voluntary accreditation are available to medical facilities and educational facilities that meet certain standards. Personnel are judged as competent practitioners based on the scope of their education and the successful completion of an examination for either licensure or certification.

Laboratory Duties and Professionalism

Some attributes that must be possessed or developed in the neophyte technician or technologist are paramount for success in completing the program of study and in a professional career. Certain intellectual abilities as well as certain physical abilities are required of the laboratorian to perform the broad range of laboratory procedures and activities. Professionalism is a less definable characteristic, but one that is gradually and necessarily learned by those who strive to provide efficiency and accuracy in their work.

Health Care Facility Organization and the Laboratory

The organization of a health care facility mirrors that of any large corporation. The laboratory falls under the general organizational chart as a separate department, with a supervisor overseeing it to provide quality, efficiency, and cost-effectiveness. Large medical facilities place a focus on departments such as the laboratory, which can help to cover the expenses of areas of the hospital that are not revenue generating. Therefore, the medical center provides for the administrative support of departments such as the laboratory on a facility-wide basis.

Safety in the Laboratory and Patient Areas

Safety is the responsibility of everyone in the laboratory, and at times it extends to the patient areas where the laboratory worker or phlebotomist might visit to collect specimens or to take possession of specimens collected by physicians and other health care workers. Safety in the laboratory includes handling of specimens and disposal of specimens after processing. The proper manner in which to dispose of specimens is thoroughly covered in this book, delineating the responsibility of the student, the instructor, and the health care workers with whom laboratory personnel interface. Not only biohazardous wastes, such as blood and other body fluids, but also bacterial growth for identification and sharp instruments must be discarded properly after use. Any accident that could include exposure to biohazardous or toxic materials must be investigated and documented properly, as well as other injuries that may occur in the course of the laboratory worker's duties. Other areas included in an overall safety plan are those related to adverse weather conditions, fire, release of toxic materials, and outbreaks of contagious illnesses that are treated in the hospital.

Infection Control

Infection control is a two-prong responsibility. Both health care workers and patients must be protected from becoming infected as a result of working with other patients or with equipment and wastes generated by providing patient care. Some of the requirements are mandated by government agencies for certain organisms called "covered" organisms (e.g., tuberculosis, human immunodeficiency virus, and hepatitis B virus). Large multidisciplinary committees within health care institutions have responsibility for developing policies and procedures for preventing and eliminating threats to those working in, visiting, or being treated in health care facilities. Representative samples from a simulated infection control manual are provided in this book to make the orientation to infection control more realistic and to avoid gaps in coverage of the topics that should be taught in this important area of health care.

Laboratory Economics

The economics of the laboratory are complex and contain a number of components. The laboratory exists primarily to serve the physician in diagnosing and treating various maladies. But in the economic scheme of the medical facility, the laboratory is mandated to be efficient and economically viable, contributing to the overhead for the entire facility. The methodology for testing, the equipment used, and even the manner in which the equipment is bought or leased are essential components of the laboratory's ability to fulfill its dual role as a major provider of diagnostic information and a "cost center."

Laboratory Mathematics

Mathematics learned during college-level prerequisites for enrolling in clinical laboratory courses provides the basis for a number of laboratory procedures requiring mathematical manipulation of raw results. An understanding of the English and metric systems, and of conversions from the "old" laboratory reporting units to the International System of Units (SI), requires a solid understanding of basic math.

Quality Assurance

The purpose of a quality assurance program in the clinical laboratory is to provide accurate and reproducible results and to enable the technical worker to troubleshoot and correct problem areas in the reporting of results. The development of quality control rules, as part of a quality assurance program, requires a thorough understanding of the terminology related to quality control and the other factors involved in the complete quality assurance program. Accreditation agencies will almost always examine the quality assurance records of not only the laboratory but also the entire medical facility.

CLINICAL LABORATORY PROCEDURES

The final seven chapters are devoted to an overview of each department of the hospital laboratory. The student should be aware of the divisions of anatomic pathology and clinical pathology and the roles and functions of each of these two major divisions. The area of testing in each of these departments is explained with an approach to aberrations in test results due to disease processes. The purpose of this book is not to train a technician or technologist to perform laboratory procedures. However, a few basic procedures are given in each area of the laboratory to learn to manipulate certain pieces of equipment and to orient the reader to the basic supplies used throughout a medical laboratory.

It is assumed that the laboratory student will have already completed courses in basic anatomy and physiology prior to delving deeply into the actual technical aspects of broad testing in all the departments found in a general clinical laboratory. The major areas where background information is presented and basic procedures are explained include phlebotomy, urinalysis and body fluids, hematology and coagulation, clinical chemistry, microbiology, immunology and serology, and immunohematology. The simple procedures demonstrated are intended to enhance the student's basic knowledge of each department and its function as a separate entity within the clinical laboratory.

ABOUT THE AUTHOR

John W. Ridley received a bachelor of science degree in zoology and a master of education degree at the University of Georgia. Earning a doctorate in health and human services, with an emphasis in psychology, and becoming a registered nurse in 1992 completed his formal education but not his practical education. During the Vietnam War, he was educated and trained in basic medical laboratory procedures at Brooke Army Medical Center, Fort Sam Houston, Texas. Military stints as a combat medic culminated in a promotion to colonel, with a position as chief of professional services and with command duty. He saw clearly that many rudimentary laboratory procedures, even when performed outside with little equipment, were extremely vital to the welfare of the troops, which whetted his desire to learn more.

Other life experiences that colored his approach to this work included working alone as a relatively untried technician while attending college and "pulling call" at a medium-sized hospital while working toward his technologist credentials. His advance from bench tech to laboratory manager and at one time part-owner of a private laboratory informed and inspired him to produce the best-prepared professional laboratory worker possible.

Upon entering the teaching profession in 1992, the author found his niche. After a few years of teaching academic science courses as well as starting two MLT/CLT programs, Dr. Ridley determined that any student for any health care program needed certain basic core knowledge in a variety of areas prior to entering or concurrent with the beginning of the medical laboratory program. His wide experience as a medical technologist combined with skills from nursing and human services contributes to a unique blend in the composition and writing style of this book.

CHAPTER 1

History and Development of Medical Laboratory Science

INTRODUCTION

There is no specific starting point when laboratory techniques were first used in diagnosing disease states in humans. Small steps were taken thousands of years ago, and occasional faltering steps have been taken throughout the centuries since, that have defined the profession and have marked progress toward formal education and training of laboratory professionals. Arguably, a comprehensive use of laboratory techniques along with other medical practices may have arisen when there was a need to screen large numbers of people who may have been harboring contagious diseases and who immigrated to the shores of the United States. Since these humble beginnings of the medical laboratory profession, when a small building was erected on Ellis Island to perform rudimentary health checks on immigrants to this country, a perceived need for screening methods for infectious diseases in such groups has been present. Although laboratory procedures were not new at this time, the processing of these groups of people with a set protocol for screening them for infectious diseases may have originated here.

The health screenings at ports of entry to the United States possibly represented the first efforts by a government agency to provide basic laboratory procedures of a broad scope. Eventually, these efforts revealed a need for the training and credentialing of medical laboratory workers to exercise knowledge and skills for detecting the presence of disease. These efforts, in a sense, initiated the first attempt to diagnose diseases in persons immigrating to the United States to prevent contagious diseases from being brought into the country and causing a catastrophic epidemic. Today, those immigrating to the United States are required to be free of certain diseases and to have undergone vaccinations before official entry.

During the early history of our country, those coming across the Atlantic Ocean to North America spent weeks and months on the high seas, sometimes confined in the holds of ships. The close proximity of the passengers was quite effective in fostering the transmission of diseases to other passengers before reaching the North American shores. The need for protecting our country against the incursions of contagious diseases that might lead to epidemics soon became apparent. So the beginnings of clinical testing and possible government influence began at that time to enforce regulations related to health. Early in the history of the United States, federal agencies became active in the quest for better health of the citizens of the United States and protection of them from infectious diseases. Discoveries by scientists of the time were incorporated into the diagnosis and treatment of diseases as they became available, and some research was funded by the federal government. An example of early efforts by the government included research by Walter Reed, whose name persists through a major U.S. Army military hospital that is named in his honor.

In the early 19th century, legions of French soldiers were attacked by yellow fever during the 1802 Haitian Revolution. Large numbers of French soldiers died as a result of infection by an organism for which the means of transmitting the disease were not understood. Outbreaks followed by thousands of deaths also occurred periodically in other locations of what is now the Caribbean and South America. Research that sometimes included and was fatal to some human volunteers led to the discovery that transmission to humans occurred chiefly by the bite of an insect vector, a mosquito, and led to the development of a vaccine and other preventive efforts in the early 20th century.

In the beginnings of clinical testing to diagnose disease states and to assess effectiveness of treatment or recovery, the physician performed his own tests in his office or in the patient's home. But as the number of diagnostic tests available and the sophistication of test methods grew, the physician was forced to rely on personnel trained to aid him in his diagnoses by performing the necessary tests, and in some instances, to interpret them, rather than just using the senses to diagnose maladies of the human body. To develop as a profession, though, appropriate training and education followed by credentialing of prospective candidates were becoming necessary. Later in this chapter, some specific milestones will be listed as important events that might have led to what we know as clinical or, if preferred, medical laboratory, technology of today.

It was not until the 1930s that a great deal of attention began to be focused on the clinical laboratory, not only for infectious processes but also for other metabolic tests for diagnosing diseases. The laboratory has now grown into a mandatory part of diagnosing a disease and monitoring its prognosis. The physician often depends on timely and accurate medical laboratory results as important and major tools for diagnosing and treating a patient. The clinical laboratory and the radiography department are the two major disciplines involved with diagnosing, confirming the diagnosis, and monitoring the prognosis for ill patients. But those simple medical laboratory procedures originally performed by the physicians themselves were not as specific as those of today nor were they sensitive enough to yield any important information of significance. However, a few of those early tests were forerunners to several of the modern test procedures performed in today's laboratory. In a few recognizable cases, the old names are still used to an extent. Some names of those early researchers will be listed later in this chapter, and will be heard again in the courses designed to teach technological procedures in the laboratory.

These early pioneers, whose research led to certain procedures and reagents used for laboratory tests, based their procedures on observable changes in body fluids, cells, and tissues. In the case of the majority of disease processes, there are changes in at least some laboratory test values. These values may be either abnormally low or abnormally high for levels of certain components of the body fluids, signifying a disruption of the body's functions. These changes enable a physician to either confirm or disprove the physical findings, as they may support an entirely different diagnosis than the initial signs and symptoms suggested. In many cases, such as in a routine physical exam, test results might provide the clinical findings diagnostic for a physical disorder when no specific clinical observations were initially found. So, in a sense, the technical workers of the laboratory are similar to clinical detectives who look for clues. Additional laboratory tests are often required to confirm earlier findings by completing different and more specific laboratory procedures.

Early History and Birth of a Profession

Laboratory testing of a very basic and simple nature began centuries ago, well before efforts to control the entry of contagious diseases into the United States. In the ancient written history of humankind, many findings have been discovered that related to diagnosing diseases by testing of body fluids, and some of these are recorded in detail. Parasites and eggs of parasites were discovered in the feces of humans thousands of years ago in the more civilized countries, and infectious diseases related to clinical signs were also observed and recorded several hundred years ago. In ancient Egypt, diabetes mellitus was diagnosed by determining if there was a high level of glucose in the urine of patients; this excreted product was known to attract ants. It is also probable that some physicians tasted the urine specimens from their patients, if spoken accounts are to be believed, to determine if the patient had an abnormal amount of glucose in the urine.

Early in the history of the United States and in other countries, blood-letting was also an acceptable treatment, as it was believed that "bad blood," or **humors** (liquids of the body), could be removed by bleeding the patient. These crude procedures were practically the only tests available for the physician for centuries. Many advances were made, including basic specimen examinations, to improve the practice of laboratory medicine, particularly during the latter part of the Middle Ages. As a multiplicity of diagnostic tests became available and more sophisticated test methods were devised, the physician in all probability found it effective to pass on his knowledge to assistants and other physicians and to rely on personnel trained to aid him in his diagnoses by performing the necessary tests, some of which required an interpretation of results.

Many of these earlier developments and discoveries were eventually incorporated into routine laboratory procedures. Some of the procedures developed by physicians were obviously shared with others, but it sometimes was years after the technology became available before the knowledge was disseminated. And, as with other types of technology, it often takes many years to develop and refine some of the equipment used to perform laboratory examinations. But today's technological advances have changed the very face of laboratory practice with regularity, although many of the basic tests from years ago, such as urine analysis and blood counts, still comprise the bulk of routine testing. In the late 1600s, a significant event occurred that provided a great deal of impetus to the diagnosis of disease. **Anton van Leeuwenhoek** (October 24, 1632–August 30, 1723) was credited with the development of the first compound microscope, although there is some evidence to the contrary, and this instrument was sufficient to enable one to observe blood cells, **protozoa**, parasites, **ova and parasites**, and some bacteria.

Marcello Malpighi (March 10, 1628–September 30, 1694), who was also working with clinical specimens in the 1600s, no doubt used Leeuwenhoek's microscope or earlier versions to begin some of the first pathological examinations so common today. During the 1800s, cell theory and bacteriology were established with the help of the microscope, and it was discovered that bacteria could cause a whole host of devastating diseases. More rapid technological advances for laboratory medicine have also become available as a result of progress in space technology and military and industrial needs, where equipment used in those areas was adapted to perform medical laboratory procedures. For example, the development of small, solid state equipment was no doubt spurred by the need to monitor physiological and anatomic changes in astronauts as they operated in a foreign environment. An example of an industrial need being adapted for the medical laboratory is that of particle counters originally used to measure the purity of industrial compounds. Electronic impedance when a particle passes through a small aperture in the instrument originally used in industry was adapted for use as blood cell counters that were eventually refined to enumerate various sizes of cells. These original developments have resulted in more sophisticated and accurate test results on thousands of constituents of the body that provide useful medical results for which tests have been developed. And it is certain that many more tests will be developed in the near future due to ongoing research.

Some other important advances that are valuable in laboratory testing include **infection control** by effective cleaning and sterilization of work areas and equipment and supplies used. A significant contributor to the field of bacteriology is **Joseph Lister** (April 5, 1827–February 10, 1912), a British surgeon. Lister determined that germs (bacteria only) could be killed by carbolic acid. It was determined at this time that many deaths in hospitals were related to the unclean conditions of the health care facilities. Lister demanded that surgical wounds be kept clean and that the air in the operating rooms be kept clean and circulating. The number of deaths related to complications of surgical procedures diminished dramatically when these changes were instituted. These practices eventually found their way to the battlefield, and the soldiers who underwent amputations in military facilities in the field began to benefit from the developing knowledge of **microorganisms**.

> **Infection Control Alert**
> **Infection and Exposure Control Measures**
> - All health care facilities are required to have a plan.
> - Plan describes what to do if an exposure occurs.
> - Hand washing is the most basic and essential measure for protection.
> - Extensive procedures in place for effective sanitation of health care facility.

Timeline for Evolution of the Clinical Laboratory

Changes in the practice of medicine roughly parallel the increasing sophistication and technological advances of the clinical laboratory for the diagnosis and confirmation of pathological conditions. Some conclude that advances in technology have dictated that medicine should become more scientific and less subjective in diagnosis and treatment, with so many tools, such as a wide range of laboratory tests, becoming more widely available. Laboratory medicine is interwoven into the fabric of the practice of medicine and cannot be separated from clinical laboratory practice because it is an intrinsic component of medical practice.

Three distinct periods of medicine parallel three different places and methods of diagnosis (Berger, 1999). The first medical diagnoses involved conditions that could be directly seen and observed through the senses of the physician, and sometimes rudimentary inspections of human specimens were involved. Early physicians, as mentioned previously, paid heed to the fluids or humors of the body, and occasionally the term *vapors* was used, based on the odors of various elements such as the breath of the patient. As early as the 1300s (Berger, 1999), physicians routinely used uroscopy, or visualization of the urine. This more than likely referred to the observation of the color, taste, and odor of the urine and had not changed much since the discovery of recordings of these practices from several hundred years BC, until the latter years of the Middle Ages. In 1684, with the advent of the microscope, Leeuwenhoek's publication of drawings of bacteria appeared, and specimens were examined for the presence of bacteria, and more than likely cells, which are much larger than bacteria and more microscopically complex, were also observed. It should be noted, however, that optics were experimented with as early as 1267 CE, when Roger Bacon may have produced the first microscope (Berger, 1999).

During the first period alluded to by Berger, substantial numbers of observations were made by physicians, including Hippocrates, who is known generally as the "Father of Medicine" (Berger, 1999). As early as 400 BC, and as mentioned before, urine was typically poured on the ground, and if it attracted ants, patients were assumed to be diabetic. Sometimes a skin condition called boils would be the first sign of diabetes. Boils are skin eruptions that heal poorly and are caused by bacteria that use the high levels of glucose in diabetic patients. Hippocrates basically advocated the use of the mind and senses as his primary tools for diagnosis, and the use of the senses extended to the study of the urine for bubbles, color, and taste, as primary laboratory tests. He also noted conditions other than those associated with laboratory testing, such as lung sounds, skin color, and any other outward physical signs that appeared abnormal as part of the assessment of the patient.

Further advances from ancient medical practices were then halted for almost a thousand years, when, in the Middle Ages, early religious figures believed that disease was punishment for misdeeds or the result of witchcraft or demon possession. Treatment consisted of religious practices such as prayer to a higher being, penitence, and praying to saints. During the Middle Ages, roughly 500 to 1450 AD, few advances were made, but the widespread and continued practice of the examination of urine persisted. However, during the latter years of the Middle Ages, investigation of diagnostic tools and the development of equipment again became more prevalent.

There are many notable advances in medical devices and other discoveries, some of which affected the laboratory, during the 17th through the 20th centuries. A few of these still bear the names of these early pioneers of medicine who blazed a path into the era of modern medicine. The developments of individual test methodologies are scattered throughout the past 100 years and are so numerous as to make it impractical to list them all (Table 1-1).

Laboratory tests were developed for the diagnosis of diseases such as cholera, typhoid fever, diphtheria, and tuberculosis and were performed by the physicians. The knowledge of these disease entities was made possible more than likely by the use of a microscope. A considerable period would elapse before specific treatment, such as the use of antibiotics for these diseases, would be available. By the 1880s, Robert Koch's studies of microorganisms led to the culture of pure colonies of organisms. He determined that epidemics may occur as a result of the spread of these organisms via water, food, and clothing under the right conditions. Many of these early discoveries greatly affected the provision of early laboratory services.

Other Factors Contributing to Technological Development

In the 1940s through the 1960s, several researchers contributed basic information that has led to sophisticated laboratory methods and to the possibility of specific treatments for curing certain diseases such as cancer that previously were only treatable through extensive surgery, chemotherapy, and radiation therapy. A wide

Table 1-1 Landmark Medical Advances Impacting Clinical Laboratory Science

Contributor	Year	Contribution
Roger Bacon	1267	Experimented with optics, possibly developed first microscope
Hans Janssen	1590	Invented compound microscope
Anton van Leeuwenhoek	1684	Published drawings of bacteria seen with microscope
Gabriel Fahrenheit	1714	Developed mercury thermometer; Fahrenheit scale still used
Josef Leopold Auenbrugger	1754	Theorized that tapping on chest gave clues to tissue health beneath
Antoine Fourcroy	1789	Chemist credited with discovering cholesterol
Gerardus Mulder	1830	Worked with chemical analysis of protein from a variety of sources
Joseph Lister	1830	Quaker physician who introduced dark-field microscopy
James Marsh	1836	Developed test for arsenic
Karl von Vierordt	1852	Developed instrument to measure blood flow; led to hemocytometry
John Snow	1854	Devised first colorimeter based on Beer's law; led to spectrophotometry
Hermann Luer	1869	Developed glass syringe with "luer" lock for needle; used today
Max Jaffe	1886	Alkaline picrate method for determination of creatinine; used today
T. W. Richards	1893	Invented the nephelometer; still in use
Ferdinand Widal	1896	Developed agglutination test for typhoid organism; name used today
Otto Folin	1900	Clinical biochemist who developed methods such as Folin-Wu glucose
Christian Bohr	1904	Bohr effect; H+, CO_2 affinity for hemoglobin, effect on pH
H. J. Bechtold	1905	Developed a procedure called immunodiffusion (Berger, 1999)
ASCP	1922	American Society for Clinical Pathology founded in St. Louis, MO
George N. Papanicolaou	1928	Developed "Pap" smear for discovering cancer from vaginal swabs
R. Gabreus	1929	Erythrocyte sedimentation rate (degree of inflammation) (Berger, 1999)
ASCP Registry	1929	Board of Registry for certifying medical laboratory technologists began
Beckman Instruments	1930	Beckman Instruments founded in Ft. Wayne, IN; now Beckman Coulter
Bernard Fantus	1937	Founded hospital-based blood bank at Cook County Hospital, Chicago, Illinois
Electronic colorimeters	1940	Replaced visual colorimeters and became forerunner of spectrophotometer
Vacuum collection tubes	1946	Vacutainer collection tube developed and sold by Becton-Dickinson
Levy-Jennings Chart	1950	Quality control (QC) chart in use today adapted from Shewhart QC charts
Technicon Corporation	1959	Initial "autoanalyzer" developed to streamline chemistry testing of blood serum
Becton-Dickinson Co.	1961	Disposable syringes and needles developed
Medicare and Medicaid	1966	Initiation of federal insurance system, greatly impacted laboratory testing
DuPont Co.	1968	First random-access autoanalyzer introduced
J. Westgard	1973	Quality control rules for acceptance of test results; in effect today
CLIA 88	1992	Final regulations implementing Clinical Laboratory Improvement Act begin
Regionalization of laboratories	1994	Large commercial laboratories form cooperative networks
Professional status	1995	National Labor Relations Board rules medical technologists are professionals

range of approaches are being developed that show promise against diseases that have previously resisted treatments to effect a total cure. Some and perhaps all cancers are known to have a genetic component, as certain families have a predisposition for developing a certain type. Gene therapy shows a great deal of promise by manipulating or replacing certain genes when defective copies are present. Laboratory tests are available that reveal certain tumor markers on cells indicating the type of cancer present, and these tests are constantly growing in number.

George Wells Beadle, Edward Lawrie Tatum, and Joshua Lederberg in 1941 were awarded the Nobel Peace in medicine for their discovery that genes act by regulating definite chemical reactions and specifically for the organization of the genetic material of the bacterium *Neurospora*. This was an apparent turning point in the understanding of the effect of genes and their expressions on gene-based diseases of living organisms. In 1962, James Watson, Francis Crick, and Maurice Wilkins jointly received the Nobel Prize in medicine or physiology for their determination in 1953 of the structure of deoxyribonucleic acid (DNA). Because the Nobel Prize can be awarded only to the living, Wilkins's colleague Rosalind Franklin (1920–1958), who died of cancer at the age of 37, could not be honored. Subsequent to this discovery, which enabled an understanding of the roles that genes play in physiology and metabolism, several other developments led to the sophisticated work in today's clinical laboratory. Current literature in the news and distributed by professional agencies for the laboratory such as the American Society of Clinical Pathologists is readily available to laboratory students and professionals. These publications provide data on a regular basis regarding recent developments that most likely will lead to a better understanding of genetic disorders. These advances may lead to the use of more genetic tests in the laboratory and may eventually become routine arsenals for the physician to use.

During the U.S. Civil War, many more deaths were caused by infection than by the severity of the wounds. Following this war, many practices that had developed during the internecine struggle, such as transportation of the wounded by ambulance for treatment behind the lines in a house, other building, or tent, were adopted by the civilian medical community. This model for quick and effective treatment persisted into World War I and evolved into rapid treatment in sanitary facilities for the wounded soldier. World War II and the Vietnam Conflict in turn contributed a great deal more of what has been learned through treatment of trauma, and these emergency techniques are being used in emergency departments and surgical suites of civilian hospitals to save many lives. Rapid and effective treatment for most trauma and for many infectious and metabolic diseases can be credited to efforts of the armed forces as they fought to preserve the fighting strength.

These major conflicts, especially the Vietnam Conflict, contributed heavily toward the development of rapid diagnostic tools, along with rapid treatment for trauma and battlefield administration of fluids and blood to save lives. Some basic laboratory testing using hand-held or portable devices was being performed in the field and in tents during the Vietnam Conflict in the 1960s and 1970s. Paramedics are now equipped with sophisticated instruments and equipment that were developed during wartime and adapted to civilian use.

Much was learned from the epidemics of diarrhea experienced during the Crimean War, where Florence Nightingale worked to provide sanitation in a humanitarian effort to achieve relief from suffering for large numbers of afflicted soldiers.

Many of these treatment practices that were borne out of necessity in times of grave danger for large groups of people have led to practical applications of medical techniques. Unfortunately, some of this knowledge of infectious diseases and toxins has also been used to develop threats of weapons of terror and mass infections of entire populations, instead of providing protection to them.

As a result of early efforts toward the development of technology to aid in diagnosing and treating diseases, large numbers of laboratories are currently available in the United States, including both general laboratories and some specialty laboratories. It is estimated that there are more than 189,000 laboratories that are licensed or regulated in a manner that allows them to come under the scrutiny of agencies that determine the competency of a laboratory. These laboratories range from small physicians' office laboratories (POLs) that perform only tests that do not require certified laboratory personnel to large commercial laboratories that perform reference testing for highly specialized tests that are expensive to perform. Hospital laboratories provide jobs for the majority of laboratory workers in the four major departments of a laboratory: hematology and coagulation, clinical chemistry, microbiology, and immunohematology (blood banking). Larger hospitals may provide a separate urinalysis department as well, although many hospital laboratories incorporate urinalysis into other departments. Some hospitals, especially those associated with schools of medicine, may have a number of highly specialized laboratories or specialized departments that may not be included in the four or five major divisions of a typical hospital laboratory.

> **Critical Reminder**
> **Regulation of Laboratories**
> - Laboratories are highly regulated.
> - Regulations may come from both federal and state governments.
> - Laboratories are licensed according to their scope of services.

Prior to World War I, there were few laboratory workers; most of those who did perform any type of medical laboratory work were usually the physicians themselves and at best possessed only rudimentary knowledge and equipment. Since the 1930s, a great deal of attention has been focused on the clinical laboratory, mainly because it has become increasingly important as a diagnostic tool. From the attempts of several professional registries that have become very active since the 1930s, to California's **personnel licensure** laws, many steps have been taken to control the entry of personnel into the medical laboratory field. Early efforts by various groups toward categorizing and determining minimum competencies of these candidates for licensure or registry in the medical laboratory profession were widely variable years ago and to an extent remain so today.

Early laboratory tests were much more cumbersome than those in use today, but due to professional activities by medical laboratory workers, the laboratories are much safer and cleaner and better equipped today than those of several decades ago. Laboratory animals were common in the past in the laboratory, as rabbits and frogs, for instance, were used for early pregnancy tests. Care and feeding of these animals were chores of the early medical laboratory workers.

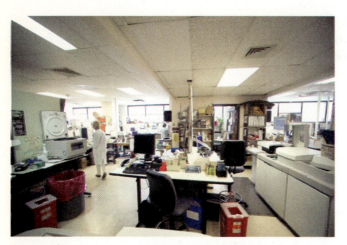

FIGURE 1-1 A modern clinical laboratory in a large hospital.
Source: Delmar/Cengage Learning.

Procedures performed today often do not require the use of animals to complete tests, except in research laboratories, as the methodology in hospital laboratories is much more sophisticated and is becoming more technically complex for most testing. The laboratory has evolved and is evolving into an even more sophisticated component of a large medical delivery system, as shown in Figure 1-1.

Lack of Recognition as a Profession

Even today, regardless of years of efforts by laboratory professionals, there is still a great deal of confusion, particularly in the general populace, as well as within health care facilities, with respect to the education, training, and hierarchy of laboratory professionals. The National Labor Relations Board (NLRB) bestowed professional status on medical laboratory technologists in 1995, but this has done little to elevate the stature of the profession. Many hospitalized patients and their families often erroneously assume that a person in hospitals who collects, transports, and processes the blood and body fluids is a "nurse" or some other unnamed medical worker. Few laypersons are aware of the diversity and numbers of laboratory tests performed on a regular basis. The duties of technologists and technicians are often the same in some facilities and further confuse the picture. Additionally, some states require personnel licensure to work in laboratories within these states, while others rely on professional registries to test and certify the competency of those entering the profession of laboratory medicine. California, as mentioned, has personnel licensure for laboratory technicians and technicians, but recently adopted the **American Society for Clinical Pathology (ASCP)** registry examination as the instrument to measure the knowledge and competency of those entering the medical laboratory profession.

States that have no personnel licensure requirements for laboratory workers are now subject to CLIA regulations. The Clinical Laboratory Improvement Amendments (CLIA) of 1988 are U.S. federal regulatory standards that apply to all clinical laboratory testing performed on humans in the United States, except for those tests performed in research laboratories with limited numbers and varieties of tests performed. A separate regulatory entity was created for administering the regulations legislated by CLIA 88. The Centers for Medicare and Medicaid Services (CMS) has the primary responsibility for the operation of the CLIA Program. In turn, CMS enforces implementation of the CLIA Program by the Center for Medicaid and State Operations, Survey and Certification Group, Division of Laboratory Services.

The CLIA Program sets standards and issues certificates for clinical laboratory testing according to the requirements of CLIA 88. CLIA defines the *clinical laboratory* as any facility that performs laboratory testing of specimens collected from humans to provide information used in the diagnosis, prevention, or treatment of disease or impairment, and for the assessment of health, such as in general physical examinations. The major objective of the CLIA Program is to ensure the accuracy, reliability, and timeliness of test results regardless of where the test is performed. Unlike some other accreditations, the CLIA Program is not voluntary, and hospitals and laboratories that collect federal funds from Medicare and Medicaid are required to fund the program. User fees collected from approximately 189,000 laboratories, as well as from physicians who accept reimbursement from Medicare and Medicaid. The majority of these laboratories are located in the United States, with a few in territories over which the United States may have a level of oversight.

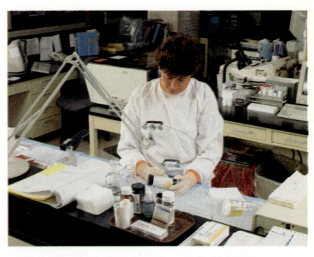

FIGURE 1-2 Performing urinalysis in a clinical laboratory. Source: Delmar/Cengage Learning.

Even the professional groups that offer voluntary credentialing of workers and that attempt to improve and to raise the standards of laboratory workers are divided as to levels of education and the length and breadth of educational processes for varying levels of workers within the laboratories. There are also differences relative to the need for ongoing efforts to ensure continuing competency throughout the career of the medical laboratory worker. Medical laboratorians in most cases work in large and well-designed facilities, as shown by a technologist performing analytical tests on urine samples (Figure 1-2). Testing personnel in the modern laboratory have a vast array of equipment and supplies at their disposal, and there is an increasing complexity of duties that seems to require an even more extensive educational background than previously. This should cause laboratory professionals on whom these increased requirements and responsibilities rest to seek more recognition.

EMPLOYMENT OPPORTUNITIES AS A MEDICAL LABORATORY WORKER

There are a vast number of areas in which one may find employment in a medical laboratory. There are also a considerable number of names or occupational specialties by which the laboratory professional may be classified, depending on where one works and the job position occupied. In addition, the various agencies and state licensing bodies will confer varying titles on the medical laboratory worker. While the majority of clinical laboratory workers are employed by hospital laboratories, there are numerous other opportunities for interesting and rewarding employment, ranging from the most common employment as a professional in the hospital setting to positions in the business sector as well as in educational institutions, and even in research or in legal categories of work such as in a state crime laboratory. Among these general categories of employment, there are numerous specialties within these overall areas.

Specific examples of some of these job opportunities are in government research laboratories or pharmaceutical companies that use medical laboratorians to produce data and compile research information for new medications and their effects on patients. Commercial reference laboratories are commonly used by hospital laboratories for seldom-requested tests and for special procedures that are not economically feasible due to the time, equipment, or supplies needed for the testing or that are beyond the abilities of the routine laboratories. To a lesser extent, POLs (which often provide for more flexible scheduling than hospital laboratories), state or federal crime laboratories, and the education setting are other avenues to pursue for meaningful employment. Laboratory professionals on all levels are gaining lucrative employment in sales for equipment and expendable supplies, product development, training of workers to use new equipment, and technical service departments of major manufacturers. An increasing need for medical laboratory workers of all specialties and designations has spurred the enrollment of greater numbers of students pursuing a laboratory vocation in the past few years and is continuing.

ESSENTIAL TASKS OR PHYSICAL REQUIREMENTS

What is meant by the term "essential tasks"? The **National Accrediting Agency for Clinical Laboratory Sciences (NAACLS)** requires a list of essential tasks from the facilities with medical laboratory programs that a medical laboratory worker must be able to perform to work in a clinical setting. The Americans with Disabilities Act (ADA) spells out the requirements for working with persons with a disability. It is against the law to discriminate on the basis of a physical or mental disability, *provided the person can perform the essential tasks of a position.* Prospective candidates for a degree in medical laboratory science cannot be denied entrance into a program based on a disability. But ADA requires that the student must be informed of the clinical work required, including tasks that may prevent the student from completing the clinical portion of the education and training. This list must be provided as part of the counseling for new students entering the program for either technician or technologist training.

Certain physical traits are required to master the broad requirements of being a laboratory professional. Good eyesight or good corrected eyesight is of absolute necessity, and normal color vision is also required, as some test results are dependent on colors that are produced in reactions and in the identification of stained cells and crystals. The ability to sit at a microscope or stand at an automated instrument, among other job requirements, may be impossible for some persons. Overall physical health is also important because the worker is in contact with both specimens from and sometimes works directly with patients who have infectious diseases. A person with an immune system deficiency would be well advised to avoid this profession for obvious reasons. Some strength is required to handle containers of reagents and solutions as well as to physically manipulate large pieces of equipment on occasion. Manual dexterity is one of the physical traits that would be at the top of the list for physical attributes.

Intellectual Requirements

Most medical laboratory training and education programs are based in community colleges, technical colleges, or universities. Generally, community colleges offer an associate's degree with an emphasis in medical technology for technician-level training; technical colleges also prepare students for the technician level. Universities or senior colleges offer a bachelor's degree in medical technology or related majors and award a 4-year degree for technologists (also called clinical scientists); some offer both types of degrees. To gain entrance to an associate's degree in many community colleges or the bachelor's (4-year) degree laboratory program, it is required that the applicant score sufficiently on an entrance examination such as the SAT or the ACT.

Some institutions require a second examination to gauge interest and ability, along with a psychological component to estimate the presence of personality traits and other abilities. An example of such a test is the one offered by the Psychological Services Bureau (PSB), which gauges the student's ability to learn materials that would equip him or her for this demanding program. Students should have an interest in a broad science curriculum as well as in mathematics to navigate the courses required to complete a program in medical laboratory technology. Licensure or registry tests of a comprehensive nature are also required on completion of the college program to work as a laboratory professional. The tests to assess the competence of the graduate of a medical laboratory program include more than the application portions of the program. Theoretical knowledge of basic procedures and a broad academic base are necessary. Programs for technologists and technicians are among some of the most challenging career fields in the health care professions.

Medical laboratory workers must be equipped mentally to pay attention to detail to be successful. Accuracy is paramount in the work, and it is not unusual to find it necessary to recheck one's work when doubts arise or the worker is questioned regarding the validity of results reported. A good technical worker must be orderly in his or her approach to the work and must be able to prioritize to organize the workload efficiently. It is not unusual for a medical laboratory worker to prioritize the workload to determine which work should be completed first when a large and stressful workload is scheduled. These workers must be able to work independently and make decisions, and have an inherent ability to know when the clinical picture does not match the results.

Much of the work is performed on automated, computerized equipment, so a good working knowledge of computer systems aids the worker in performing preventive and routine maintenance as well as performing repairs when necessary. This set of abilities enables the worker to avoid large periods of downtime when equipment is malfunctioning or to troubleshoot problems while under the stress of needing to report results as quickly as possible. Patients' well-being depends on the diligence and high level of integrity and responsibility the technician or technologist must possess. Laboratory work ranks high in the list of stressful occupations by demanding high levels of accuracy in performance while being under extraordinary time limits in some cases. A high level of stress invariably results when equipment is not working satisfactorily, the laboratory is short-staffed, and the physicians and the other clinical workers are demanding results on an immediate basis (called "stat"). Even under the stressors listed, laboratory workers are expected to produce accurate results in a timely manner.

Image Projected by Laboratory Professionals

Social status is often associated with one's profession. Few laypersons and medical workers, including phlebotomists, are aware of the knowledge required to become a medical laboratory worker. Many patients and visitors are unfamiliar with the role a medical laboratory technician or technologist plays on the health care team. Pharmacists and nurses, to name a couple of medical professions, have done a great deal to raise their stature as professionals, but laboratory professionals have not accomplished as much in that area. Fragmentation of educational and training standards have possibly harmed the progress of the profession and the raising of the public's consciousness regarding the value of medical laboratory workers. The various registry bodies that provide certification for laboratory workers sometimes still appear to be at odds with each other, even while purportedly pursuing the same goals. During the past 30 years, little progress has been made to cure these ills, despite the efforts of many laboratory professionals and sometimes politicians (CLIA 67 and 88) to push for consistent standards and requirements for this important component of the medical care industry.

Some of the reasons for the lack of progress in moving the profession forward lie in the apathy of many of the workers themselves. There are still some medical laboratory workers who were "credentialed" by the old government programs initiated by the U.S. Department of Health, Education and Welfare, which has evolved into the Department of Health and Human Services. Others attended a 1-year program decades ago that credentialed them as "technologists" with no college-level academic preparation. Some credentialing agencies maintain that certain academic requirements are unreasonable obstacles to some persons aspiring to become laboratory workers. Regardless of whether these issues are real or perceived, some activity must be taken to provide consistency between the differing factions for credentialing or licensure. Most professions require a college degree, so many consider this to be a precondition for entering the training portion of a clinical laboratory program. For the past few years, the American Society for Clinical Pathology (ASCP) and the **American Society for Clinical Laboratory Sciences (ASCLS)** have worked with the **National Credentialing Agency for Laboratory Personnel (NCA)** to form a unified front in dealing with these problems. In December 2008, an agreement was reached that resulted in several committees beginning work to resolve any differences between these groups. But until these groups and their members grow to such proportions that collective efforts will produce positive results, the situation will likely not change.

Advances in the Laboratory for the Future

As the medical detective of the health care industry, the laboratory worker has an almost unlimited range of opportunities for employment. Laboratories are growing dramatically in physical size as well as in the level of technology offered and the equipment available for efficient and accurate results. The real growth of medical laboratory work began following World War II, and since then, the level of technology for laboratory procedures has become increasingly complex and technical in nature, calling for even more well-trained and educated workers. Laboratory tests now are as essential as the specialized radiological and surgical procedures available in modern facilities. Advances are occurring, with the laboratory evolving and changing in response to the new discoveries that were at first possible only in university and government research laboratories facilities but then were quickly tailored to be provided in hospital laboratories and other treatment centers around the country.

Some of the most exciting advances are being made in **molecular biology** and **nanotechnology**. Some sophisticated methods in these fields are already making their way into general hospital laboratories. Laboratory scientists will soon be performing more genetic testing than was ever dreamed possible. Medications will be tailored to the **genetic predisposition** of the patient with regard to allergies and amounts of medication needed. The numbers of receptors on individual cells of the body are under genetic control and may dictate the amounts and types of specific medications needed. Immunological testing and treatment involving the stimulation of or production of specific antibodies against cancers and other maladies are likely in the near future. Continuing education and retraining will be commonplace in the modern medical laboratory.

More testing is done today than was ever performed previously. This is made possible by automation, which allows fewer workers to perform more procedures and to perform them more efficiently and accurately than in the past. It was initially thought that automation and the advent of robots, as well as **point-of-care testing (POCT)**, would put many medical laboratory workers out of a job, but the opposite is true. More sophisticated and more highly trained and educated practitioners in the medical laboratory are required to perform these highly skilled procedures, which in many cases require some interpretation and critical thinking in their performance. The job outlook for medical laboratory practitioners appears bright, and the field is projected by some to be one of the most in-demand occupations in the country, with shortages forecast for the next several years.

PERSONNEL CERTIFICATION

What is meant by the term "personnel certification?" *Certification* itself is a word that indicates a legal document that is designed by an official office or agency to indicate a person or facility has met certain published standards. For a person, this would mean that a prescribed course of study or training is required and perhaps culminates in an examination to document that certain competencies have been achieved. For a facility, policies are established and procedures are developed based on the policies, and these processes result in the meeting of standards developed by an accrediting authority for facilities, such as a health care facility.

In medical education and training, there are three levels of education and training, all of which result in certification of individuals. The first and primary level is that of the certificate, which is earned for a lesser level of training and education than for those of the next two categories of certification—the diploma and, ultimately, the college degree. Examples of the three levels of certification most often seen are as follows:

	Category of Certification
Certified Nurse Assistant	Certificate
Licensed Practical Nurse	Diploma
Medical Laboratory Technician	Associate Degree

Certification is a term, therefore, that can be ascribed to those who complete a *certificate*, those who attain a *diploma*, and those who attain a college *degree*. Other terms also apply to becoming certified. Registered nurses were once "registered," which indicates they appeared on a registry indicating they had met the requirements for becoming a registered nurse. This term persists even though registered nurses are now *licensed*, another form of certification. Nurses are licensed by the states, but the states generally use the same professionally developed exam for documenting competency as a professional nurse. Professionally developed tests are often the same from state to state and are used to determine demonstrated knowledge, rather than each state developing its own test. Some states require personnel licensure of laboratory workers, while others require that the workers be registered laboratory workers. Issues involved with becoming registered or licensed will be explored fully in this section.

Official Regulation of Medical Laboratories and Workers

For an occupation to develop as a profession, education and training are required. In reality, some so-called professions are actually trades that require only technical skills with little or no educational background. It was not until the late 19th and early 20th centuries, in large part, that it was realized that credentialing of prospective candidates was becoming necessary. It is generally agreed that the first medical laboratory and teaching of pathology occurred at Johns Hopkins Hospital during the late 19th century. Only relatively recently, during the 20th century, did the growing push toward credentialing of medical laboratory workers receive attention. Since the 1930s, when California adopted personnel licensure laws for laboratory workers, a great deal of attention has been focused on the clinical laboratory by both government agencies and professionals within the field. Much of this attention was fueled in the 1950s and 1960s, when public money began to be expended for laboratory reimbursement, causing governmental oversight to increase, and erroneous laboratory results were brought to light. With the increasing importance of laboratory tests, it became increasingly important to ensure the accuracy and effectiveness of laboratory testing for health care professionals who are treating patients. This focus led to the implementation of CLIA 67 and the final regulations, entitled CLIA 88.

In 1922, the first formal recognition of the medical laboratory profession came when a group of 39 physicians laid the groundwork for the American Society for Clinical Pathology (ASCP) with the objective "to promote the practice of scientific medicine by a wider application of clinical laboratory methods for the diagnosis of disease." This seems to have spurred the efforts in California to require licensure of laboratory workers before other states focused on the need for ensuring competence of laboratory workers. It was widely reported on April 20, 1999, that poor training of a phlebotomist had led to a situation where an uncertified health care worker had exposed several thousand patients to used needles. At that time, California legislators began efforts to require certification of phlebotomists because of an incident when a person performing phlebotomy was found to be rinsing out used needles and reusing them. Because laboratory workers and phlebotomists have a great deal of job interrelationship and both professionals may be responsible for collecting specimens, certification of phlebotomists is also important to clinical laboratory workers. Following the lead of California, three other states (West Virginia, Connecticut, and Kentucky) introduced bills requiring certification of phlebotomists, but none of the bills made it out of committee. Massachusetts has a bill to establish a board of registration for phlebotomists, and efforts are continuing with active involvement by residents of that state. A bill in Missouri was introduced in both the Missouri House of Representatives and Senate, but never made it out of committee in 2008 (Ernst, 2008).

Credentialing and Certification of Medical Laboratory Technical Workers

As opposed to laboratory personnel licensure, which is a nonvoluntary process required predominantly by state governments, most states (with several exceptions) do not require licensure of medical laboratory personnel. This issue will be covered in other areas of this book. Certifying or credentialing bodies operate independently of government agencies but do require knowledge of government regulations and laws in the administering of examinations to determine the competency of candidates for credentialing.

The major agencies that provide for testing of those who have completed educational and training programs are the American Society for Clinical Pathology (ASCP), the American Medical Technologists (AMT), and the National Credentialing Agency for Laboratory Personnel (NCA). Along with the American Society for Clinical Laboratory Sciences (ASCLS), a professional society that does not provide for testing of personnel but focuses on professional matters affecting medical laboratory workers, ASCP and NCA have joined forces and ASCLS is a partner in these collaborative efforts to form a united front for certifying, testing, and supporting the profession. Titles differ between the major agencies, with AMT and ASCP using the titles "medical technologist" (MT) and "medical laboratory technician" (MLT), while NCA currently uses the titles "clinical laboratory scientist" (CLS) and "clinical laboratory technician" (CLT) (Table 1-2). In October of 2009, a merger between NCA and ASCP was completed. The new professional designations will be MLS for Medical Laboratory Scientist, a bachelor's level educational program, and MLT for Medical Laboratory Technician, an associate's degree program.

Table 1-2 Comparison of NCA Certification Categories and Equivalent ASCP Categories

NCA Designation	ASCP Designation
CLS, clinical laboratory scientist	MT, medical technologist
CLT, clinical laboratory technician	MLT, medical laboratory technician
CLSp, clinical laboratory specialist	S, specialist
CLSup, clinical laboratory supervisor	DLM, diplomate in laboratory management
CLPlb, clinical laboratory phlebotomist	PBT, phlebotomy technician

Issues Related to Licensure

Professional credentialing agencies and state governments may differ in the standards required for laboratory workers. In extreme cases, some authorities question whether any standards at all are needed that lead to any sort of certification. Laboratory professionals who are aware of the importance of educational and performance standards do not subscribe to this sentiment, which is espoused mostly by administrative personnel. Obstacles to "defining" professionals that are either real or perceived abound. There is a school of thought by some laboratory managers and directors that no educational and training standards are necessary. The contention is that technology has provided the means by which to perform sophisticated procedures merely by manipulating equipment, and the operators need no professional level of knowledge or credentialing. Individual perceptions even by some candidates entering the profession of laboratory medicine obscure their view of the value of academic and theoretical knowledge provided by educational programs. This group may include some state government officials who, instead of developing a body of knowledge, focus solely on the practical, hands-on skills, but this view is not as prevalent today as it was in the past. Some of the concerns of employers with health care facilities and others regarding certification are as follows (NAACLS, 2008):

- Fear of increasing salaries and thereby increasing costs of operation
- Perception of utilization of overqualified personnel
- Perception that minimally skilled persons can run tests by merely "pushing buttons"
- Fear of upsetting salary and wage schedule for other health care professionals
- Lack of understanding of laboratory functions and personnel qualification levels and responsibilities
- Threat of licensure as contributing to loss of control
- Belief that a qualified medical director can oversee laboratory operations and therefore more-skilled and higher-level personnel are not needed
- Fear of encroachment on physicians' turf by more highly educated workers

As laboratory procedures became more important in making a diagnosis, the laboratory professionals seized the initiative and began to take basic steps to ensure competency of laboratory technical personnel, with some efforts beginning at the end of the 19th century. Several agencies have become very active since the 1930s, when California initiated personnel licensure for medical laboratory professionals. Attempts from the beginning by professional groups ranged widely in their approaches and state and federal government offices were not consistent in applying standards developed by professional registering agencies. State government regulations requiring licensure of clinical laboratory workers exist in a relatively small number of states. Some of these states will accept those registered by the major registering agencies as being equivalent to licensure, while others do not and require a licensing exam even for those who have been certified for a number of years.

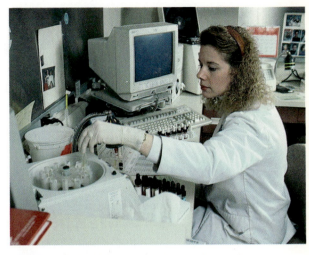

FIGURE 1-3 Clinical laboratory professional at work. Source: Delmar/Cengage Learning.

Since the earliest efforts, many steps have been taken to control the entry of personnel into the medical laboratory field. Work positions in the laboratory (Figure 1-3), standards for excellence in education and training, and scope of practice regulations that categorize and determine minimum competencies of candidates for licensure or registry have become increasingly stringent in the medical laboratory profession. Clinical laboratory personnel are now recognized as professionals in an ever more complex field by the National Labor Relations Board (NLRB).

DUTIES OF THE MEDICAL LABORATORY WORKER

The typical laboratory worker may work in a variety of settings, ranging from large commercial laboratories that are sometimes specialized to hospital and clinic laboratories, crime laboratories, or physician's office laboratories. Many POLs do not perform tests of sufficient complexity to be required to use only registered or licensed laboratory personnel. The simple tests they conduct are termed "waived" and are basic tests that require little or no interpretation. They are allowed under federal regulation to be performed by personnel with minimal training and education. These categories of testing will discussed later in this book.

Most laboratory workers find employment in hospital laboratories. Hospital and clinic laboratories contain four general departments: hematology and coagulation, clinical chemistry, immunohematology (blood banking), and microbiology. Simple and routine slide tests and examination of urine samples may be performed in separate departments in larger facilities or may be incorporated into one of the four major departments. Some large laboratories may have a dozen or more departments where specialized testing is done in specialized laboratories areas by qualified personnel.

There are two major categories of laboratory worker in the United States who perform medical laboratory procedures. The MLT may also be known as a CLT depending on the work-site policies or the credentialing agency that certified the worker. Some government agencies also have their own set of descriptive job titles for laboratory workers.

This profession demands the ability to move from task to task, attention to details, and the ability to work well under pressure with samples of the various body fluids, such as blood, sputum, feces, and tissue specimens. With supervision by medical technologists, MLTs perform complex examinations on body fluids and waste products.

Major categories of tasks performed routinely by MLTs and CLTs in the majority of medical facilities are the preparation and staining of a variety of slides with various types of stains designed to stain specific components of body fluids. They perform routine chemistry tests on blood, tissues, and fluids and perform counts of various cell types. MLTs keep official records of results and perform quality control procedures to ensure accuracy of results. They use a variety of laboratory equipment such as computers, microscopes, and analytical equipment to gather data used to determine the absence, presence, extent, and cause of diseases. As they gain experience, MLTs are often given more responsibility and may progress to performing more complex tests. Technicians generally are associate-degree–level personnel who have completed an academic and clinical course of study leading to a specialized degree. Almost all states require that the technician successfully complete a major credentialing test or that the technician be licensed by the state, if licensure is required by a particular state where personnel licensure laws have been adopted. Technicians most often perform routine tests that are repetitious and must work under the direct supervision of a technologist. Areas of specialization in the medical laboratory include clinical chemistry, hematology and coagulation, immunohematology, microbiology, serology, and urinalysis.

The MT may also be known as a CLS for the near future, again dependent on the policies of the work site and credentialing agency. At least a bachelor's degree based on both academic studies and clinical training are required to become a technologist. The technologist must be organized and work independently while supervising other categories of laboratory workers such as technicians (MLT or CLT). Good problem-solving skills with critical thinking are required, and the ability to work well under pressure is important. Medical technologists must be able to recognize abnormalities in the functions of instruments during the analysis of patient specimens. They are responsible for monitoring, screening, and troubleshooting analytical systems for calibration, quality control results, and constant monitoring of results. To maintain the integrity of the entire laboratory process, the medical technician or technologist must be capable of recognizing factors or errors that could be or have been introduced into the test results and rejecting samples and reagents that are contaminated or not performing properly.

MTs and CLSs are the technical experts who have great input into the functions of nearly every laboratory. They ensure a well-run operation by providing reliable results and controlling the quality of results obtained. These technical experts also provide training and supervise laboratory technicians and laboratory technology when students are assigned to their facility during clinical practice. They provide data so that physicians and researchers can determine the presence and extent of disease as well as evaluate the effectiveness of treatment.

Technologists use microscopes, a variety of laboratory analyzers, computers, and various pieces of complex equipment for certain procedures in the course of their duties. MTs and CLSs may also prepare and study body tissues and fluids, although there is a category of worker, either a histologist or cytologist, who is responsible for preparing and testing surgical specimens and some cellular preparations as a separate professional category. Laboratory professionals test for the presence of bacteria, therapeutic drugs, and drugs of abuse and for diseases, such as leukemia, diabetes, cancer, and HIV/AIDS. They possess the theoretical and scientific background necessary to understand the reasons for performing specific tests and the significance of the results. Laboratory professionals who have a bachelor's degree often choose specialty areas such as microbiology, clinical chemistry, immunohematology (blood banking), immunology, drug testing, therapeutic drug monitoring, and biogenetics, among others. These professionals work in a variety of settings, often as supervisors of technician-level workers. Certain professional levels of education and training for specialization are available for the technologist. These specialty programs often require a master's or doctoral level of education for special procedures.

SCOPE OF PRACTICE

What is meant by the term "scope of practice?" The term is used by state licensing boards and by certifying agencies, such as those who "register" medical laboratory workers, for various professions to define the procedures, actions, and processes that are permitted for the licensed individual (American Society for Clinical Laboratory Science, 2001).

The scope of practice is limited to what the law allows for a person with specific education and experience and specific demonstrated competency. Professionals are expected to perform only those tasks for which they have been trained and for which they are responsible. Otherwise, there may be legal ramifications if a professional is operating outside his or her specific scope of practice. Each state has laws, licensing bodies, and regulations that describe its requirements for education and training, but not all states have the same limitations or scope of practice for certain professions. Governing, licensing, and law enforcement bodies are generally at the state level. In some cases, federal guidelines or regulations exist.

Why Differentiate between CLS/MT and CLT/MLT?

Not all employers attempt to differentiate between the various levels of laboratory professionals (National Accrediting Agency for Clinical Laboratory Sciences, 2008). Depending on the certification of the laboratory worker, different nomenclature for job titles is used. A laboratory worker with an MT designation is equal to the worker who is called a CLS. Requirements for these two categories are essentially the same. Laboratory professionals called CLTs or MLTs are likewise equal in status. In some medical facilities, a CLS/MT and a CLT/MLT have essentially the same duties and perform essentially the same functions.

Are the two levels of laboratory worker interchangeable, because some employers believe that they are and hire workers based on that premise? Or, regardless of level, should they be used for the same levels of tasks? These questions may seem simple on the surface, but they are difficult to answer and vary depending on the facility in which the worker is employed and, to an extent, on state in which the worker is practicing. And to further complicate the nomenclature used, in some areas of the country, a CLS/MT is called a CLS and a CLT/MLT is called an MLT, to differentiate between the level that requires an associate's degree (MLT) and the one that requires a bachelor's degree (CLS). In answer to these questions, CLIA 88 regulations differentiate between levels of tests and between the category of laboratory that will perform them, as laboratories are classified as being qualified to perform "waived tests" only or moderate- and high-complexity tests. In some cases, a procedure for one type of test may be of a waived classification, while the same test using another methodology may fall under another classification.

Laboratory classifications are based on the difficulty of the tests performed, which is based on the complexity of the procedure, and laboratory personnel standards differ for each of the categories of testing. More complex tests require more training than do those that are of the waived variety. Each laboratory is classified and receives a CLIA certificate stating the category for which it is classified. There are five different certificates (Table 1-3).

Who Differentiates between CLS/MT and CLT/MLT?

Accreditation agencies that inspect health care facilities may review scope-of-practice requirements and determine what level of worker is assigned to various tasks. The agencies and organizations listed on the next page observe scope of practice policies.

Table 1-3 Types of Certificates Issued through CLIA 88 Regulations and Activities Performed under Each Category of Certificate

Certificate	Activity Permitted
Certificate of Waiver	Permits a laboratory to perform only CLIA-waived tests
Certificate of Registration	Permits the laboratory to conduct moderate- or high-complexity laboratory testing (or both) until the laboratory is determined by survey to be in compliance with CLIA regulations
Certificate of Compliance	Issued to a laboratory holding a Certificate of Registration after an inspection finds the laboratory to be in compliance with all applicable CLIA regulations
Certificate of Accreditation	Issued to a laboratory that has been accredited by a CMS-approved accrediting organization
PPMP	Issued to a laboratory in which a physician, mid-level practitioner, or dentist performs no tests of complexity other than the microscopy procedures; this certificate also permits the laboratory to perform waived tests

- Certification agencies' (NCA and ASCP) boards of registry differentiate.
- Many employers do not differentiate between CLS/MT and CLT/MLT for entry-level generalist positions.
- Accreditation agencies for education (NAACLS) differentiate the levels.
- CLIA differentiates the levels "beyond the bench."
- State licensing bodies differentiate between all levels of medical laboratory professionals.

Employment advertisements in professional journals recruit either a CLS/MT or a CLT/MLT for many generalist positions. During shortages of certain professionals, this may be done to provide hiring flexibility. It may not be feasible for an employer to hold a position open for a subsequent applicant with the appropriate certification level. The employer may decide that either level would qualify to meet the job requirements.

The level of education attained appears to be the prime factor in differentiation between levels in many institutions and not the actual categorical status. The job tasks for entry-level bench positions are the same regardless of certification level. On September 9, 2007, the governor of California signed the Aanestad Medical Technology Bill (SB 366) that is intended to provide for improved health care for California patients. A licensed CLT/MLT will be permitted to perform waived and moderate-complexity testing. Some employers also limit the worker to certain departments. For instance, the CLT/MLT may not be allowed to perform microscopic analyses and immunohematology tests, as some health care facilities make a distinction between levels by not employing a CLT/MLT for blood bank (immunohematology) work although this subject is taught in CLT/MLT programs. Major differences are outlined as follows (Table 1-4).

Testing for Credentialing of Various Levels of Laboratory Workers

Certification agencies have written professional-level definitions that differentiate between the CLS/MT and CLT/MLT. Content outlines and test items for certification examinations are derived from the professional-level descriptions. Certification agencies validate these categorical examinations by conducting practice examinations that provide a link between job performance and examination content. The results of the practice analysis for CLSs/MTs, CLTs/MLTs, and phlebotomists conducted in 2001 by ASCP's Board of Registry shows an overlapping scope of practice for many tasks performed by CLTs/MLTs and CLSs/MTs in the United States. In some clinical laboratories, though, only the CLSs/MT is allowed to perform the more-advanced technical tasks as a policy for that facility.

Accrediting agencies such as NAACLS, the premier agency for medical laboratory educational programs, write the educational and professional training requirements and standards for clinical laboratory science programs. The program standards delineate the level of training with specific content differences. CLIA is responsible for defining several routes for personnel specifications that qualify an individual for several positions within a clinical laboratory (i.e., laboratory director, clinical consultant, technical consultant, technical

Table 1-4 Differences in Technologist (CLS/MT) and Technician (CLT/MLT) Duties

	Medical Technologist/Clinical Laboratory Scientist (CLS/MT)	Medical Laboratory Technician/Clinical Laboratory Technician (CLT/MLT)
Education	Minimum of bachelor's degree	Associate's (2-year) degree
Duties	Clinical laboratory technologists may evaluate test results, develop and modify procedures, and establish and monitor programs, to ensure the accuracy of tests. In many laboratories, technologists supervise clinical laboratory technicians. Some states require that a technologist be available for technicians to report independent test results.	Clinical laboratory technicians perform less-complex tests and laboratory procedures than do technologists. Usually these are repetitive in nature and do not often call for subjective interpretation. Technicians often prepare specimens or operate automated analyzers with detailed instructions provided. Technicians may perform manual tests in accordance with detailed instructions. They most often work with supervision by medical and clinical laboratory technologists. Just as technologists do, clinical laboratory technicians may work in any of the several areas of the clinical laboratory or may specialize in one area.
Certification	Certification is provided by a number of agencies (e.g., AMT, ASCP, AAB)	Certification is provided by a number of agencies (e.g., AMT, ASCP, AAB)
Teaching	Accreditors of educational programs require instructors who are technologists/laboratory scientists. Some agencies require a minimum of a master's degree for a program director and for teaching.	Technicians are not qualified to teach the academic portions of medical laboratory programs by accrediting agencies for educational programs.
Specialization	Categorical specialization is available; these require a master's degree in most instances	Not available for technician-level medical laboratory personnel; requires MT certification; often a master's degree
Complexity of Testing	Perform tests of moderate- and high-complexity (CLIA rules)	Depends on facility; most technicians do not perform high-complexity tests
Supervisory Role	Departments supervised by MTs or CLSs	Technicians are not assigned supervisory roles in an official capacity

supervisor, general supervisor, and testing personnel). While CLIA has specified the qualifications for different personnel roles within a clinical laboratory, it does not differentiate the CLS/MT from the CLT/MLT. NAACLS revised the CLS/MT program standards in 1995, and again in 2001, to ensure that CLS/MT programs are preparing graduates to possess the skills set for the consultant and management job specifications as defined by CLIA.

NAACLS hosted a futures conference in September 2000 to profile laboratory professionals of the future and to differentiate the future roles of the CLS/MT and the CLT/MLT. The Executive Summary of the conference outcomes defines some of the responsibilities expected of the CLS/MT graduate in 2005: "Management opportunities will include laboratory supervision and coordination, laboratory finance issues and roles in compliance and reimbursement." "CLS/MTs as educators will educate the CLT/MLTs, staff, patients and the public. CLS/MTs will have opportunities in consultation, wellness programs, and public health. In 2005, will our CLS/MT graduates be prepared for the manager and educator roles? "

Many exceptional CLS/MT programs are preparing graduates with the advanced skills set needed for technical performance as well as management roles (National Accrediting Agency for Clinical Laboratory Sciences, 2000). When the new graduates arrive in the workplace, will managers provide positions so graduates can use these skills in addition to their technical skills, or will the basic core job tasks still be the province of the new graduates? In July 2000, the ASCP Board of Registry's prospective study of career patterns reported that in the first 5 years of practice, CLSs/MTs did acquire more advanced technical and management tasks but were still assigned mostly core tasks. Many CLS/MT programs have an introduction to management and education course(s) in their curricula. But is it sufficient to prepare them for the future, or is a generous amount of technical work a valuable component of preparing an advanced laboratory worker for a management role? With the CLT/MLT performing the majority of bench tests, it is possible that many MT/CLS personnel will eventually move to administrative roles early in their respective careers.

SUMMARY

Medical laboratories have evolved over a span of several thousand years beginning with simple observations by the physicians who also performed their own rudimentary laboratory "procedures." Mass screening of immigrants also lead to an understanding of infectious and chronic diseases and the awareness of tests to rule out a variety of illnesses. As laboratory procedures increased in number, a new profession was born in the early 1900s that required training and education. Inventions and research leading to improved methodology persists to this day that were initiated by early innovations and observations by scientists and physicians. The laboratory of today is one of the most technologically advanced departments within a major medical facility.

Clinical laboratory workers have a myriad of opportunities within the laboratory profession. The four major departments of the clinical laboratory afford the professional a choice of the basic types of work that are performed in a typical laboratory setting. An additional possibility lies in the histology and cytotechnology sections of the pathology laboratory, in which tissue specimens and cell preparations, respectively, are evaluated. These two choices usually require additional specialized training, and it is possible for technicians to transition into the pathology department, as some of the skills practiced by technicians and technologists are directly transferrable to the pathology section.

Most job opportunities exist in hospitals and clinics. Other good job opportunities exist in government and pharmaceutical research laboratories and in the armed forces laboratories, where both civilians and military personnel work side by side. Reference laboratories (where smaller laboratories send seldom-performed tests) and POLs are other potential sources of employment. Education, sales, and training for users of manufactured equipment offer good job opportunities with excellent pay and benefits.

Basic nomenclature for the two major levels of technical personnel of the laboratory differs, based on which accrediting body or registry is being used. MLTs registered in one agency may be known as CLTs in another. The same is true for MTs; they will be called CLSs by one agency and medical technologists by other accrediting agencies. There is also a blurring of the edges between duties performed by the two basic levels of personnel, and the job tasks depend on the clinical facility and its interpretation of personnel standards. Some states even license laboratorians and mandate what each category can or cannot do in the way of producing laboratory reports. Still other states have few or no regulations regarding the practice of laboratory personnel. This has resulted in years of competition between "registering" authorities and their own interpretation of laws and provisions.

Some laboratory tasks are physical and have certain essential tasks to perform that may hinder or keep some people with physical or mental disabilities from achieving a position in the laboratory. Accuracy is vital, and the ability to concentrate for long periods and to pay attention to detail is a must. The work may be stressful, and the ability to organize the work flow and to prioritize the tasks is essential. The laboratorian must also maintain a professional decorum as it is important for work with other health care professionals as well as with patients and family members. Few members of the public are aware of the hierarchy of workers, such as technicians and technologists, within the laboratory, or even of the existence of such a program of study. Even among health care workers, there is little knowledge of the extent of education and training the laboratory workers acquire. For this reason, is important that all laboratory workers be ambassadors for the profession.

REVIEW QUESTIONS

1. Name several locations where personnel may perform laboratory procedures. Not all who perform laboratory procedures will be clinical laboratory technicians and technologists.
2. Name the four general departments in the clinical laboratory.
3. What level of laboratory worker is required to supervise a department?
4. What are some attributes a medical laboratory technician or technologist must possess in order to be effective in the workplace?
5. What are some of the reasons that there is no consistency in the credentialing of laboratory workers?

CHAPTER 2

LABORATORY PERSONNEL CREDENTIALING AND FACILITY ACCREDITATION

LEARNING OBJECTIVES

Upon completion of this chapter, the reader will be able to:

- List the two types of pathologists.
- Describe a Ph.D. scientist and his or her role in the laboratory.
- Compare the duties of cytotechnologists and histotechnologists.
- Contrast the duties of cytotechnologist and histotechnologists with those of medical laboratory workers.
- Differentiate between the duties of the technician and the technologist-level laboratory professional.
- Compare the terms *licensure, certification,* and *professional registration.*
- Name the organizations chiefly concerned with the education of medical laboratory workers.
- Compare and contrast the requirements for medical laboratory technicians and technologists.
- List the reasons for seeking facility accreditation.
- Provide some of the components necessary for credentialing of medical laboratory workers.
- Discuss voluntary versus involuntary processes in licensure, accreditation, etc.
- List and discuss federal regulation of medical laboratories.
- Explain the licensure procedures that states use to regulate medical laboratories and provide examples.
- Discuss why some professional organizations might be against personnel licensure for laboratory workers.

KEY TERMS

Accreditation
American Board of Pathology
American Association for Clinical Chemistry (AACC)
American Association for Respiratory Care (AARC)
American Medical Technologists (AMT)
American Society for Microbiology (ASM)

American Society for Clinical Pathology (ASCP)
Anatomic or clinical pathologist
Association of Surgical Technologists (AST)
Cerebrospinal fluid (CSF)
Certification
Clinical Laboratory Improvement Act of 1967 (CLIA 67)

Clinical Laboratory Improvement Amendments of 1988 (CLIA 88)
Clinical Laboratory Management Association (CLMA)
College of American Pathologists (CAP)
Commission on Accreditation of Allied Health Education Programs (CAAHEP)

Commission on Colleges (COC)
Cytotechnologist
Director (medical laboratory)
Doctor of osteopathy (D.O.)
Equivalency testing
Health Care Financing Administration (HCFA)
Histotechnologist
Illinois Society for Microbiology (ISM)
Licensure

National Accrediting Agency for Clinical Laboratory Sciences (NAACLS)
National Credentialing Agency for Laboratory Personnel (NCA)
Occupational Safety and Health Administration (OSHA)
Pap smear
Pathologist
Physician office laboratory (POL)
Pleural, pericardial, peritoneal, and synovial fluids

Point-of-care testing (POCT)
Registration
Registry
Southern Association of Colleges and Schools (SACS)
The Joint Commission (TJC; formerly JCAHO)
U.S. Department of Health and Human Services
U.S. Department of Health, Education, and Welfare
Waived tests

INTRODUCTION

Laboratories have become complex and valuable assets for a medical facility. Organizational charts are needed for administration and for accrediting agencies, which require that lines of authority and of communication be formally established. Laboratories were originally only loosely organized, with the "technicians" working directly under a doctor of medicine. If a hospital laboratory was available at the turn of the 20th century, formal training and education of physicians practicing pathology and the technical personnel working within the facility were practically nonexistent. The laboratory was merely a minor tool in aiding in the diagnosis and treatment of diseases until roughly the first quarter of the 20th century.

Pathology training was not widely practiced in a formal manner until most likely the early 20th century. Massachusetts General Hospital (Mass General) has documentation of autopsies being performed as early as 1811 by surgeons and other physicians. However, it was not until James Homer Wright, director of the Department of Pathology at Mass General in 1896, came into the forefront of what we know as the practice of pathology that this field was embraced as a distinct medical specialty and that most hospitals established a pathology department that also encompassed the clinical laboratory as an adjunct to autopsies and tissue examinations (http://www2.massgeneral.org/pathology/history.htm). In today's laboratory, the pathology department includes the clinical laboratory and falls directly under the CEO of the medical facility, as shown in the organizational chart in Figure 2-1, which closely resembles the structure of most hospital laboratories today.

Clinical and Anatomic Pathologist/Director

The **director** of a medical laboratory is usually a **pathologist**, who has either an M.D. or a **doctor of osteopathy (D.O.)** degree and who is typically board certified by the **American Board of Pathology** as an **anatomic or a clinical pathologist**. Pathologists perform specialized procedures on tissues and cells from organs of

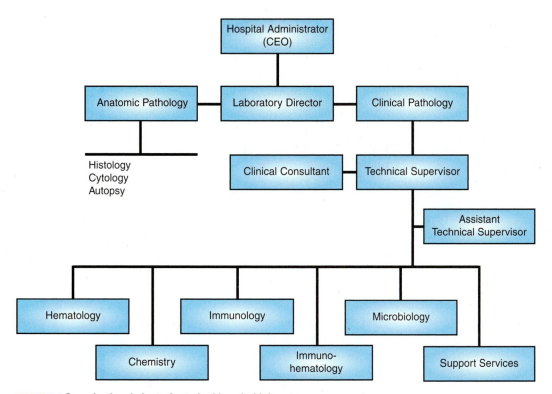

FIGURE 2-1 Organizational chart of a typical hospital laboratory.
Source: Delmar/Cengage Learning.

the body, as well as some of the more routine work such as evaluation of bone marrow. But an extremely important role of the pathologist is to explain clinical test results and their meanings to patients, family, and other physicians. A pathologist may function as either an anatomic pathologist or a clinical pathologist, or as both in smaller laboratories. A Ph.D. scientist may also serve as the laboratory director in most states, but pathologists must also direct the histopathological and cytological departments of the anatomic laboratory, as well as perform tissue and cell examinations.

Anatomic pathologists are responsible for the examination of all surgical specimens, including those from postmortem examinations. Quick tissue examinations from frozen sections while a patient is still in surgery is often performed by the anatomic pathologist and gives the surgeon an answer as to the probability of a tissue being malignant (cancerous), allowing more extensive surgery while the patient is still under anesthesia. The anatomic pathologist often works closely with **cytotechnologists** or **histotechnologists** in the preparation of and staining of cell specimens such as those from **Pap smears** and in finely slicing and staining tissue sections for examination to look for cellular inclusions or to assist in the diagnosis of cancer. Early diagnosis of cancer is made possible by the quick evaluation of these specimens, which often saves lives with early detection.

Some pathologists are trained in and practice a specialty called *clinical pathology*, which is also known as *laboratory medicine*. This is the medical specialist who coordinates the diagnosing of diseases by examinations and analyses of all body fluids, mainly plasma and serum. But urine, stool, respiratory or mucosal secretions, exudates from inflammation, and fluids from body cavities such as **pleural, pericardial, peritoneal, and synovial fluids,** as well as **cerebrospinal fluid (CSF),** are also important specimens used in the diagnosis of disease conditions. Clinical pathology focuses on the clinical laboratory rather than surgical specimens, which histotechnologists, cytotechnologists, and anatomical pathologists study. In modern clinical laboratories, most of the routine studies are automated and large amounts of data are quickly produced, requiring comparison and correlation of laboratory test results.

The clinical pathologist is responsible for overseeing the work of laboratory technologists and technicians. Quality assurance and, in particular, quality control programs are analyzed by select section supervisors under the direction of the clinical pathologist to ensure the validity of test results. Some clinical pathologists exhibit more individual interest in this area than others and review quality control results on a regular basis. These specialized physicians often perform interpretations of highly complex studies, but their chief role is to serve as a consultant to practicing clinicians to guide the treating physician in the proper laboratory examinations and to provide an interpretation of the results. Efficiency dictates that appropriate studies should initially be performed for both the diagnosis of a condition or the evaluation of a patient's prognosis or his or her current condition. In some areas, nonpathologists, such as other physicians or those with Ph.D. degrees, may conduct or supervise clinical laboratory tests and perform administrative and clinical activities within the medical laboratory, functioning in a role similar to that of a board-certified clinical pathologist.

Doctor of Laboratory Medicine (D.L.M.)

As a relative newcomer to the field, the doctor of laboratory medicine (D.L.M.) requires a Ph.D. in which many of the courses required of physician students are also required of this professional. The D.L.M. is knowledgeable in all areas of clinical laboratory medicine and operates in a consultative manner with practicing physicians in the interpretation of sophisticated laboratory tests.

Clinical Sciences Specialist

Clinical chemists, and clinical microbiologists in particular, are increasingly achieving a higher role than previously and are found in larger laboratories, research laboratories, and medical centers. These specialists often have a Ph.D. degree in a scientific area such as clinical chemistry and biochemistry, immunology, or microbiology. These specialists are sometimes hired at a master's degree level in their area of expertise, and then they pursue a 3- to 5-year doctoral program that requires a research project that is incorporated into a published dissertation. These scientists direct, manage, and supervise their particular departments since they have a greater body of knowledge about their respective fields than any other laboratory worker, including providing consultation with the pathologist. These

Critical Reminder

Job Opportunities

- Broad scope of practitioners in the laboratory
- Good career mobility within a clinical laboratory
- Technical personnel range from assistants to doctoral scientists
- Some professional positions require extensive education

specialists often consult with the attending physicians regarding the interpretation of laboratory findings in their department.

Laboratory Manager

In most instances, a laboratory manager has worked his or her way up the career ladder within the laboratory. The laboratory is usually a clinical laboratory scientist who has years of experience working with technical aspects of the laboratory and often has served as a departmental supervisor before becoming the manager. The manager of many of the larger laboratories has a master's degree, often in business management or a related field. The laboratory manager creates and manages budgets for all departments, with feedback from departmental supervisors. The laboratory manager ensures that scheduling is appropriate to cover all the departments for each day of the week. Input from the technical chiefs and the section supervisors provides appropriate departmental data to enable the managers to make well-informed decisions. The laboratory manager reports directly to the director, who is generally a pathologist, as stated earlier.

Clinical Laboratory Scientist/Medical Technologist

At this time, these titles are interchangeable and the particular title used relates to the agency certifying the worker or the facility in which the holder of the title is employed. Each department has a general supervisor or department head who is generally the most senior person in the department and holds the highest professional credentials and degrees. In the larger facilities, there are general supervisors on each of the three shifts. The clinical laboratory scientists supervise medical laboratory technicians and provide expertise in troubleshooting of equipment and procedures. They make decisions on the best methods to use based upon sensitivity, specificity, ease of performance, and economy. In moderate-sized to large laboratories, each department has a specialist such as for clinical chemistry, microbiology and immunohematology (blood banking). These are the specialists in the general practice of laboratory medicine and they provide training and orientation to new personnel but may also be able to perform most of the routine laboratory procedures in all the major departments of a laboratory. This category of medical laboratory worker will have at least 4 years of education and training before becoming certified or registered.

The clinical laboratory scientist (CLS), who is also known as a medical technologist (MT), possesses at least a bachelor's degree and is often required to be registered with one of the major organizations providing registration of medical laboratory workers. This level of worker is able to provide critical analysis, assimilating information and providing solutions to problems. He or she is able to confirm results based on instrument function records and able to correlate and interpret groups of test results as they fit the clinical picture. A technologist-level employee is generally by state regulations required to be present in any department when technicians are performing laboratory procedures. The technologist reviews and approves work by the technicians whom he or she is supervising. The establishment of effective quality control programs and the oversight of proficiency testing are important tasks for this category of medical laboratory worker. Technologists generally have the knowledge to work in all general areas of the laboratory if necessary but may confine themselves to one department and assume responsibility for their work as well as for those whom they supervise, the technician-level employee.

Technician-Level Medical Laboratory Worker

Technicians as Medical Laboratory Professionals and technicians employed in the medical laboratory generally possess at least an associate degree in medical laboratory science. They perform most of the routine laboratory testing and may work in any department. Technicians perform mostly repetitious tasks that do not require any modification of the procedures and are not responsible for making judgments as to any changes in organization of the laboratory or in choosing methodology. In many facilities they provide services as a basic "**bench tech**" and perform many of the same functions as the technologist level but without the decision-making responsibilities. They do not supervise other workers except in the case of laboratory assistants who perform no laboratory procedures but only ancillary duties such as clerical and inventory functions. Technicians work closely with phlebotomists, however, and may provide direction to them. Continuing education from outside organizations and inservice programs are required in most medical facilities for all categories of laboratory worker.

Phlebotomists

The name "phlebotomist" literally means *vein cutting*. The first basic step and perhaps the most important step is to attain a specimen that is adequate and appropriate for the required testing. A phlebotomist should be trained in a number of techniques for collecting blood. Phlebotomists usually are graduates of an approved phlebotomy program and the current trend is to require **certification** of the graduates of a formal program. Some of the agencies of **registry** for medical laboratory technicians and technologists, such as AMT, also provide for certification of phlebotomists but some are dedicated to certification of only phlebotomists. They must have a high degree of manual dexterity as well as good communication skills and considerable knowledge of laboratory tests and the specimens required, along with institutional policies. But some facilities provide on-the-job training in which a high school graduate is paired with an experienced phlebotomist, and most of the knowledge is of an informal nature through the gradual attainment of experience and practice. Most agencies require continuing education each year to maintain certification.

JOB DESCRIPTIONS FOR TECHNOLOGISTS AND TECHNICIANS

Broad lists of general responsibilities and duties that may be performed by technologists and technicians have some overlap in duties, and in most general laboratories job descriptions are the same or similar in the tasks performed. The profession demands the ability to move from task to task, paying attention to details, and working well under pressure while not having an aversion to body fluids, such as blood, sputum, feces, and tissue specimens. With supervision by medical technologists, medical laboratory technicians (MLTs) perform complex examinations on body fluids and waste products. They stain slides and perform routine tests on blood, tissues, and fluids. MLTs keep official records of results and perform quality control procedures to ensure accuracy of results. They use microscopes, computers, and other laboratory equipment to gather data used to determine the absence, presence, extent, and cause of diseases. As they gain experience, MLTs are given more responsibility and perform more complex tests. Possible areas of specialization in the medical laboratory include clinical chemistry, hematology, immunohematology, immunology, microbiology, and urinalysis.

The MT must be organized and be able to work independently while supervising other categories of laboratory workers. A combination of good problem-solving skills coupled with critical thinking, along with the ability to work well under pressure, is important. MTs are the supervisory personnel and technical experts of nearly every laboratory. They ensure a well-run operation by providing reliable results and controlling the quality of results obtained while training and supervising laboratory technicians. They provide data so that physicians and researchers can determine the presence and extent of disease as well as the evaluation of the effectiveness of treatment. MTs (also called CLSs) are skilled in the use of sophisticated equipment, most of which is computerized, and requires a knowledge of computer applications. The MT is a professional who performs diagnostic analytic tests on specimens, including blood, urine, stools, sputum, cerebrospinal fluid, and miscellaneous body fluids, such as pericardial, peritoneal, and synovial fluids.

Most technologists find employment in hospital laboratories, but other areas of employment include **physician office laboratories (POLs)**, commercial reference laboratories, research laboratories, and various positions within the biotechnology realm. Technologists most often work as generalists and are skilled in all areas of the clinical laboratory. MTs understand the theory behind the performance of specific tests and the significance of those results. MTs often choose specialty areas such as drug testing for therapeutic drug monitoring and drugs of abuse, biogenetics, immunohematology, microbiology, and biochemistry. MTs are the specialists in many departments of the laboratory and may possess graduate degrees pertinent to their field of expertise. Those who possess specialty credentials may use acronyms such as "SBB" for "specialist in blood banking" following their basic registry status of, for instance, MT(ASCP)SBB.

INTRODUCTION TO ACCREDITATION FOR EDUCATIONAL PROGRAMS, FACILITIES, AND PERSONNEL PROGRAMS

Accreditation groups are responsible for sanctioning both the medical facilities and educational programs. Accreditation is not focused toward individuals but toward entire facilities and programs. However, to be accredited, many of the accreditation agencies also require that any personnel working in or completing educational programs as students must have met certain standards—thus, the reason for combining these two separate entities. Although facility accreditation and personnel certification are separate entities, facility accreditation may require that personnel hired in various departments of the facility are certified, licensed, or registered, depending on the field in which the personnel are employed. Professional agencies exist for all medical professions, and they provide for some sort of evidence, usually by examination, that the various individuals have achieved a certain level of competence. Such documentation serves as evidence that the professional has met certain requirements to protect the public. This is a form of self-policing where the public can be assured that the accredited medical institution is examining the credentials for all workers at a health care facility.

Facility accreditation is entirely different from the certification of personnel due to the scope of services in a complex health care facility, which covers all aspects of the operation of the entire institution that is staffed by multiple professional employees performing in a wide range of departments. However, there are some parallels and some blurring of distinction between personnel **licensure** or registry and facility licensure or accreditation due to similar standards. Accreditation of facilities and educational programs is a voluntary act certifying adherence to certain standards espoused by the various accreditation bodies.

Although the accreditation process is "voluntary," the programs and facilities are not allowed in many cases to enjoy certain privileges and rights unless they "voluntarily" choose to become accredited. So, in some instances, the voluntary process of becoming accredited may be in essence an involuntary act. Most professionals in the health care field must personally hold certain credentials regardless of any other factors in effect such as overall accreditation of the facility. Typically, if professional agency standards are more stringent, for instance, than state personnel licensure, the stronger of the two sets of standards may take precedence. All of these categories of credentialing are similar in scope, with the exception of personnel licensure, which is most often mandated by the state government. For instance, some states have laboratory licensure but not personnel licensure for laboratory workers. These states may require that laboratory workers be formally certified to work in the licensed laboratory as one of the requirements leading to licensure of the laboratory. This would accomplish the same results as would personnel licensure.

Medical laboratory educational programs may operate under several facility-wide accreditation offices because the program includes clinical practice most commonly in a hospital laboratory, while the education portion of the program occurs on a college campus. The major accreditation body for facilities such as hospitals is **The Joint Commission (TJC; formerly the Joint Commission on Accreditation of Healthcare Organizations [JCAHO])**. This major accrediting body covers all of the departments and areas of hospitals that are accredited by TJC. Hospitals other than federal facilities most often require state licensure in addition to accreditation. As a further restriction, new hospitals can exist only after receiving a Certificate of Need from the appropriate government office, meaning that a survey was performed with an identified need for the facility before it is allowed to be built.

Educational Program Accreditation

Educational programs are also separately accredited as a type of facility accreditation. The agency responsible for the accreditation of most of the medical laboratory training programs in this country is the **National Accrediting Agency for Clinical Laboratory Science (NAACLS)**. A nonprofit agency called the **Commission on Accreditation of Allied Health Education Programs (CAAHEP)**, also accredits a number of medical programs while the NAACLS is responsible for accrediting educational programs for laboratory workers only. Several groups exist that specifically accredit each of the various medical programs around the country and are responsible for ensuring that the programs of training adhere to high standards set by members of the profession. Table 2-1 lists the agencies that accredit educational programs for clinical laboratory personnel.

There are many examples of other agencies that accredit or license departments other than the medical laboratory within the hospital and in educational institutions. The **Association of Surgical Technologists (AST)** provides accreditation for programs of surgical technology, and the **American Association for Respiratory Care (AARC)** exists for the education of respiratory therapists. Some educational facilities are accredited by regional branches of the **Commission on Colleges (COC)**, a *facility-wide form* of accreditation that covers the entire scope of operations for southern colleges and universities.

Regional Institutional Accrediting Agencies

Middle States Association of Colleges and Schools (MSA)
Middle States Commission on Higher Education

New England Association of Schools and Colleges (NEASC-CIHE)
Commission on Institutions of Higher Education

New England Association of Schools and Colleges (NEASC-CTCI)
Commission on Technical and Career Institutions

North Central Association of Colleges and Schools (NCA-HLC)
The Higher Learning Commission

Northwest Association of Schools, Colleges and Universities (NWA)
Commission on Colleges and Universities

Southern Association of Colleges and Schools (SACS)
Commission on Colleges

Western Association of Schools and Colleges (WASC-ACCJC)
Accrediting Commission for Community and Junior Colleges

Western Association of Schools and Colleges (WASC-ACSCU)
Accrediting Commission for Senior Colleges and Universities

Table 2-1 Examples of Agencies That Accredit Programs for Clinical Laboratory Workers

CAAHEP	Commission on Accreditation of Allied Health Education Programs (formerly CAHEA)
NAACLS	National Accrediting Agency for Clinical Laboratory Sciences
NCCA	National Commission for Certifying Agencies

This differs from the agencies that may require that individual programs be separately accredited by agencies such as AST, NAACLS and AARC even if the educational facility is also COC accredited. It should be noted that in the case of laboratory educational programs, some certification agencies such as ASCP for laboratory workers will only provide for certification of candidates who have completed an NAACLS-accredited program.

Facility and Departmental Licensure and Accreditation

Health care facilities and educational institutions are accredited and licensed separately and independently of laboratory personnel credentialing. In most, if not all, states, hospitals and medical clinics as well as physician's offices must be licensed. And sometimes individual and specialized departments within the health care facility must be separately licensed based on state or federal regulations. In addition, a veritable host of other organizations will provide accreditation for individual departments within the hospital. As an example, the medical laboratory is almost always required by most states to be licensed or is at least in some way regulated through state agencies.

But some departments within the clinical laboratory might also be required to become licensed, such as those performing nuclear medicine procedures. In addition, departments may seek voluntary accreditation for increased status on a categorical basis (Table 2-2). And quite frequently, the laboratory as a whole will also be accredited by the **College of American Pathologists (CAP)** with its own set of professional standards. Some federal agencies such as the **Occupational Safety and Health Administration (OSHA)** enforce regulations and inspections by local fire departments designed to protect the health of workers. These two

Table 2-2 Accreditation Agencies for Health Care Facilities and Educational Programs

Acronym	Title
AABB	American Association of Blood Banks (blood bank accreditation)
CAP	College of American Pathologists (laboratory accreditation)
CAAHEP	Commission on Accreditation of Allied Health Education Programs
COC	Commission on Colleges (regional [southern] accreditation for higher education)
COLA	Commission on Office Laboratory Accreditation (physician's office laboratories)
CHEA	Council for Higher Education Accreditation (nonprofit organization of colleges and universities serving as the national advocate for voluntary self-regulation through accreditation)
TJC	The Joint Commission (evaluates and accredits hospital laboratory services and freestanding laboratories)
NAACLS	National Accrediting Agency for Clinical Laboratory Sciences (international agency for accreditation and approval of educational programs in the clinical laboratory sciences and related health professions)
NCCA	National Commission for Certifying Agencies (accreditation of a variety of certification programs/organizations that assess professional competence)

agencies have little to do with personnel requirements or facility accreditation except that certain types of annual training may be required of the employees as a condition of employment under the category of inservice education.

While facilities voluntarily ask for accreditation to present themselves as abiding by a certain set of standards associated with given professions, becoming accredited does not substitute for licensure when a license is required by a government agency. The accreditation process for facilities that mostly includes hospitals may require that the facilities adhere to both institutional and state standards. These standards encompass a number of occupational areas in which they mandate that all personnel be certified in some manner by professional agencies. In a typical hospital, there will be specialized workers, of whom some are certified, some are registered, and some are state licensed.

Examples of these differing methods of documenting competence of the workers would include licensure laws for registered nurses, pharmacists, and many other professional groups working in a hospital. Medical laboratory workers are most often registered with a major body such as ASCP or **American Medical Technologists (AMT)**, although in a number of states, personnel licensure for laboratory workers is required. As of this writing, the following states require personnel licensure or require that licensed laboratories hire only credentialed personnel: Florida, Hawaii, North Dakota, Rhode Island, Louisiana, Tennessee, Nevada, New York, West Virginia, Montana, and Georgia. Some health care positions only require certification, in which the training program is normally shorter than those requiring college degrees. An example of a certified worker is the certified nurse assistant (can).

Personnel Certification or Licensure

It would be wise at this time to be reminded that the term "certification" may include achieving personnel licensure, meeting the requirements through a registry examination, or mere certification, which indicates a certain level of training but is something less than an academic diploma or degree. Merely attaining a certificate for laboratory workers is no longer an option, but it is possible for a limited number of health care workers other than clinical laboratory employees. The clinical laboratory assistant (CLA) position was an option at one time but is no longer available as a laboratory training program for entry-level laboratory workers.

Another reason that professional registries for medical personnel exist stems from a desire by members of the various professions to control their own destinies rather than a governmental agency licensing them through a licensing board composed in part of non-medical professionals. The term "registered nurse," or RN, stems from just such a train of thought, and even though nursing licensure is now mandatory in all states, the term has persisted.

Registering agencies often will not allow any medical program graduates to take a registry examination unless they have graduated from a program that is accredited by an approved agency, but some proprietary for-profit schools will often advertise themselves as being "accredited." However, the accrediting body may have no credibility, as the system sanctioning the program may be an invention of the company that owns the school! So, as a precautionary note, the student who wishes to receive a diploma or certificate in an area of health care should ensure that any private school attended is accredited by a professional organization with national standing. A school that is not accredited or advertises that the program is accredited but "certifies" the completer of a program as a professional in a very short period of time and for large sums of money should be suspect. In the past, some schools even certified students as professional laboratory technicians in a program of only a few months' duration.

Disparities in Personnel Standards

The credentialing process becomes further muddied when there are differences between facility accreditation bodies and other professional accreditation groups that require the employees of the facility to meet certain standards. **These two types of groups** offer credentialing from entirely different vantage points, where one focuses on the needs of the facility, and the other has the professional employees' interest at heart. In the best of worlds, all of the standards, whether they are from licensure, registry agencies, or accreditation bodies for both facilities and educational programs, would be the same, but this is not always the case. However, most accreditation organizations for facilities will accept personnel qualifications as satisfactory when the laboratory workers have met the requirements for competency that are acceptable to the state licensure office or the facility itself.

There are some areas of the country where states are weak in their requirements for certification of medical laboratory workers. In those states where obtaining credentials such as certification and registration is somewhat voluntary, the accreditation process for the facility may require stronger credentials than either the institution's standards or state laws may have established. Then, the requirements for the facility accreditation agency would take precedence. As stated previously, in most states there are no personnel licensure laws and these states normally accept registry by one of the previously mentioned agencies as being equivalent to having a license.

Those states not requiring personnel licensure typically accept technicians and technologists registered by ASCP and AMT, among other certifying groups, as workers who are essentially licensed. For instance, graduates from an educational program for medical laboratory students accredited by NAACLS and registered by one of the major agencies such as ASCP or AMT would be acceptable. The ASCP, for example, will only administer the registry examination to those who are graduates of an NAACLS-accredited program. States without personnel licensure will then accept these registrants as being qualified to work in the medical laboratory. As one can see, all of the processes relating to facility accreditation and certification such as registry and licensure are interwoven and it is difficult to separate the three entities. Table 2-3 shows the agencies that currently certify laboratory personnel along with others that either collect samples or provide basic tests of a variety called *waived procedures*, such as those accrediting POLs. This will be discussed more fully later in this book.

Most colleges and universities require an additional level of accreditation for the institution such as regional accreditation through COC. These are regional accreditations from units that are branches of the COC, such as the **Southern Association of Colleges and Schools (SACS)**. All of these requirements stem from an attempt to standardize the training, educational. and clinical components of a program. This is to ensure that all laboratory workers will possess the same entry-level assets that have been determined as being important for the level of skills the workers will be practicing. It is also due to a publicly displayed claim of protecting the public from unqualified practitioners. The significant number of professional societies listed in Table 2-3 illustrates the competition that may arise among agencies that certify competency for laboratory education and training.

The reality is that such a fragmentation of credentialing agencies for medical laboratory workers will make it difficult to achieve any consistency in the requirements for credentialing laboratory workers. Even states requiring licensure and a set of standards for education of laboratory workers may differ from state to state as to the level of education and training a technician or a technologist should attain and which programs provide acceptable licensing or credentialing examination before they deem a laboratory worker qualified or competent.

Certification, Registration, or Licensure of Personnel

While most states do not require personnel licensure, states that do not require personnel licensure usually require that all laboratory professionals attain some sort of certification acceptable to the individual states before they may be employed as laboratory technical workers. Professional credentialing is available through a number of agencies including the ASCP, American Medical Technologists (AMT), **National Credentialing Agency for Laboratory Personnel (NCA)**, American Association of Bioanalysts, and other lesser known credentialing bodies. Hospitals

Table 2-3 Partial List of Agencies for Credentialing Laboratory Personnel

Acronym	Title
AAB-BOR*	American Association of Bioanalysts Board of Registry
AAMA	American Association of Medical Assistants (point-of-care testing only)
ABB	American Board of Bioanalysis
AMT	American Medical Technologists
ASCP	American Society for Clinical Pathology
ASPT†	American Society of Phlebotomy Technicians
DHHS‡	Department of Health and Human Services
ISCLT	International Society for Clinical Laboratory Technology (now AAB)
NCA	National Credentialing Agency for Laboratory Personnel (laboratory workers only)
NPA	National Phlebotomy Association

NOTE: Not all health care facilities accept credentials from all of these agencies.
*Formerly International Society for Clinical Laboratory Technology (ISCLT).
†Credentials phlebotomists.
‡DHHS no longer certifies new laboratory personnel.

in most states that are licensed to provide medical care and accept insurance reimbursement are required to hire registered MTs and MLTs to perform laboratory tests.

Phlebotomists and laboratory assistants may be certified or registered but are <u>not</u> authorized to perform and report laboratory tests, but they may provide services such as collecting and accessioning laboratory specimens and clerical duties such as logging of samples and the physical acts of sending out reports either by computer or by hand. Information regarding professional organizations that provide avenues for becoming registered as a professional laboratory worker or to promote the profession may be found on the Internet. All of these agencies have codes of ethics specific to the agency, but all are similar. An example of this code is one by the American Society for Clinical Laboratory Science (ASCLS) (Table 2-4), which is a professional organization and does not itself credential workers but works to advance the profession.

Categories of Medical Laboratory Workers for Certification

Although a number of different forms of nomenclature are used for workers in the laboratory in different locales, those certified by any agency to work in medical laboratories are basically divided into two major groups. Each of these two groups may be known by several names (Table 2-5). The MLT may also be known as a clinical laboratory technician (CLT) based on the job position and the type of credentialing obtained by the technician. A technician level usually requires an associate's degree, which includes both academic components and training involving technical skills and the practice of the skills. The next category is that of the technologist, which requires a bachelor's degree. The MT is also known as a CLS, depending, again, on the organization granting the credential and, in some cases, the workplace that uses particular job titles for the technologist. Pathologists are not discussed with medical laboratory workers as they are in a separate category as medical doctors, who are licensed by the state and who also often belong to professional registries. Table 2-5 shows equivalent titles between two major credentialing agencies. Some technologists will be certified by more than one organization.

An MT/CLS technologist may choose to become specialized in a particular area of the laboratory. Some of these specialties may require a master's degree

Table 2-4 ASCLS Code of Ethics to Which Clinical Laboratory Members Ascribe

As a clinical laboratory professional, I acknowledge my professional responsibility to:

- Maintain and promote standards of excellence in performing and advancing the art and science of my profession;
- Preserve the dignity and privacy of patients;
- Uphold and maintain the dignity and respect of the profession;
- Contribute to the general well-being of the community; and
- Actively demonstrate my commitment to these responsibilities throughout my professional life.

Table 2-5 NCA Certification Categories and Equivalent ASCP Certification Categories

NCA Designation	ASCP Designation
CLS, clinical laboratory scientist	MT, medical technologist
CLT, clinical laboratory technician	MLT, medical laboratory technician
CLSp, clinical laboratory specialist	S, specialist
CLSup, clinical laboratory supervisor	DLM, diplomate in laboratory management
CLPlb, clinical laboratory phlebotomist	PBT, phlebotomy technician

and successful completion of specialized testing to be designated a specialist in an area of the laboratory. Technologist-level workers are allowed to work independently without supervision in most states, with some varying requirements. Technologists may supervise technicians, and in most cases technicians are not able to work independently, except with supervision of a technologist who is on the premises, when a technician performs and reports results of laboratory tests. Many of the procedures are performed by both technicians and technologists, but a number of tests of moderate or high complexity require that they be performed by a technologist. The general division of labor allows technicians to perform repetitious and routine procedures, while a technologist is expected to be able to exercise more critical thinking and is allowed to modify the steps of a procedure if necessary.

Specialty Designation for Categories of Clinical Laboratory Scientists

Specialty registries exist under the auspices of the major credentialing agencies. For instance, ASCP has specialties in histotechnology and cytotechnology, blood banking, and microbiology, to name a few. A number of professional societies also exist for the purpose of advancing the various specialties, and to provide for input into the profession by the members of the societies. Continuing and inservice educational opportunities are available at annual national and international meetings. Note that some major accrediting agencies also provide for continuing education for their members along with professional societies, as well as providing for credentialing and personnel certification. Table 2-6 is a list of societies that are active in providing for their members in matters of certification and in promoting the profession, often providing lobbying efforts to gain favorable government action. These organizations, for the most part, provide categorical specializations in the major departments of the laboratory.

There are certain levels of knowledge that students must reach before entering into clinical practice. This ensures a basic level of knowledge necessary to protect the public. Workers employed by a facility should in some form be registered, certified, or licensed, as appropriate for the position of employment or the state in which the worker is employed. Most states do not require licensure for medical laboratory workers but most often do require that all laboratory professionals be registered by certain agencies. Hospitals in most, if not all, states are required by regulation to hire only registered MTs and MLTs to perform laboratory tests.

REQUIREMENTS FOR CREDENTIALING OF LABORATORY WORKERS

Several professional registries have become very proactive in recent years with efforts toward making medical technology more visible as a highly skilled profession. In the 1930s, California adopted personnel licensure laws, making public the need for credentialing of laboratory workers, but relatively little progress toward an overall effort to unify the profession has occurred in recent history. Other states have since adopted laws requiring personnel licensure, but there is often a disparity between those states in the educational and training requirements for becoming licensed as individuals.

Over the intervening years since California began to require personnel licensure, some steps have been taken by professional agencies to control the entry of personnel into the medical laboratory field. These groups have categorized and determined minimum competencies for candidates for licensure or registry in the medical laboratory profession. There are also professional societies for specialties that uphold certain standards for laboratory managers, microbiologists, blood bank specialists, and clinical chemists, along with other societies that address the needs of all areas of the medical laboratory. Many laboratorians believe it is best for the profession to be associated with an agency composed of other medical laboratory workers on a voluntary basis than to have legislation requiring licensure that might not be as effective. But others favor the opposing view in that state licensure in all states would be the best solution for addressing the disparities in education and requirements for entry into the profession. Most professional organizations set forth that standards for the titles used in the

Table 2-6 Professional Societies for Clinical Laboratory and Related Professions

AAB	American Association of Bioanalysts
AABB	American Association of Blood Banks
AACC	American Association of Clinical Chemistry
AAMA	American Association of Medical Assistants
AMT	American Medical Technologists
APIC	Association of Practitioners in Infection Control
ASCLS	American Society for Clinical Laboratory Science
ASCP	American Society for Clinical Pathology
ASM	American Society for Microbiology
ASPT	American Society of Phlebotomy Technicians
CLMA	Clinical Laboratory Management Association
NPA	National Phlebotomy Association

clinical laboratory should be similar and perhaps mandated by government agencies, same as in the nursing profession.

To date, a number of reasons for credentialing as well as methods of credentialing medical laboratory workers have been identified. The main reason for requiring credentialing concerns the obvious inconsistencies in the present system. Not all accreditation agencies, whether licensing bodies or registry agencies, are in agreement with each other regarding standards for entry level credentialing. There are well-founded charges that some professional organizations as well as government agencies have attempted to remove or weaken any existing current regulations toward strengthening requirements for entering the profession. In recent years, there has been a general movement toward merging of several of these agencies, and it is possible that eventually there will be only one certifying body for medical laboratory workers. If this does not happen, it is highly probable that most, if not all, of the states will eventually adopt their own licensing process for the laboratory personnel. Purposes for credentialing, forces behind credentialing, approaches to credentialing, competition between credentialing agencies, confusion of job titles, vague regulations, and miscellaneous issues are all areas that are manifestations of the problem that should be discussed and acted upon by the entire medical laboratory profession.

Regulation of Medical Laboratories and Laboratory Professionals

Because issues related to certification have not been settled as far as a consistent approach to regulation of medical laboratory professionals, there is still a great deal of confusion and controversy concerning which current agency, if any, should have the responsibility for dictating personnel and facility requirements. There are some medical laboratory personnel registries that various institutions will accept as ensuring competence in the field, while others may not accept that same credential. There is confusion even in the general populace. The medical laboratory as a whole is largely misunderstood by the consumer of medical care. Students in science majors are often not aware that a program such as medical laboratory technology even exists, even though it is a field that will require the infusion of a large number of new employees within the next few years.

But even within health care facilities, other medical professionals are often not knowledgeable as to the education, training, and hierarchy of laboratory professionals. Many patients and families of those being treated assume that the person who collects, transports, and processes the blood and body fluids of diverse patients is a "nurse," an "intern," or some other unspecified allied health worker. In some areas of the country where identification of the various workers within the health care facility is not as obvious, this type of assumption is probably more prevalent. But for general laypersons, the scope and importance of laboratory specimen collection and processing are less well known than the work performed by nurses, pharmacists, radiographers, and other ancillary departments of the hospital. This is particularly true because there will likely be little contact between the patient and a medical laboratory worker, except for the phlebotomist.

And as discussed previously, state licensure is required to work in laboratories in several states, while others rely on professional registries to test and certify the competency of those entering the profession of laboratory medicine. This often leads to a considerable disparity between the requirements and standards for those requiring state licensure and the major agencies that currently certify medical laboratory workers, so it is no wonder there is so much uncertainty for everyone else. Even the professional groups and the government agencies that attempt to improve and to raise the standards of laboratory workers are strongly divided as to levels of education and training that are required to document and ensure competency for those entering the medical laboratory profession. At issue is the lack of agreement as to the appropriate length of the educational process for varying levels of workers within the laboratories. Another basic question is whether there is an actual need for continuing efforts to ensure continuing competency throughout the career of the medical laboratory worker through mandated continuing education. With the rapid evolution of medical laboratory technology, and the potential for becoming even more technologically advanced as a profession, it appears that the view that continuing education is not necessary would further harm the profession as it seeks to gain more recognition.

ROUTES FOR CREDENTIALING OF MEDICAL LABORATORY WORKERS

There are four separate methods for credentialing medical laboratory workers, one of which is no longer used. Remember, as stated earlier, that the term "certification" is sometimes used to include licensure requirements, fulfillment of registry requirements, and the earning of a certificate. In addition, at one time (1970s and early 1980s), the **U.S. Department of Health, Education, and Welfare (HEW)** (which later became the **U.S. Department of Health and Human Services [HHS]**) administered equivalency tests that allowed anyone with laboratory experience to take a certifying examination in some cases without regard to any formal educational requirements or any assessment of the clinical experience a candidate may have had. The four types of credentials are as follows:

1. **Certification** is the process by which a *nongovernment* agency or association recognizes an individual's educational competence predetermined by that group. Programs leading to certification are usually of less duration than diploma programs. Standards employed usually include a written examination with emphasis on *either* theoretical and/or practical knowledge.

2. **Licensure** is the process by which a *government* agency gives permission for a person to engage in a particular activity requiring a certain body of knowledge. This would presumably enable him or her to perform functions impinging upon the public health, safety, and welfare. The process usually includes a period of education and training under the supervision of practitioners who assess the abilities of the individual before he or she is allowed to sit for the examination. Standards for ensuring suitability of a candidate to complete an examination include both theoretical education and clinical training where students are monitored and taught technical aspects of laboratory medicine. Licensure laws are almost always a function of state government, and many require a college degree. Most states require licensing

for a variety of health care professions, while others accept certification or registry as an official means of ensuring competency of a number of practitioners. There are basically two types of state licenses:

a. Personal Licensure for Individuals
b. Facility Licensure (may be for a department or for an entire institution and does not cover individual practitioners, but may require employment of only registered personnel)

3. **Registration** is the process by which an association of professionals places an individual on a list (registry) of persons who are in possession of minimum competencies necessary to perform a group of related tasks. In cases where state licensure is not required, this process includes the medical laboratory worker. To qualify for the registry examination, there are both educational and training requirements, and in some cases supervised experiential aspects of preparation for entering the medical laboratory profession.

4. **Equivalency testing** is a relative newcomer to the medical laboratory field. A number of states began to accept College Level Entrance Proficiency (CLEP) examinations in lieu of registry examinations in the 1970s. Some states have now dropped the acceptance of the CLEP tests as a substitute for registry examinations in qualifying personnel for medical laboratory work. In this way, a candidate for a position in the laboratory could at one time take a categorical examination in one of the specialties such as hematology, clinical chemistry, microbiology, or blood banking and work in this area as a technologist, or could take the entire set of specialty examinations offered and then work as a generalist technologist.

The most dramatic example of equivalency testing occurred in the 1970s and 1980s when HEW (now HHS) offered an equivalency examination, which was given four times in the 1970s and once time in the 1980s. This test was given to aid hospitals in fulfilling the Medicare regulations, which stipulated that laboratory workers must have certification, registry, or a license for the health care facility to receive reimbursement from Medicare and Medicaid. Only a few laboratory workers of this category of technicians and technologists currently remain in the workplace as medical laboratory workers; most workers of these categories have retired.

FEDERAL REGULATION OF MEDICAL LABORATORIES

After many committee hearings in both the U.S. House of Representatives and the U.S. Senate during the 1960s, the federal government entered into the arena concerning the competence of workers in the medical laboratory field. Some of the concerns voiced were aimed at ensuring that quality results were obtained on federally funded testing through Medicare, but some were prompted by citizens who had been damaged through erroneous laboratory results. Erroneous Pap smear evaluations were the most visible of the problem areas that caught the attention of federal lawmakers. HHS still recognizes those who completed the equivalency examinations given in the 1970s but, as alluded to previously, the numbers are so small as to be insignificant.

The federal government's first attempt to improve the situation centered on the **Clinical Laboratory Improvement Act of 1967 (CLIA 67)**. Those who were qualified under previous regulations were "grandfathered" on a permanent basis. But then ways were sought to credential laboratory workers who were supposedly already deemed qualified to work in a medical laboratory through a hodge-podge of on-the-job training, various obscure registries, and sometimes on a self-regulating basis. Problems continued to erupt, and the **Health Care Financing Administration (HCFA)** developed the final regulations called **CLIA 88**. This act attempted to deal with the competence and credentials of medical laboratory workers but it has done nothing if not worsened the scene. HCFA, under CLIA 88, now states that all personnel performing high complexity testing must have had a minimum of 2 years of college by 1997. Critics of this provision, on both sides, argue that it places an undue burden on those who were previously qualified, while other interest groups say that at least a baccalaureate degree is necessary to be a supervisor. HCFA claims that personnel standards are so intertwined with complexity models and other sections of the law that modifying one aspect could lead to other complex adjustments and would give various interest groups, including private registering agencies, more grounds for appeal.

Those who were deemed qualified and worked before March 14, 1967, were permanently "grandfathered" in the first version of CLIA. But the final rule of CLIA 88 states that those with only a 1-year program of training must not perform high-complexity testing without supervision. And to keep their jobs, they must have completed an associate's degree by 1997. This requirement has sometimes been conveniently overlooked by individuals, institutions, and governing bodies. Debate still rages from those who say the personnel requirements are too strict. And there are those who say that the educational requirements have been gutted by all of the interest groups. Some of these groups have much to gain by maintaining their status quo. These groups often resist efforts requiring that their members expend more educational effort but may insist that their constituents maintain the same level of employment as their peers who have 4-year college degrees and should earn the same salary with essentially on-the-job training and no advanced formal education.

These final regulations have done nothing to enhance the profession from the personal viewpoint of most medical laboratory workers. It has also not served as a means of added protection to the consumer. The medical laboratory profession would do well to adopt the stance of the various nurses' and pharmacist's associations. In an informal show of unity by the various licensing boards and professional associations, nurses and pharmacists have greatly advanced the stature of their respective professions. State licensure even includes specialty boards for various nurse practice acts; for example, for a certified nurse anesthetist (CRNA), the nurse with this specialty education is licensed separately from those practicing basic nursing care. The nursing and pharmaceutical professions also appear to have achieved somewhat consistent standards from state to state, with standardized tests that are the same, regardless of the state issuing the license. And for medical technology workers, CLIA 88 was a classic example of a movement that started out with extremely lofty goals and then was gradually weakened by the attempts of special interest groups or by ignoring the provisions by many.

A law mandating high-quality testing no matter where the tests are performed and strict personnel standards is a worthy law. But it was ineffective in the final analysis for the CLIA regulations. It is an almost certainty that further efforts will follow in the future to achieve the intended goals.

COMPETITION BETWEEN AGENCIES FOR PERSONNEL CREDENTIALING

The major credentialing agencies in reality compete with each other in promoting their respective registries. One of the major agencies that is controlled by pathologists believe that this particular agency should be the one that regulates the medical laboratory field, including personnel standards. The other agencies are somewhat controlled by the medical technologists themselves who think they should be the masters of their own destiny, and were formed based on that main premise. There also seems to be a strong sense of self-survival by these registries, as well as a belief that they are performing the proper service and are the best credentialing agencies for the medical laboratory worker.

Due to the inaction of the states providing any meaningful regulations of the medical laboratory, action, by the federal government, through its Medicare licensing acts, has attempted with its equivalency tests to legislate some sort of competency standards in competition with the existing credentialing agencies by entering yet another version of a credentialing examination as occurred in the 1970s and 1980s. This act essentially made those without any sort of educational preparation equivalent to a college-degreed technician or technologist by virtue of mainly experience and basic on-the-job training. The desire for operating funds and for sufficient political clout through numbers of registrants seems to have led the registries to broaden and dilute their registry. Through selective choosing of registries, almost any aspirant for a medical laboratory career can find an examination for which he or she qualifies, regardless of educational or experiential level. The sentiment among some of the more cynical medical laboratory technicians and technologists is that the main function of some professional registries is to merely collect an annual fee from its members.

Credentialing Agencies

The current array of state licensure and major registry choices available to the candidate for registry or licensure makes it almost impossible for a new graduate to determine the best choice for registry if the goal is to enhance one's career and to improve the profession. However, if one's state has a personnel licensure law, there is no choice as to whether to take a licensure examination to qualify for employment in the medical laboratory. And it is virtually impossible to objectively compare the knowledge or qualifications of one worker with those of another, each of whom may be duly "registered" by one of the major organizations. This is because of the differences in areas of emphasis or difficulty of the various requirements for credentialing due to the different levels of academic preparation and the taking of a certification examination.

To be prepared for any differences in required credentials, some medical technicians and technologists decide to take different registry examinations from each of the several registering agencies in case they move from one state to another or from one facility to another. Potential employers may subjectively view one of the professional organizations with more favor than any of the others and may hire only those who possess registry credentials from one particular professional body. Most of the registries and state licensing agencies require a formal period of formalized on-the-job training, and some allow for a "grandfather clause" that grants certification to personnel who were working in a particular capacity before an arbitrarily established date. The "grandfather clause" sometimes enables those who have no training or academic credits to perform medical laboratory work, even at a supervisory level.

Laboratory Testing by Those Other Than Professional Laboratory Workers

Laboratory procedures may be legally performed in both hospitals and medical offices by those with minimal training. And even with the availability of situations where certain tests may be performed by other than laboratorians, there are still occasional attempts by some pathologists, physicians, and hospital officials to remove the often minimal constraints currently placed on the appropriately credentialed technician-level worker. This is explained more thoroughly in the section dealing with efforts to gain state licensure. The menu of laboratory tests that may be performed in POLs or by hospital workers for monitoring inpatients by those with no formal training in laboratory medicine has broadened from only 11 low-complexity tests to a somewhat wide range of tests as technology improves and becomes more foolproof. These tests are called **waived tests** and they are not required by CLIA 88 regulations to be performed by credentialed personnel.

Point-of-care testing (POCT) includes a menu performed by nurses and in some facilities even by patient care technicians to monitor a patient's condition, such as the measurement of a finger-stick glucose to determine if insulin should be administered. Certain laboratory tests for patients by other than medical laboratory workers in the home or in a hospital bed are possible due to these rules allowing low-complexity testing by minimally trained personnel. These training requirements must be documented, however, before a non–laboratory worker is allowed to perform even these waived tests. And in some hospitals and clinics, noncredentialed personnel performing POC testing must be monitored periodically by a laboratory professional. It is common in many facilities for the laboratory to provide technical expertise in calibrating the instruments used for POC testing on a daily basis and to document and record quality control results. These are areas that may be examined by site visitors performing facility inspections for continued accreditation of the health care facility.

POLs represent an area where non–laboratory personnel may perform certain laboratory tests. In some cases, to their credit, a POL with several physicians who practice in a large clinic may insist on a laboratory that is established with high standards and that performs more than tests of the "waived" variety.

The training and supervising of personnel, maintenance of equipment, document-ing of quality control results, and record-keeping for test procedures require a medical technologist as the supervisor. But in some states, a laboratory with this scope of practice may require a site license by the state agency responsible for ensuring competence and accuracy of results produced, as well as establishing adherence to state laws and regulations. Requirements would most likely include a site license, which would result in periodic site visits to inspect the operations to ensure compliance with policies and procedures for a full-scale laboratory.

Laboratory professionals at the technician level are currently legally allowed by most states to perform only those tasks that are routine and repetitive. This provision would also be consistent with the requirements by CLIA 88 that match the complexity of the procedures with the level of technical personnel required for laboratory testing. In most states, this level of worker must be supervised at all times by a technologist. The technician is often not allowed to perform emer-gency work or to do work that requires a great deal of interpretation and subjec-tive judgment as determined by most regulatory agencies. One argument against this requirement preventing certain processes by a technician is that some of the requirements are too stringent and that automation removes some of the variables that would require troubleshooting or the interpretive skills of a highly trained professional such as the technologist.

At one point several years ago, a dramatic attempt was initiated by certain special interest groups to require that only the supervisor had to have formal training or to possess any kind of credentials. He or she would then be able to hire any applicant, regardless of the level of or lack of training, and simply vouch for the results produced, certifying that they were accurate. It appears this would create a dangerous precedent, and a step backward for the laboratory profession, since an environment would be created in which the bench worker would have little or no training, and the work would be performed in a fragmented manner, with each person trained to perform only a few specific tests or to perform only some of the steps of a laboratory test. Fortunately for medical laboratory profes-sionals, this suggestion has apparently been abandoned.

The laboratory seems to be the only allied health profession that allows so many and varied alternate routes to credentialing. In contrast, the pharmacy does not allow its pharmacy technicians to eventually take the pharmacy board examinations following a certain level of experience. The ward clerks and nurs-ing assistants do not automatically qualify to take the registered nurse examina-tion with no further training by virtue of having worked in the nursing field for a given period of time. Although they do inspect all departments and functions within the hospitals, another important organization that is vitally interested in the credentialing of health care professionals is TJC. TJC, as well as other agen-cies that inspect and accredit health care facilities, does not certify the compe-tence of personnel. However, TJC usually leaves the matter of credentialing of personnel to the local facility or the respective state governments, if there are any regulations governing these professions in a certain locale. TJC does not man-date any specific level of training and education but merely ensures that state requirements for the credentialing of medical laboratory workers as well as all of the other professionals working in the facility are met. But because there are so many societies involved in the credentialing of laboratory personnel, it is currently extremely difficult for any consistent standard to be used in evaluating the competencies of medical laboratory personnel by accreditation site visitors.

STATE LICENSURE FOR LABORATORY PERSONNEL

In the *Journal of American Medical Technologists* (McBride, 1978), no fewer than seven agencies were listed as being involved in evaluating by examination the competencies of medical laboratory personnel. This did not even include the states that now require licensure of laboratory personnel. These states— California, Hawaii, Florida, North Dakota, Rhode Island, Tennessee, Louisiana, Nevada, West Virginia, Montana, Georgia (facility-only license), along with the Commonwealth of Puerto Rico—have their own licensure examinations and standards. By 2005, New York State passed a revised requirement for personnel licensure in facilities that employ medical cytotechnologists, laboratory technicians, and technologists. The standards imposed by these states and one territory (Puerto Rico) are acceptable to the federal government as they meet or exceed the standards imposed by Medicare and Medicaid.

Over the past few years, efforts to require personnel licensure in other states have continued or renewed, but most states and territories with existing personnel laws have had these laws since 1978 or earlier. If it is difficult for laboratory managers or hospital administrators to know about all of the agencies that offer credentialing, how much more difficult is it for third-party payers or the consumer to determine if the personnel performing the diagnostic testing are competent? On the surface, it apparently costs no more for laboratory testing in a laboratory where only well-qualified personnel work than in one where marginal or questionable credentials are held by the laboratory technical staff.

State Personnel Licensure Efforts

The term *licensure* is generally authority given to a state by legal permit from a constituted body. Only a few licenses are granted by the federal government, such as licensing of airline pilots under the Federal Aviation Authority (FAA) and the Federal Communication Commission (FCC). But it is mostly a function of the state government in most cases for the purpose of protecting the public from potential harm from unscrupulous or incompetent practitioners. In states where licenses are required, it is illegal to practice a profession covered by the licensing regulation without a license. Penalties may be severe, and not being certified by licensure makes it more difficult, if not impossible, to get a job in the field of work in question.

Some states and some medical facilities also require certification in addition to licensure to fulfill continuing education and professional advancement issues. This is because some personnel credentialing agencies and some professional organizations also require continuing education to maintain professional accreditation. For specific information, it may be necessary to contact the state in which you wish to work for specific requirements for employment in the laboratory. Most states require documentation of certification from agencies sanctioned by the state as being acceptable in their standards. Some states even have educational standards to include the amount and types of practical clinical training for institutes of higher learning that make the requirements more consistent throughout the state. Other states give reciprocity between those with personnel licensure, meaning the license may be transferred from another state or even country to another if the standards are similar. At the end of this book, there is a list of state agencies with personnel licensure laws. The list provides information for contacting the proper authority for specific information. (See Appendix A, States and Territories with Laboratory Personnel Licensure Requirements.)

Several efforts to require personnel licensure by each state have largely fallen by the wayside. During the 1970s, a host of states formed committees to pursue laboratory personnel law following the highly publicized federal government efforts beginning in 1966–1967 that culminated in CLIA 88. Even today, an occasional sensationalized news story will surface, revealing horror stories of the results of erroneous laboratory results and the incompetence of laboratory worker(s) that led to the incorrect treatment or lack of treatment. It is usually only then that the weaknesses of some of the licensure and credentialing methods currently used will come to the surface.

Then, consumers and legislators will raise a hue and cry as medical mistakes by laboratory personnel are revealed that possibly led to the needless death of a child, for instance. But with the publicity from the past few decades, as of 1995, only the states listed on the prior page, along with a few others, have been successful in enacting legislation. This has been achieved only after much effort and often against great odds due to resistance by special-interest groups, which includes some agencies offering registry examinations that are practicing turf protection. These organizations believe that if all states required licensure, some of the registry agencies either would be without business or would be forced to change the manner in which they would support the profession.

In a unique situation, New York City had its own laboratory personnel licensure laws for years while the state of New York had a separate licensure law for those not residing or working in New York City. On January 30, 2005, New York City dropped its unique licensing law requiring licensure or certification of clinical laboratory technologists and technicians, as well as cytotechnologists, in favor of the newly passed state personnel licensure law. However, it is not easy to accomplish the task of attaining laboratory personnel licensure laws. A number of states have sought personnel licensure for medical laboratory personnel for several decades. Some were successful and other attempts have ended in failure or in a temporary halt to attempts.

Louisiana fought this battle for 5 years before the passage of a law requiring laboratory personnel licensure—another issue on which significant differences prevail between registering agencies and state licensure. A frequent difference in opinion is the disparity between academic and training requirements between credentialing bodies and states that require licensure. State licensure that is similar between states such as that for other professions would do a great deal to minimize this problem.

A common analogous statement used by those advocating state licensure for laboratory personnel licensure is that plumbers, barbers, cosmetologists, electricians, and other tradesmen, along with health care personnel such as physicians, emergency medical technicians, dentists, and physical therapists, must be licensed. But in a profession such as medical laboratory technology, with the potential to do great harm to an individual, some states do not require licensure or even formal education and some sort of credentialing, such as by examination. Economic factors that are cited by higher-level administrators (CEOs of hospitals) and loss of control cited by pathologists seem to be the crux of the arguments against personnel licensure. This is more of an emotional statement by some than a fact, but the argument for personnel licensure does in many cases hold some merit.

CLIA 88 as federal legislation attempted to address problems in the quality of laboratory services as opposed to quality of personnel. CLIA is more convinced that the laboratory director is able to judge competency and that adequate proficiency testing would remedy poor practice in the medical laboratory. However, results of proficiency testing for accuracy can be performed by the best-trained and most competent personnel in the laboratory, yet do not necessarily address incompetent and poorly trained or untrained personnel. CLIA on the surface tended by this position to weaken (relax) staffing rules, and this occurred at the same time that more POC testing was being performed by untrained or ancillary health care personnel. Bedside testing with more portable and sophisticated equipment is an area toward which medical laboratory personnel are usually adamantly opposed as an encroachment on their territory, particularly in light of their quest for more professional recognition and for personnel licensure.

Through use of pressure by both influence and lobbying, special-interest groups such as the manufacturers of these instruments designed for bedside testing are of kindred mind with CLIA, intimating that extensive training is not necessary for performing many of these tests. Of course, manufacturers would like to sell more of the expensive portable machines. Although revenue would be taken from the laboratory, and laboratory technical personnel are the experts who calibrate and document results and perform preventive maintenance (without any reimbursement to the laboratory), the actual procedures of this sort are easily performed by properly trained personnel other than medical laboratory technicians and technicians. It is not just turf protection for some professionals, as they do not see any shifting of specialized work to other less-trained personnel occurring to any great extent in other health care professions, such as nursing.

Current Efforts to Gain State Personnel Licensure

An example of the hurdles that must be overcome to legislate state licensure of personnel is given by Nebraska. Nebraska does not currently have personnel licensure regulations, but an extremely difficult and rigorous process is required to ascertain the need for personnel licensure before a legislative bill can be proposed. Requirements that must be met require the following proofs. There must be sufficient potential harm to the public by the practice of procedures by unlicensed personnel in the given profession. Practitioners must be independent and not require strict supervision. And finally, the scope of practice must be clearly defined so it is readily distinguishable from the scope of practice for another profession.

Two agencies that support the efforts of medical laboratory technologists and technicians are the ASCLS and the ASCP. Both of these organizations support laboratory personnel licensure since accurate testing by medical laboratories is not possible without practitioners who have been deemed competent, from the technician to the technologist level. One might use the oft-repeated analogy that a chain is only as strong as its weakest link, and weak personnel standards result in poor end products. These professional societies would still function as advocates for the profession of laboratory medicine by pushing for consistent and stronger personnel requirements, even if they were no longer responsible for examining and registering medical laboratory workers. There is a need for these societies to provide professional development and to provide a forum for discussion and action by those who work as medical laboratory professionals. Regional meetings for medical laboratory personnel, exposure to literature and new technology, and opportunities for continuing education would be valid reasons for their continued existence.

A slightly different form of an argument previously listed is the old debate between those in favor of personnel licensure and those against it. Those in favor state that even hairdressers have to be licensed to apply their skills professionally, which are not in general life-threatening in its practice. But currently only 11 states and territories have laboratory personnel licensure even though they perform tests that have the potential of directly affecting the lives and well-being of patients. Most states have a highly vocal group of medical laboratory workers who support the process of personnel licensure, but few of these are pathologists. State branches of professional societies have made repeated efforts to achieve personnel licensure in a number of states, but none have been successful in the past several decades except for Montana, whose law was approved in 1993, and New York, in 2005, through the efforts of the state societies. Efforts in the early 2000s were aimed toward personnel licensure in several other states. Licensure efforts were renewed during this time period in Illinois, Iowa, Massachusetts, Missouri, Minnesota, New York, and Pennsylvania. State leaders are renewing their efforts in all of these states toward achieving their goal for licensure.

Not all of the provisions of New York's state licensure laws were met with unbounded enthusiasm, even by those in favor of licensure in the state. As in most other licensure endeavors, when new legislation is proposed, enacted, and then implemented, there are special provisions that must be addressed and that often only relate to a small number of individuals. In 2005, when New York State enacted its new laboratory personnel licensure regulations, a number of issues either were not addressed or were not palatable to professional organizations such as ASCP and ASCLS.

Legislation is usually written to cover those who were previously considered "qualified" or to allow a timeframe in which to meet the new requirements. "Grandfather clauses" allow those who have worked in the field for an arbitrarily set number of years to have a route for becoming licensed even with few or none of the requirements for becoming licensed by formal means of education and training. New York's law included provisions for both of these routes to licensure. There were a number of "grandparenting" provisions for gaining licensure, as well as two controversial provisions for granting licensure to those with a bachelor's degree and 2700 clock hours of experience by September 1, 2006. In addition to "grandfather" laws, a person who has worked 7200 clock hours, even with no formal college education or additional training other than on-the-job, can still qualify for licensure as a technologist in New York. And those who are currently pursuing educational requirements have until September 2011 to complete these requirements.

Much opposition from both local and national groups is focused on professional licensure for all the categories of laboratory medicine professionals. Hospital associations, state medical societies, laboratory managers, and a number of pathologists are averse to any changes in the way laboratory professionals are categorized and their competence is verified. Many of these groups work behind the scenes with their state representatives from the position that work is progressing in a satisfactory fashion so there is no need for licensure. This type of opposition is probably responsible for the complicated, cumbersome, and difficult process of documenting the need for licensure, as in Nebraska's case. Even some doctoral scientists who are directors of laboratories state that they do the hiring and firing and believe they can determine the competence and certify the quality of the work performed in their respective laboratories without further laws. They maintain that no harm is coming to the public as things are now, so licensure is not necessary.

In a rare display of unity, several Illinois state societies, with support from the national offices of some of the professional organizations, began meeting in 1999 on issues of common concern such as personnel licensure. ASCP, ASCLS, **American Association for Clinical Chemistry (AACC)**, **Clinical Laboratory Management Association (CLMA)**, **Illinois Society for Microbiology (ISM)**, and AMT were all in attendance. This is not to say that all were in favor of laboratory personnel licensure, but at least contemporary issues of interest to the medical laboratory community were mutually discussed. A bill was eventually written and introduced in the Illinois legislature, but there was opposition from the Illinois Society for Pathologists, whose official organization is the College of American Pathologists (CAP); the American Association of Bioanalysts; the Illinois Hospital Association; the Illinois State Medical Society; and the Illinois Department of Professional Regulation. In the face of such pressure from powerful groups with lobbyists, the bill did not pass. However, it was hoped by those in favor that the bill would be reintroduced at a later date.

Others states that have recently mounted a strong campaign for laboratory personnel licensure include Massachusetts, which had a personnel licensure bill "stuck" in legislative committees in 2004. But strong efforts through ASCLS continue currently in Massachusetts. Minnesota is trying to educate the population and to identify those who would oppose legislation for personnel licensure. A coalition of supporting organizations will work toward that end. Pennsylvania's effort failed and efforts were not renewed for a number of years following strong efforts in the 1990s. In 2004, a coalition of ASCLS Region II states met, seeking to organize a regional approach from the states of Delaware, New Jersey, Virginia, and Maryland, and from Washington, DC. West Virginia is also in Region II but has recently succeeded in obtaining personnel licensure.

In February 2008, efforts were renewed to gain licensure for personnel in Massachusetts. Pathologists from Massachusetts successfully persuaded the legislators not to consider the bill in a House floor vote to establish state licensure of clinical laboratory personnel. The CAP and the Massachusetts Society of Pathologists (MSP), along with the Massachusetts Hospital Association, Massachusetts Medical Society, Massachusetts Cytology Society, American Association of Bioanalysts, and American Clinical Laboratory Association, all opposed the bill. The CAP and the MSP, in a letter to members of the Massachusetts Committee on Ways and Means, stated, "The personnel qualifications established in the legislation are arbitrary, overly stringent, excessive and not commensurate with the demands of the clinical laboratory positions for which licensure is contemplated." The Massachusetts bill died a slow death and no further efforts have been reported to pursue a new version of the bill. This is the opposition most often encountered by laboratory professionals who seek to advance their profession.

There is a shortage of qualified laboratory workers, and laboratory managers are rather reluctant to further shrink the pool of persons who might be working in their facilities. Rightly or wrongly, many of these managers think that would be the case if personnel licensure became a fact. Many believe they know how to hire qualified personnel, but the charge has been made that in reality they do not want to pay more for personnel with some sort of documentation of their competence such as licensure. In actuality, if licensure became a requirement in each state, the initial shock would wear off and the personnel shortage would most likely begin to abate. The publicity might bring more students into the profession, as occurred in the nursing profession, thereby alleviating the shortage through more concerted recruitment efforts. In addition, the use of more qualified and educated workers could serve to offset the increased personnel costs by improving efficiency and productivity. But there is one thing of which medical laboratory professionals can be sure. The battles on various playing fields will undoubtedly continue into the foreseeable future, based on current negotiations between ASCP, ASCLS, NCA, and AMT.

SUMMARY

Although there are differences, accreditation, certification, and licensure are similar in that they provide formal recognition of facilities, institutions, and personnel through standards that have been established to ensure competence and effectiveness in meeting responsibilities to the public. In fact, all of these methods have one goal in mind—to protect the public. There have always been those who, for their own personal gain, would circumvent the system for ensuring competency of professionals, even if the patient is harmed.

Most often a health care facility is accredited, and tenets of the accreditation require that the facility only hire personnel who are licensed or registered by professional organizations. Certification and accreditation are voluntary, while licensure is required by the government. This function of credentialing professional employees retained in most cases in the state in which the facility exists or where the professional is employed.

Educational institutions also have a number of accreditation bodies; some are institution-wide and others affect programs only. However, the entire institution is affected by individual program accreditation, as the institution is ultimately responsible for enabling program officials to meet the program requirements. In some states, personnel licensure of professionals, including laboratorians, is required, while other states accept registered personnel as being "licensed." To further complicate the situation, some states have few or no requirements for various professions, including laboratory workers.

In addition, some of these states will accept registry as laboratory workers by one professional organization and not by another such agency due to differences in the standards of each. The graduate of a clinical laboratory program must choose an acceptable route to become qualified to work as a professional, based on state, local, and institutional requirements. The administrators of various schools of laboratory medicine around the country should be able to aid the graduate of an accredited program in determining the qualifications needed to work in the area where the laboratory worker seeks employment.

Some signs of cooperation have occurred relatively recently. Some states have adopted personnel licensure and have accepted the examinations from an accreditation agency as the official licensure test. The fragmentation that has been rife in the laboratory field since the early 1900s has changed very little. There is much work to do for the professional who works in laboratory medicine. Each new graduate should become involved in local, state, and national organizations to enhance and advance the profession.

Hundreds of years ago, clinical or medical laboratory technology began its climb toward its present status as one of, if not the most, important diagnostic and prognostic tools possessed by the medical practitioners. From early observations of ants eating sugar in the urine of diabetic patients and the idea that the blood of sick patients could contain impurities and poisons, the profession has evolved into an extremely sophisticated and technologically advanced career choice.

From the contributions of the fledgling scientists of yesteryear to the efforts of biomedical engineers and innovative practitioners has come the base of knowledge that we take for granted today. All components of laboratory practice, from the preanalytical aspects of collection of specimens and treatment of them along with proper documentation of identification, are the first basic steps of providing accurate and useful clinical information. In some cases, these tasks fall on the phlebotomist, before the specimens are presented to the laboratory technologists and technologists. Laboratory professionals then become involved in the analytical portion of the process of providing clinical data. A great deal of knowledge, diligence, and attention to detail is necessary to provide the best possible results. The third dimension of providing this service is the postanalytical portion of the entire process, where the results are produced in an intelligible format and provided to the right person.

We have seen from the previous introduction that the laboratorian's daily duties have changed dramatically. With current advances in the laboratory arena, the work will become even more important as well as more sophisticated. Terms such as *nanotechnology, molecular biology,* and *genetic manipulations,* as well as the use of genetic information, will be ever more prevalent in the diagnosis and treatment of virtually all diseases. There is still much to be done in the area of credentialing of laboratory workers, and training and retraining these professionals will be necessary as their roles in the positions they occupy change, as they certainly will. It is incumbent on all laboratory workers to become a part of these areas that need to be addressed.

Clinical laboratory workers have a myriad of opportunities within the laboratory profession. The four major departments of the clinical laboratory afford the professional a choice of the basic types of work that are performed in a typical laboratory setting. An additional possibility is in the histology and cytotechnology sections of the pathology laboratory, in which tissue specimens and cell preparations, respectively, are evaluated. These two choices usually require additional specialized training, and it is possible for technicians to transition into the pathology department, as some of the skills practiced by technicians and technologists are directly transferrable to the pathology section.

Most job opportunities exist in hospitals and clinics. Other good job opportunities exist in government and pharmaceutical research laboratories and in the armed forces laboratories, where both civilians and military personnel may work side by side. Reference laboratories, where smaller laboratories send seldom-performed tests and physician office laboratories, are other potential sources of employment. Education, sales, and training for users of manufactured equipment offer good job opportunities with excellent pay and benefits for many of these businesses.

Basic nomenclature for the two major levels of technical personnel of the laboratory differ, based on which accrediting body or registry is being used. MLTs registered in one agency may be known as CLTs in another. The same is true for MTs, who may be called CLSs by one agency and medical technologists by other accrediting agencies. There is also a blurring of the edges between duties performed by the two basic levels of personnel, and the job tasks depend on the clinical facility and its interpretation of personnel standards. Some states license laboratorians and mandate what each category can or cannot do in the way of producing laboratory reports. Still other states have few or no regulations regarding the practice of laboratory personnel. This has resulted in years of competition between "registering" authorities and their own interpretation of laws and provisions that are in some cases local based.

Some laboratory tasks are physical and require that certain essential tasks be performed; this may hinder or keep some with physical or mental disabilities from achieving a position in the laboratory. Accuracy is vital, and the ability to concentrate for long periods and to pay attention to detail is a must. The work may be stressful, and the ability to organize the work flow and to prioritize tasks is essential. The laboratorian must also maintain a professional decorum as it is important to work with other health care professionals as well as with patients and families. Few members of the public are aware of the hierarchy of workers such as technicians and technologists within the laboratory or even of the existence of such a program of study. Even among health care workers, there is little knowledge of the extent of education and training the laboratory workers acquire. For this reason, it is important that laboratory workers be ambassadors for the profession.

A modern hospital laboratory more closely resembles a business with a CEO (pathologist) who directs and manages a laboratory manager or managers; it sometimes includes a technical chief who is also a technologist and works directly to solve technical issues. Laboratories have evolved over a period of a little more than 100 years to highly sophisticated and automated facilities.

The organization of a laboratory is affected for the most part by the size of the hospital and the laboratory. Many of these laboratories complete thousands of analyses per day and are staffed by technologists who may also have specialty degrees, licenses, or other certification. Laboratories are highly regulated departments that employ large numbers of clinical scientists who are highly skilled and educated. It is estimated that 70% to 80% of the diagnoses for patients with diseases are diagnosed on the basis of laboratory tests. The future is bright for this profession, and the laboratories will continue to advance along with medical science.

REVIEW QUESTIONS

1. In your opinion, list some factors that contribute to contracting infectious diseases.
2. Name some things that may be visualized by observing them microscopically.
3. What are some basic differences between a modern laboratory and an early laboratory?
4. Why is it important that the laboratory worker of today be recognized as a professional?
5. What has occurred on a number of occasions that has led to increased awareness of the value of laboratory procedures and the value of being able to practice medicine in the field around the world?
6. Name several locations where laboratory procedures are performed. Not all those who perform laboratory procedures will be clinical laboratory technicians and technologists.
7. Name the four general departments in the clinical laboratory.
8. What level of laboratory worker is required to supervise a department?
9. What are some attributes a medical laboratory technician or technologist must possess to be effective in the workplace?
10. What are some of the reasons that there is no consistency in the credentialing of laboratory workers?
11. In your own words, describe the hierarchy of a medical laboratory in a hospital setting.
12. Compare the roles of the clinical and the anatomic pathologist positions.
13. Name the major types of specimens that are tested in a clinical laboratory.
14. In your own words, why are the functions of the phlebotomist extremely important as the first step in performing a procedure?
15. What are some important decisions that may be required of a technician or technologist with regard to the methodology to use for performing tests?

16. What are the basic differences and similarities between accreditation and licensure?

17. What are the four ways in which a medical laboratory worker may be deemed qualified in performing professional duties in the laboratory?

18. Name two or more professional organizations that serve to register or certify laboratory workers.

19. What is the chief purpose for becoming credentialed as a laboratory worker?

20. What group should work to improve the laboratory profession? What areas should be addressed?

CHAPTER 3

MEDICAL LAW, ETHICS, AND MORAL ISSUES OF HEALTH CARE

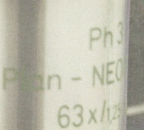

LEARNING OBJECTIVES

Upon completion of this chapter, the reader will be able to:

- Identify the meaning of the word *ethics*.

- Compare ethics and morality.

- Discuss whether moral and ethical concerns may involve a legal component.

- List some components of moral and ethical treatment of patients.

- Discuss the medical laboratory worker's responsibilities toward the patient and the family.

- Name several formal documents related to professional practice and ethical treatment of the patient.

- Discuss the difference between legal and ethical standards.

- Discuss the impact of HIPAA on a medical practice.

- Identify some ways in which medical information could be unintentionally made public.

- Discuss the misuse of a computer by a medical professional and how disciplinary action against the employee might ensue.

- List several methods of protecting a patient's records.

KEY TERMS

Breach
Causation
Damages
Department of Health and Human
   Services (HHS)
Duty
Ethics

Health care clearinghouse
Health Insurance Portability and
   Accountability Act (HIPAA)
Health maintenance organizations
   (HMOs)
Morality
Nurses Creed

Oath of Hippocrates
Patient's Bill of Rights
Preferred provider plans (PPOs)
Professionalism
Risk management
Tort

INTRODUCTION

Medical law and ethics are inseparable in their approach to the rights of patients. Patients have an inherent entitlement to certain expectations in their medical care. Their rights as citizens do not end at the doors of medical facilities. There is a document that is publicly displayed in most hospitals and clinics that formally lists elements of what a patient can expect when presenting for treatment. This publication is called the **Patient's Bill of Rights** and a sample of the form from the American Hospital Association will be provided in this chapter. The intention of this form is to inform patients of their rights when they are receiving medical care. Legal issues may arise and medical workers may be held liable if a patient's rights are violated.

Ethical, moral, and legal aspects of the health care system are inextricably interwoven. Legal matters are closely related to and evolve from morals and ethics. Ethical and moral issues are treate as interchangeable as there are many commonalities. The material presented here depicts the inseparable components of morals, ethics, and legalities involved in the delivery of health care. For example, hospital documents are legal documents, and the confidentiality of patients limits the distribution of medical documents to those treating the patient. Some ethical standards have become law, as will be shown.

The medical worker or student should know, through appropriate education and training, how to treat patients humanely, legally, and ethically and how to avoid any legal entanglements, before being assigned to a clinical facility. Role playing is a strategy often used in educational facilities to acquaint students with situations in which they may become involved. A well-informed practitioner will avoid many of the pitfalls such as negligence and malpractice that may lead to litigation. An important component to be considered in the treatment of patients is that of confidentiality and privacy of records and any other personal information about the patient. Privacy and confidentiality of patient records are of sufficient importance that a federal law was created to provide consistent standards for issues dealing with handling, storage, and transmission of records to other offices. A section is provided in this chapter to inform the student of the importance of treating a patient and his or her records in a confidential manner.

Legal, Moral, and Ethical Concerns

Ethical practices and **morality** are the basis of most dealings between persons who may be practicing medicine, operating a business, or working in the legal system. One of these entities, that of law, cannot be separated from morals and ethics. Law is based on and derived from both moral and ethical treatment of our fellowman and evolved from the early history of mankind and the collective experiences of various groups of people. In addition, most major religions have a common basis in morals and ethics. The common origin of many of our laws went through an evolutionary process where rules of behavior now set in legal codes were handed down over many centuries. Laws came from common behaviors that developed from a realization that moral and ethical treatment of others was necessary to enable humans to coexist in a community.

The behaviors that became laws were eventually codified and served to provide a climate where trust and a sense of security could come about for everyone, not just the privileged class. Areas of civilization initially were clusters of persons of similar heritage, which then became neighborhoods, and then grew into towns with perhaps a number of neighborhoods. Eventually, larger collections of towns became organized as states with a governing system that covered a geographic region, and entire countries with common laws for everyone were then born out of these collections of people with common pursuits. The legal, ethical, and moral components of our existence work together inextricably and produce an environment in which all the citizens can live with a measure of security and well-being.

What is Meant by the Term *Ethics*?

A dictionary definition of **ethics** shows it stems from the word *custom*. The meaning of the word *custom* is a set of generally accepted practices or types of behavior associated with a specific group of people. This meaning has eventually evolved to that of a meaning more closely associated with "doing the correct or proper thing." The use of the term *ethics* is frequently associated with medical or business practices. In the medical arena, we view care of the poor and elderly, the newborn or unborn children, and handicapped persons as an ethical responsibility. Denial of certain procedures because a patient falls into categories such as age or medical conditions, along with a myriad of other conditions, would be measured by standards in the ethical realm. The term *morality* is associated with actual conduct, from which the *Patient's Bill of Rights* originates. *Morality* refers to a system of conduct that is right and wrong, or what is virtuous. The science of morality relates to the principles of proper professional conduct concerning the rights and duties of health care professionals, their patients, and their colleagues.

Ethical Delivery of Medical Care

Providing medical care in an ethical manner has many tenets that are necessary to provide an overall system that works to the patient's advantage. All patients desire and deserve to have their treatment delivered in a confidential and professional manner. As a significant factor in health care, federal laws such as the Health Insurance Portability and Accountability Act (HIPAA) have been enacted to delineate the responsibilities of health care providers and the manner in which medical information is to be handled. There are three basic components of the rights of the patient receiving care. These fundamental rights of the patient regarding personal privacy of self and records are:

1. The patient's condition or his or her medical data should not be revealed to anyone other than those who have a valid right to obtain the results.
2. No tests should be performed unless ordered through proper channels by the physician or his or her designees. Positive tests for certain diseases often have connotations of wrongdoing by the patient and could bring great embarrassment to the patient whose results are revealed to others.
3. Results of tests are never given directly to patient without guidance from the attending physician(s), as patients are often poorly equipped to understand, interpret, and to handle critical test information.

The *Patient's Bill of Rights* is an important component of the duty of the health care facility to provide adequate care. This document will typically be posted conspicuously in the hospital in areas where patients check into the facility or are treated as an outpatient, such as in the emergency areas. This document is based on the responsibility for ethical and moral treatment of the patient, regardless of his or her station in life. The *Patient's Bill of Rights* is an institution-wide document and has some application to the medical laboratory, where there might be some contact with patients and with sensitive records of medical testing. All people deserve appropriate health care and the ability to enjoy a sense of well-being, regardless of their respective stations in life or their status related to having a disease, whether chronic or acute. Those who are stricken by an illness or permanent or temporary condition should expect to be treated by health care providers who possess not only professional competence but also the appropriate compassion and caring needed to ensure comfort during illness or recovery from illness. In other words, all health care personnel should be professional in all matters related to a patient and the care rendered. Social issues, ethnic issues, and those of psychological or religious matters should be treated with due respect.

Organizations for the various medical professions have been founded over the years to ensure that health care providers have attained the credentials necessary to perform certain duties in a medical facility. These organizations may be on a state or national level, as previously discussed. They always involve members of their own professions who play a role in governing these professional organizations. Almost all health care professions require a certain level of credentialing and adherence to standards, as will be discussed in a following section. This is typically done by licensing or by a registry examination developed by the organization dedicated to a particular profession. All of these organizations exist to protect the public from unscrupulous and unprofessional practices. All medical professions have components in both their education and training that deal with the sensitive issues of personal facts related to the patient.

It is also part of a patient's rights to be treated by a practitioner who is knowledgeable in the area in which he or she is employed. The professional organizations were at least in part established to have input into the education and training processes for students seeking a career in one of these health care professions. That is why there is an organization for most of the health care professions that accredits educational programs; in some cases the same organization may administer a registry or licensure examination to ensure competency when state licensure is not required.

As a general statement, professional groups and accrediting bodies require certification or registry to become members, while government organizations require licensure. Certification and registry may be viewed as somewhat of a quasi-legal requirement, since most health care organizations will not hire unqualified and uncertified personnel. Processes leading to certification, registry, or licensure usually require an examination developed to ensure competency by meeting certain standards established by a particular professional organization or a professional testing agency. These examinations are administered to qualified candidates to determine competency of the individual prior to the person performing professional duties in a health care facility. Medical organizations, which exist to document that standards of care have been achieved to their satisfaction, also have codes of ethics by which they operate and to govern behavior of its members. Personal and institutional practices and standards of behavior exist, often in formal documents, which are to be adhered to by each member of the professions represented within a medical care facility. Professional organizations that govern medical facilities support a mission statement that provides at a minimum the tenets of a patient bill of rights. It should outline the meeting of certain patient expectations, including the right to privacy for records and person, and the right of self-dignity, in which the patient is treated respectfully.

Relationship of *Ethics* and *Professionalism*

Just as *ethics* and *morals* cannot be separated, *ethics* and *professionalism* cannot be separated. There is a blending or blurring of distinction for these two words. These words may be used in adjective or adverb forms and often mean different things to different persons. Sometimes a code of ethics is contained along with the *Patient's Bill of Rights* as a vital part of the structure. Compiling of an organized set of ethical issues is sometimes a legal matter and might include, but not be limited to, the expectations of the patient for competent and adequate care.

Ethics is more than a set of rules, and practicing ethics while treating patients should become an affective part of the medical worker's life. The term *affective* is a psychological term meaning that the individual worker should arrive at a point that ethical practice is such a part of the life of being professional that it cannot be separated from the worker. Cosman and Bissell (1991) state, "Ethics consists of far more than abiding by rules, procedures, and guidelines. It represents an expression of conscience," which might be summed up in the word professionalism. But the practice of ethical behavior includes much more than the surface actions of a health care practitioner. In the health care arena, there is a responsibility for all health care workers to treat people as they should be treated, as well as for the careful handling of private information that should not be disseminated to the general public, or even to another person, without a need to know. Laws related to the treatment of patients and the protection of patients and their privacy are established and at times modified as society and procedures change.

Appearance and grooming of the professional are the first visible signs of professionalism that a patient may be aware of. Perhaps the next thing a patient would recognize in the professional would be the manner of speech and the behavior exhibited by the worker. Patients regard the health care practitioner or other medical worker as more "professional" and place more trust in the health care employee if he or she is dressed and groomed in a professional manner. A clean and properly dressed health care worker does a great deal to engender confidence in the patient and his or her family members and visitors as to the medical worker's abilities. Some safety issues are also involved; as an example, consideration is given to dangling jewelry and artificial fingernails, which may interfere in the performance of medical procedures and entangle in equipment. Long hair that is hanging loose may also pose a risk for transmitting infections to patients, as hair is often covered with organisms and other materials.

Critical Reminder

All Patients Have a Right to Certain Expectations of Health Care Facilities

1. Bill of rights for the patient
2. Right to privacy
3. Right to self-dignity

Formal Statements of Professionalism

Physicians have the **Oath of Hippocrates**, nurses recite the **Nurses Creed** when they are formally capped, and facilities have mission statements that incorporate core values and beliefs of society at large with respect to medical

Critical Reminder

The *Oath of Hippocrates* Is a Formal Statement of Core Values and Beliefs

- Do not harm anyone intentionally.
- Perform according to sound ability and good judgment.
- Do that for which training has occurred, and not more.
- Do not become involved in anyone's care out of curiosity; only deal with those to whom assigned. Only information that is needed to provide the appropriate level of care is to be disseminated to or obtained or solicited by those who do not have a professional need for the information.
- Facts about patients are not to be part of personal conversations but are to be kept confidential.

Critical Reminder

Health Care Professionals Should Not:

- Be impolite to a patient or his or her family and should always treat the patient with respect and in a professional manner.
- Discuss a patient's ailment with him or her. This is the role of the physician or his or her assistant or other designated person.
- Discuss various types of therapy chosen for treatment.
- Prescribe or suggest changes in medication or means of treatment.
- Discuss patient's physician or his or her designated assistant with the patient or his family or yield information of a confidential nature to anyone except those who need to know.

treatment. Other medical professions that incorporate the process of "pinning" as a traditional rite of passage into a profession also incorporate a statement of values and beliefs essential for the profession the student is entering. The Critical Reminder box (upper left) sets out a modern version of the Oath of Hippocrates.

Professional Societies

Professional societies, in most cases, are composed of professional groups restricted to a particular area of expertise and most, if not all, have a statement or statements governing the ethical practice by their respective associations and members. These groups generally reflect in their codes or creeds the major themes of reliability, accuracy of procedures, assessments, and confidentiality. Hospital and most medical clinics have a formal code of ethics that may be included in other documents, such as a code of ethics, which may include the *Patient's Bill of Rights*. Basic tenets of the *Patient's Bill* statements such as those shown in the Critical Reminder box (lower left).

PATIENT EXPECTATIONS AND RIGHTS

In the past few years and as mentioned earlier in this chapter, health care facilities have begun to publish a *Patient's Bill of Rights* and a mission statement. Many of the components of the bill of rights (Table 3-1) relate to morality, ethics, and legality as they apply to providing health care. Mission statements based on corporate models that most large companies embrace have also become a focal point of providing proper services to patients. These two official documents support and enhance each other. Since medical care workers are in direct contact with the patients and their families, as well as becoming aware of personal information related to the person, it is necessary that ALL health care workers be trained as to their responsibilities. This would include ways to deal with patients, their families, and any information they are knowledgeable of that would be pertinent to the patient's treatment.

Basics of Patient's Right to Informed Consent

One of the major patient's rights is the requirement for "informed consent" documentation. The patient has the right to be informed of hospital policies and practices that relate to patient care, treatment, and responsibilities. The patient has the right to be informed of available resources for resolving disputes, grievances, and conflicts, such as ethics committees, patient representatives, or other

Table 3-1 Excerpts from the American Hospital Association Patient Bill of Rights

This Bill of Rights is provided by the American Hospital Association (AHA) and is usually used in a similar form and with the following provisions by health care facilities. These rights can be exercised on the patient's behalf by a designated surrogate or proxy decision maker if the patient lacks decision-making capacity, is legally incompetent, or is a minor.

1. The patient has the right to receive considerate and respectful care.

2. The patient has the right to and is encouraged to obtain from physicians and other direct caregivers relevant, current, and understandable information concerning diagnosis, treatment, and prognosis.

    Except in emergencies when the patient lacks decision-making capacity and the need for treatment is urgent, the patient is entitled to the opportunity to discuss and request information related to the specific procedures and/or treatments, the risks involved, the possible length of recuperation, and the medically reasonable alternatives and their accompanying risks and benefits.

    Patients have the right to know the identity of physicians, nurses, and others involved in their care, as well as when those involved are students, residents, or other trainees. The patient also has the right to know the immediate and long-term financial implications of treatment choices, insofar as they are known.

3. The patient has the right to make decisions about the plan of care prior to and during the course of treatment and to refuse a recommended treatment or plan of care to the extent permitted by law and hospital policy and to be informed of the medical consequences of this action. In case of such refusal, the patient is entitled to other appropriate care and services that the hospital provides or transfer to another hospital. The hospital should notify patients of any policy that might affect patient choice within the institution.

4. The patient has the right to have an advance directive (such as a living will, health care proxy, or durable power of attorney for health care) concerning treatment or designating a surrogate decision maker with the expectation that the hospital will honor the intent of that directive to the extent permitted by law and hospital policy.

    Health care institutions must advise patients of their rights under state law and hospital policy to make informed medical choices, ask if the patient has an advance directive, and include that information in patient records. The patient has the right to timely information about hospital policy that may limit its ability to implement fully a legally valid advance directive.

5. The patient has the right to every consideration of privacy. Case discussion, consultation, examination, and treatment should be conducted so as to protect each patient's privacy.

6. The patient has the right to expect that all communications and records pertaining to his/her care will be treated as confidential by the hospital, except in cases such as suspected abuse and public health hazards when reporting is permitted or required by law. The patient has the right to expect that the hospital will emphasize the confidentiality of this information when it releases it to any other parties entitled to review information in these records.

7. The patient has the right to review the records pertaining to his/her medical care and to have the information explained or interpreted as necessary, except when restricted by law.

8. The patient has the right to expect that, within its capacity and policies, a hospital will make reasonable response to the request of a patient for appropriate and medically indicated care and services. The hospital must provide evaluation, service, and/or referral as indicated by the urgency of the case. When medically appropriate and legally permissible, or when a patient has so requested, a patient may be transferred to another facility. The institution to which the patient is to be transferred must first have accepted the patient for transfer. The patient must also have the benefit of complete information and explanation concerning the need for, risks, benefits, and alternatives to such a transfer.

9. The patient has the right to ask and be informed of the existence of business relationships among the hospital, educational institutions, other health care providers, or payers that may influence the patient's treatment and care.

10. The patient has the right to consent to or decline to participate in proposed research studies or human experimentation affecting care and treatment or requiring direct patient involvement, and to have those studies fully explained prior to consent. A patient who declines to participate in research or experimentation is entitled to the most effective care that the hospital can otherwise provide.

11. The patient has the right to expect reasonable continuity of care when appropriate and to be informed by physicians and other caregivers of available and realistic patient care options when hospital care is no longer appropriate.

Source: Reprinted with permission from The American Hospital Association.

mechanisms available in the institution. The patient has the right to be informed of the hospital's charges for services and available payment methods.

The following sections provide information related to ethics, organization of the health care delivery system, and terms widely used in documenting the meeting of medical standards established for health care facilities. Both government and professional groups have taken measures to ensure that health care institutions and practitioners of various medical professions are effectively trained and monitored. In the following sections, specific training areas are also addressed to acquaint the student with the proper information and expertise needed to provide quality care for those in his or her care.

Legal Action against a Medical Facility or Worker

It will be helpful to understand a few legal terms associated with the medical profession to grasp a thorough understanding of this section. A **tort** is a wrongful act that is a civil matter rather than a criminal one, arising from negligent or intentionally wrongful behavior that results in harm. A tort occurs if a person, including a health care worker, does not meet customary, established, and expected standards of care in a given situation. Many types of torts are possible in medical facilities. Malpractice is the one that is most often levied against a medical practitioner, but torts can include negligence, assault and battery, invasion of privacy, abuse, and defamation of character, although the latter category is rare.

A health care worker has a **duty**, or a moral obligation, to the patient. The moral commitment requires action that is in the interest of the patient and not just a condition of the mind of the medical worker. Usually, duty involves some sort of sacrifice on the part of the worker, who is committed to act in the best interest of the patient. A failure to act in the prescribed manner is a breach by the health care worker of a commitment. **Causation** is the "causal relationship between conduct and the result derived from that conduct." As a consequence, causation provides a means of connecting a manner of conduct with the resulting harm or resultant element. Causation is only applicable where a result has been achieved. Compensatory **damages** are paid to compensate the claimant if he or she is successful in proving in court a loss, injury, or harm suffered by another's breach of duty.

Risk management is a health care approach in which a specialist addresses the prevention and containment of liability by documenting critical or unusual patient care incidents. There are university programs that prepare working professionals in health care or law to enter the field of health care risk management and patient safety. After completing the program, graduates will have an understanding of general risk management techniques; standards of health care risk management administration; federal, state, and local laws; and methods for integrating patient safety and facility risk management into a comprehensive risk management program.

The objective of risk management is to reduce different risks related to an act or a failure to act to a level acceptable to the facility. It may refer to various types of threats caused by the environment, technology, and humans. The risks that are most likely to occur are prioritized and management attempts to reduce the risks by appropriate supervision and training of the workers. Some level of risk is inherent in the health care industry, and strategies for dealing with this risk involve transferring the risk to another party through insurance coverage. This coverage aids the health care facility in avoiding the risk, reducing the negative effect of the risk, or accepting some or all of the consequences of a particular risk.

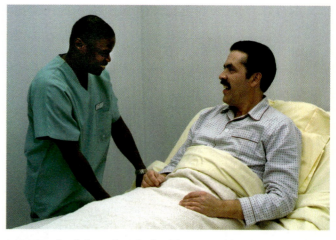

FIGURE 3-1 Any information obtained from the patient is considered confidential.
Source: Delmar/Cengage Learning.

MEDICAL LAW AND PRIVACY

Medical law and *privacy* are also interwoven, similar to the inseparable relationship between *morality* and *ethics*. Privacy, however, is not the only aspect of medical law but is of sufficient importance to have warranted a federal law to protect the confidentiality of patients and their records from intrusion by those not involved in the direct treatment of the patient, or for use in solicitation of sales, or for stealing the privacy of a patient.

Confidentiality of Medical Information and Records

Any information obtained by the medical facility from a patient or any privileged information about the patient is considered confidential (Figure 3-1). This information includes the patient's history, diagnosis, and plan of treatment or current condition. The medical worker is not even allowed to reveal that a patient is being treated, in most cases. The only time this information may be shared with others is when a signed release statement has been prepared or when imparting information to another medical care provider who has the need to know the information. Information for insurance purposes and information transmitted to another medical care professional for continuity of care is allowed within established guidelines. HIPAA guidelines covering confidentiality will be discussed later in this chapter. The medical care worker should never discuss anyone's condition or treatment or any personal information with anyone who does not have the right to know, even family members. The only time to discuss a patient's medical condition with family members is when a patient has given written permission for family members to act on his or her behalf, as with a living will. It is quite easy to disclose that a patient was treated in your facility without intentionally revealing any pertinent information. However, even this is not acceptable under the provisions of federal law.

Critical Reminder
Legal Aspects of Records Protection

1. Hospital documents are always legal documents and must not be altered except as policy allows. Some types of records are never disposed of, but kept in an electronic format.

2. Legal requirements require that the categories of who, how, and when work is done, and by whom it was ordered are documented. Often, insurance reimbursement will be denied in the absence of this information.

3. Dispensing of results to the patient is normally done only by the physician or his or her designated practitioner.

Basic Rules to Observe for Confidentiality

1. Never discuss the patient or his or her condition with family and friends. On a practical basis, a medical care worker should not be involved in matters that are not directly related to the performance of his or her specifically assigned and reasonable duties for his or her position.
2. Never discuss a patient's illness in the patient's presence or with another worker or family member unless it is within the scope of practice. There is evidence that patients may hear everything that is said, even when in a comatose state. At best, the patient may misinterpret what you have to say.
3. Refer questions by the patient regarding his or her disease and treatment to the physician in charge of the patient's care. The patient and his or her physician are the only persons legally and ethically able to divulge information of any type to another party. A medical laboratory worker should not discuss test results and the clinical significance of them. The technician or technologist may tell the patient he or she is collecting blood for tests to assist the patient's physician in the diagnosis or treatment of the patient. The laboratory worker is not aware of the patient's condition in many instances and may give innocent but erroneous information that may be misinterpreted.

Standards for Legal and Ethical Issues

Legal and ethical standards are developed to provide safe medical care for the patient and to protect the caregiver. Ethical or moral activities and laws that have been developed to govern the legal aspects of care are often the same, and are inextricable. In fact, this country's legal system and those of many other countries evolved from ethics and morals that often were spawned by various religious groups. The medical worker may be faced almost daily with decisions to make about what is the morally or legally correct thing to do. Often, there is an attorney on the hospital board, or an attorney on retainer, to provide input into questions of legality when policies and procedures are being developed and implemented. Slight differences between legal and ethical standards are:

Legal standards

Legal standards are developed within the legislative and judicial departments of our country. If a worker fails to follow the legal standards and does not work within the scope of practice established for his profession, he may be liable for legal action against him.

Ethical standards

Ethical standards are based on moral standards and are in some cases based on religion or customs. Many laws have been traditionally developed based on the religious practices of various groups of peoples.

Sample Legal and Ethical Questions

Arguments often arise in the discussion of legal and ethical dilemmas by persons who have an interest, perhaps even emotional or cultural, in a particular issue.

An example of this difference of opinion is the issue of the right to life. Questions regarding this issue involve more than the rights of one person. Examples of some of these legal and ethical questions are as follows:

- Do all of our citizens have the right to life and the pursuit of happiness?
- What are the rights of the unborn and of the newborn?
- Should the tissue of an aborted fetus be used to provide medical treatment for persons suffering illnesses that might be aided by transplantation of tissue from a fetus?
- Is euthanasia ever legally justified, such as in assisted suicides as performed by Dr. Kevorkian, the Michigan pathologist?
- Should a person have the right to refuse water and food in order to die if a disease or condition is terminal, and should medical intervention be used to force the person to eat and drink?
- Does a person on public assistance (Medicare or Medicaid) deserve to have continuous treatment for an incurable condition, as opposed to one who has insurance that has a limit on the amount of treatment that may be received?
- Does a person of a lower socioeconomic class without financial resources deserve the same treatment as a person of a higher status?

STANDARDS OF CONFIDENTIALITY

Most medical workers, particularly those with direct patient contact, will be faced with at least some of these questions as well as others of their own in the course of their duties. Many medical facilities have ethics committees that include clergy, legal personnel, and interested citizens to develop standards to use in the workplace. Some of these committees may even be state-wide or national in scope. Most assuredly, we will hear about more of these issues in the next few decades, as technology evolves and personal information becomes more widely available. Health care workers should be aware that a record of accessing a patient's or an employee's records by computer leaves a trail that may be followed. Disciplinary action for unwarranted intrusion may follow an attempt to gain access to private records, and in many cases workers have been surprised by a visit from computer services personnel, asking for verification of the need for various persons to have accessed certain files. Laws are strict as to who can access a patient's records and the conditions under which this is done (Figure 3-2).

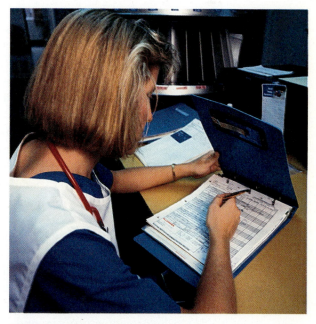

FIGURE 3-2 A patient's right to privacy must be maintained when a patient's medical records are accessed.
Source: Delmar/Cengage Learning.

Health Insurance Portability and Accountability Act (HIPAA)

In 1996, an act of Congress established the Health Insurance Portability and Accountability Act (HIPAA). This legislation took effect on April 14, 2002. In reaction to intrusions into personal lives, the purpose of the legislation is to protect the privacy of patients' health information and records.

In the past, many agencies such as health care insurers had routinely purchased or otherwise obtained individual patient records to determine premium charges based on medical conditions or to deny insurance coverage for certain patients and their families. Also, commercial efforts for mass distribution of contacts and for companies that wanted to establish a base of customers and private information for sale to certain businesses had become prevalent.

HIPAA regulations protect medical records and other individually identifiable health information, whether on paper, in computers, or communicated orally for recording. There are also offshoots of this legislation affecting institutions other than the health care industry. One example of this is the Family Education Rights and Privacy Act (FERPA), which provides students with certain rights with respect to their educational records. It is designed to protect the records of students enrolled in any training or educational institution and is designed to protect the privacy of individual students. The rules for FERPA are similar to those of HIPAA.

Although HIPAA was the first attempt to protect private information, others will surely follow, to establish federal privacy standards to protect patients' medical records and other health information provided to health plans, physicians, hospitals and other health care providers. The plan was developed by the U.S. Department of Health and Human Services (HHS), and in addition to protecting patient records, provides patients with a process for accessing their own medical records and gives them more control over how their personal health information is used and disclosed. A consistent format is provided for privacy protections for consumers of medical care throughout the nation. In instances where current state laws already provide protection, or are more stringent than federal law, the state laws are not affected by the federal law.

In 1996, Congress asked HHS to provide a plan for patient privacy protections as part of HIPAA. As a means to transfer health information from provider to provider, and for insurance reimbursement, HIPAA encourages electronic transactions and provides requirements to safeguard the security of health care information when sharing that information between medical facilities and any agency with a need to acquire individual patient records. Health insurance plans, including health maintenance organizations (HMOs) and preferred provider plans (PPOs), and health care providers of all types have a mammoth task in protecting the privacy of patients and other consumers of health care.

Maintenance of records may be contracted to a company that specializes in the storage and disseminating of medical records to third parties. For efficiency and economy, there are health care clearinghouses that specialize in maintaining medical records for large institutions as well as for other medical care providers by providing financial and administrative transactions. Duties such as collecting enrollment information, billing of patients and plans, and ensuring eligibility for family members and verifying enrollment are accomplished electronically in large computerized offices. It is easy to see that these records could easily be misused if they fell into the wrong hands. HIPAA prohibits the sale of records without the patient's permission. The sale of databases with personal information about private citizens has turned into big business in this country; businesses can target certain individuals who fit their profile as a potential consumer, and medical records have been no exception to this practice. Insurance companies might also seek to deny coverage to those with chronic or genetic medical problems.

On April 14, 2003, almost all health insurers, pharmacies, physicians, and other health care providers were required to begin complying with HIPAA regulations. A number of agencies requested exemption from the timeline, and Congress allowed some small health plans to have an additional year to comply. HHS provides assistance to health care providers to assist them in transitioning to a more structured manner of obtaining, using, and transmitting information. An HHS website is provided for medical providers to ask questions about the rules and to obtain explanations and descriptions about specific components of rules. These materials are available at http://hhs.gov/ocr/hipaa.

Provisions of the HIPAA Regulations

Privacy rules enacted by the federal government describe the patient's right to privacy as well as the situations where patient information can legally be shared. Each employee who handles patient information is required to receive instruction and training on the policies and procedures under which information is gathered and transmitted to other persons or facilities. The patient must sign an agreement that he or she understands the conditions under which information may be shared.

Access to Personal Medical Records

Patients may see and obtain copies of their medical records, and they may request corrections where errors and mistakes are found and receive assurance that the records have been corrected. Copies of records should be available within 30 days of receipt of a request in writing. Patients may be charged for the cost of copying and sending the documents.

Notice of Privacy Practices

Patients must be advised in writing of their rights after the first visit on or following April 14, 2003, the date when compliance will be required. Patients must acknowledge receipt of notice of their rights under HIPAA, as they will be apprised of their rights, usually when they make an initial visit to a health care practitioner for assessment or treatment. Patients are usually asked to sign a form indicating their understanding of the HIPAA regulations and how those regulations are used to limit the amount of information imparted to a third party (Figure 3-3).

RELEASE AND ASSIGNMENT

Date _____

To _____
INSURANCE COMPANY

_____

Group No. _____ Certificate No._____

I hereby authorize Dr. _____

to release to your company or its representative, any information including the diagnosis and the records of any treatment or examination rendered to me during the period of such Medical or Surgical care.

I also authorize and request your company to pay directly to the above named doctor the amount due me in my pending claim for Basic Medical, Major Medical and/or Surgical treatment or services, by reason of such treatment or services rendered to:

_____
PATIENT

_____
SIGNATURE OF INSURED

_____   _____
WITNESS   ADDRESS

FIGURE 3-3 Official form that provides a release of medical information as approved by patient.
Source: Delmar/Cengage Learning.

Limited and Specified Use of Personal Medical Information

There are limits as to how information may be used and what information will be shared, which does not include personal information or the patient's entire medical file. In the past, many facilities sold information to companies performing research or those interested in marketing a product and desired a population that used a particular product. Personal information not related to health care issues may be provided to outside entities, but the patient must authorize release of medical and/or personal information to other health care facilities, providers, insurance companies, or financial institutions. Facilities must reveal dissemination of demographic information to other agencies that are studying a region of the country or a particular population group.

Prohibition on Marketing

Information released to pharmacies, pharmaceutical firms, health plans, and so on must be authorized by the patient, as stated previously, before the information may be transmitted. As an example, many pharmaceutical firms use patient data for research purposes related to treatment with medications developed for the treatment of specific diseases. Patients are asked to sign a release allowing specific information to be passed to an insurance carrier or another agency needing such information.

Stronger State Laws

These federal privacy standards give states that have laws requiring privacy protections for patients a minimum standard to ensure that effective protections are in effect. One area where this requirement would affect state laws is in the reporting of infectious diseases to state health departments. Certain protections of this information would be in effect for the states in their reporting, tracking, and use of information for surveillance purposes. Most states have laws requiring the reporting of certain contagious and communicable diseases. This type of surveillance is necessary to provide more protection for the entire population. Sexually transmitted and foodborne diseases comprise the major portion of reportable diseases as required by law.

Confidential Communications

Patients may request that physicians, their health care plans, and other involved offices enact practices that ensure that communication with the patient is kept confidential. A patient may ask that any medical consultation be done at his or her home or in a private office where access is limited to those performing the consultation or procedure (Figure 3-4). Most medical treatment facilities and professionals take the responsibility of safeguarding private information from their patients most seriously, as they could be successfully sued if they are careless with the information. There have been cases of suits against a medical office or facility when records were carelessly discarded in waste containers in a form that could easily be read and where others could retrieve the records.

Consumer Complaints

Patients may file complaints where they suspect that violation of privacy has occurred. These concerns may be made in writing directly to the covered provider or health plan or to HHS's Office for Civil Rights. Even large corporations, such as pharmaceutical manufacturers and government agencies, are subject to sanctions for violations of personal privacy issues. Only information that is necessary to process medical claims for insurance purposes and, in some cases, for research to determine the usefulness of certain medications and procedures may be solicited from medical professionals. In

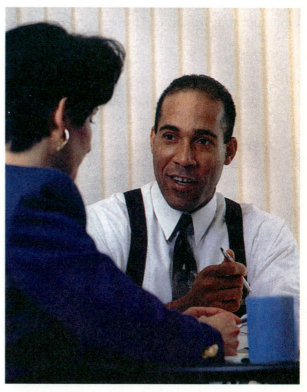

FIGURE 3-4 Importance of the practice of confidential communication.
Source: Delmar/Cengage Learning.

most cases, patients give their permission for dissemination and use of their personal information, with or without identification of the patients. Patients are under no requirement to release any of their information if they choose not to do so.

SUMMARY

Ethics, morals, and legal issues are all intrinsically interwoven. It is difficult to separate the three entities entirely. Laws were originally based on morals, so they often were of a religious basis, such as the Ten Commandments. It appears that ethics evolved from customs in many societies, so the approach to ethics between ethnic and cultural groups differs widely. Some theocratic countries have a legal system that is based on religion. As society advanced, the distinction between religion and law became slightly more defined, but culture and religion remain the bases of the legal system. Health care is based on the worth of the life of the individual and is considered a right for everyone by some politicians and average citizens.

Law is based on ethics, and medical law is no exception. There are a few legal issues related to medical law that one would do well to remember. First, all hospital and other medical records are legal documents. They should not be disposed of or altered. Each piece of documentation is required to be identified as to time and date, who performed the work, and any relevant notes. The patient's records should be guarded as confidential, and results of a patient's medical treatment are to be shared only with the patient's physician, who dispenses results to the patient. A release statement is required if records are to be sent to another facility or person.

Only the patient's physician can discuss the treatment plan with the patient. A medical worker should never discuss a patient's diagnosis or treatment received by the patient. Any health care worker who accesses a patient's records without a valid reason may be sanctioned or even brought to court. All patients deserve the same treatment without regard to financial or social status. Patients' personal records cannot be marketed to other companies and only that patient information necessary for processing an insurance claim may be disseminated.

Formalized statements are found in health care facilities and even in the official positions of professional organizations who certify health care professionals. Hospitals and medical clinics usually are required to hire only practitioners deemed competent by their professional accreditation agencies. Most hospitals and a number of large medical clinics will have a *Patient's Bill of Rights* prominently displayed in the facility. This document outlines general positions the facility adopts as to what a patient can expect when presenting for medical treatment. The *Oath of Hippocrates* and the *Nurses Creed* are formal statements that the medical and nursing professionals are expected to adhere to as professionals.

Ethics and professionalism go hand in hand. Professionalism is expressed outwardly as an appearance of cleanliness, orderly behavior and manner, and assured self-confidence in one's abilities. Sometimes professionals are expected to participate in a formal adoption of the various oaths and creeds, by a public ceremony. An example of this is the "pinning" or "capping" of nurses as they graduate, marking the transition from student to professional. Patients generally hold health care professionals in high esteem and expect selfless and competent care when they present themselves for treatment. They should expect and accept no less, and they should be made to feel comfortable and at ease, knowing their privacy will be observed when they communicate with you. This instills confidence in the health care worker as a professional (see Figure 3-1).

REVIEW QUESTIONS

1. Name some formal statements that certify that a profession or institution will provide the best care possible.
2. How do ethics and morality affect legal issues?
3. Should a health care employee provide medical information to the patient? If not, why?
4. What is the basic tenet of the *Oath of Hippocrates*?
5. What are a person's personal rights when hospitalized?
6. What two federal laws spell out the rights that a patient or a student has to privacy?
7. Who has the right to see a patient's medical records?
8. Who has the right to at least basic medical care, regardless of ability to pay?
9. What is the purpose of an ethics committee? Give some examples of those who serve on them.

CHAPTER 4

HOSPITAL AND LABORATORY ORGANIZATION

LEARNING OBJECTIVES

Upon completion of this chapter, the reader will be able to:

- Provide the former title for the administrator of a medical facility before adoption of the business-oriented title of chief executive officer (CEO).

- Discuss how the role of the hospital or health care facility CEO has changed.

- List the order from CEO down to the medical laboratory personnel on the organizational chart.

- Explain the six major departments of the hospital laboratory and the major duties of each.

- List three typical committees found in the health care setting and their functions.

KEY TERMS

ABO grouping
Activated partial thromboplastin time (APTT)
Antibodies
Antigens
Bone marrow
Chief executive officer (CEO)
Clotting time
Direct test

Fungi
Gel technology
Immunologic hormones
Indirect test
Infection Control Committee or Exposure Control Committee
Leukemias
Prothrombin time (PT)
Retroviruses

Rh type
Rickettsiae
Safety Committee
Serology (immunology)
Thrombocytes
Tissue Committee
Treponema pallidum
Viruses

INTRODUCTION

For the past several decades, at least, the hierarchy of a hospital organization has been well entrenched, although some of the names for certain offices within the facility have changed over the years, and a variety of differences exist between facilities. A worker's or professional's position within the framework of the organization usually depends on the level of education and responsibility given to the individual in the health care facility. The **chief executive officer (CEO)**, who is often known as the health care administrator, is the highest ranking official of the hospital. With increasingly complicated business systems within a hospital, this official is now generally awarded a title with the same terminology as that used in most business enterprises. This reflects the greater demand on health care institutions to be more cost conscious and to use good business practices. In past years, this was not generally the case, when traditionally a physician with no business training held this position. Many of the other officers of the various departments within the hospitals are frequently called assistant administrators and are often categorized by the area over which they exercise authority and responsibility. For example, larger hospitals may have an administrator for finance, computer services, clinical services, support services, and so on.

Professional organizations for individual employees and for the institution itself play a major role in the functioning of a health care facility. Facilities voluntarily ask for accreditation to present themselves as abiding by a certain set of professional or institutional standards. A hospital would encompass a number of occupations that could be addressed by these accrediting agencies. This meeting of the requirements for accreditation assures the public that the institution is seeking to provide a high standard of care; it is also a form of self-policing. Hospitals are dedicated to providing the best care possible, and they should seek to employ only qualified personnel to meet their responsibility to their patients. Accreditation agencies monitor the credentials of workers in a facility. In communities with more than one major health care facility, there is often competition for the better employees and, with personnel shortages, less-qualified personnel may be hired out of necessity.

Since hospitals are accredited and also licensed in most, if not all, states, they must meet regulations and standards required to be in good standing with government and accrediting agencies. Most job positions in a hospital require that personnel be registered, licensed, or certified in their respective field. As a condition of the hospital accreditation and licensure, employees must meet the standards for entry into the profession when they present themselves to the public as practicing professionals. Most often there are continuing requirements for remaining in good standing with the respective accrediting bodies, and the health care facility will either furnish training or aid the employee in efforts to maintain skills and certification. While most states require both facility licensure and accreditation for medical facilities, the requirements for accreditation and licensure are often similar, and in fulfilling a requirement for one agency, the other's requirements may be satisfied.

Hospitals are highly organized entities with various levels of supervisory managers existing in every department. The CEO provides coordination for the various areas within the hospital. In the larger facilities, the assistant administrators, who focus on broad areas such as finance, nursing, ancillary service, etc., report to a CEO. The lines of authority in a large hospital are typically complex and are based on the number of ancillary services and satellite clinics associated with the medical center. Some hospitals are

Critical Reminder
Organization of Health Care Facilities

- Board of directors includes chief of staff, administrator or CEO, attorney, business leaders, and in some cases committee chairs and representatives from the major departments within the hospital
- Chief of professional services
- Department supervisors for all ancillary departments, such as laboratory and pharmacy
- Section supervisors of areas within a major department
- Shift supervisors who report to section supervisors
- Staff (considerable ranking among staff, with the professional staff of persons who are licensed, registered, or certified at the top of the group in their scope of duties and responsibility)

components of a larger medical center or health care system, and this provides for even more complex organizational charts.

Anatomic Pathology

The clinical laboratory is usually organized under the pathologist in a department called pathology services, for example. The anatomic section would include anatomic pathologists, histotechnologists, and cytotechnologists, who perform studies of surgical specimens and cellular differentiation of cancerous cell types and their morphology. The anatomic pathology section differs from the clinical pathology section, which would include all the departments of the medical laboratory where body fluids and samples from the body are processed. Both the anatomic and the clinical pathologists have a M.D. or D.O. (doctor of osteopathy) degree; in some very large facilities, there are anatomic as well as clinical pathologists. If there are both clinical and anatomic pathologists, the clinical pathologist would be the chief officer of the clinical laboratory, separate from the pathology department. In the lines of authority established under the CEO, the chief pathologist would be found on an organizational chart at the same level as the chief of professional services in most instances.

Clinical Pathology

In larger facilities, supervision of the clinical departments of the laboratory may be provided by a pathologist who will often be a clinical pathologist, rather than an anatomic pathologist. There will then likely be a laboratory manager at the top of the laboratory organizational chart who supervises the day-to-day operations of the laboratory. The laboratory manager may or may not be a medical laboratory professional; some hold graduate business degrees and are concerned mainly with the monetary flow of the laboratory and the effectiveness and economy of providing services. In some laboratories, a chief technologist coordinates the daily functions of the laboratory for the laboratory manager. The chief technologist would manage department supervisors, such as the supervisor of hematology and coagulation. The department supervisors may have supervisors for each shift, because the laboratory is most often open 24 hours per day, 7 days per week. Then the technologists would be under the direction of the department supervisor and would in turn supervise the other technologists and technician-level employees.

DEPARTMENTS WITHIN THE LABORATORY

The organization of departments within the medical laboratory is as varied as the number of hospitals and clinics that contain clinical laboratory entities. Sometimes departments are combined; as an example, hematology and coagulation are often performed within the same department. Serological testing may be spread out among various departments, with no specific department that performs all of the serological tests. Often the department in which the procedure is performed is the area where other, related tests are performed. An example of this departmentalization would be the performance of serological testing for identifying bacterial organisms, which would be performed in the microbiology department where organisms are also grown and biochemically tested for identification of some strains of organisms.

Virology and parasitology are usually incorporated into the microbiology department unless the hospital is extremely large and provides a full range of all services. Routine urinalysis tests are often performed in other departments rather than having a single department to perform only urine analyses. For example, biochemical tests on urine samples may be performed in the clinical chemistry department. Urinalysis is often performed in hematology unless a large number of specialized urine analyses are performed, in which case there would probably be a separate urinalysis department. If the facility is large enough, there might be a special chemistry department that would perform all biochemical tests except the basic chemistry procedures from blood samples. Most often, a laboratory is divided into several major departments, some of which may be combined.

Hematology

Descriptively, *hematology* means "study of blood." The Greek word root *haema* literally means "blood," and the suffix *–ology* means "study" or "science" of a particular clinical site or body part. An adult human has 5 to 6 liters of blood in the body. Human blood and the blood of other vertebrates is composed of a liquid portion called plasma and a solid component composed of formed elements such as red blood cells (erythrocytes), white blood cells (leukocytes), and platelets (thrombocytes).

Most laboratory examinations are performed on blood samples and may include the liquid or the solid portion. Blood carries nutrients for the cells and oxygen for delivering needed materials to the cells; blood also removes toxic waste products and carbon dioxide from the body. Specialized proteins derived from the immune system are also found in the plasma. The function of white cells is chiefly as a defense against bacteria, viruses, fungi, and protozoa that invade the body.

The basic test performed in the hematology laboratory is the complete blood count (CBC). The CBC procedure is used to analyze a sample for the number, size, and shape or type of both white and red blood cells. It is useful in determining various types of anemia, infection, and abnormalities of the bone marrow where the cells originate. There are a number of methods for determining and calculating values for a CBC, ranging from totally automated systems to manual counts. Other tests commonly completed in the hematology department would include cell counts from cerebrospinal (CSF) fluid, pleural fluid from around the cavity containing the lungs and heart, parietal fluid from the abdominal (peritoneal) cavity, dialysate fluid (from dialysis), and synovial fluid from the joints.

Many major diseases may be determined from the CBC. In some cases, cancer may be discovered or overwhelming infections of either viral or bacterial infections are found. Dietary and genetic types of anemias may be diagnosed from red blood cells, and cancer of the bone marrow (leukemias) of many types may be found here. Also, deficiencies and abnormalities of the platelets (thrombocytes) that aid in clotting may be evaluated. These are but a few of literally hundreds of hematological tests that may be performed on whole blood. Many of these are extremely sophisticated and complex in the methodology used.

Coagulation

Coagulation is often combined with the hematology department, but coagulation testing is extremely important for treating a number of chronic diseases, so it will be treated as a separate department in this book. Coagulation tests are performed by using the liquid portion of blood, and the specimen requires that an anticoagulant be added to the sample to prevent clotting. The clotting factors, of which a number remain in the plasma, enable the laboratory worker to determine abnormalities in clotting of the blood.

Bleeding and clotting problems may be genetic or environmental or may be created by medically treating a person to prolong the **clotting time,** to prevent clots that lead to stroke or heart attack. The body also is in a precarious position as blood must be maintained as a liquid but must be able to clot in regions where tissue damage may cause bleeding. While there are a number of tests to determine abnormalities of clotting or to monitor the medication of a patient to prolong the coagulation time, there are two tests that are performed on a routine basis: the **prothrombin time (PT)** and the **activated partial thromboplastin time (APTT)**. These tests may be performed both manually and at varying levels of automation depending on the instrumentation used.

Advances over the past few years have led to more sophisticated testing. One of these lines of testing involves the use of extremely potent anticoagulants that may be injected in an extremely small area of the brain, lung, or heart to dissolve clots that may be life threatening. If treated quickly enough, emboli (clots) that can cause certain strokes and heart attacks and emboli of the lungs may be quickly dissolved, thereby minimizing tissue damage to these organs.

Immunohematology (Blood Banking)

The blood bank provides for a safe blood supply for patients requiring transfusions. Units of blood are screened for communicable diseases and are stored in conditions making contamination of the blood unlikely. Some diagnostic tests are performed by the blood bank, but its chief tasks are to store and test blood for compatibility before transfusing it into the patient. Blood products are also a vital part of a full-service blood bank. Some patients require transfusions of white blood cells as well as red blood cells. Platelet transfusions for patients who are deficient in levels of platelets (thrombocytes) required for forming a functional clot may receive platelet-rich plasma. Certain clotting factors are also concentrated for use by patients with abnormal clotting mechanisms.

Units of blood are tested for the **ABO grouping** and the **Rh type**, as well as for the presence of HIV or hepatitis infection. The basic tests for determining if a unit of blood is compatible with a patient are blood group and type. A type-specific unit is the best choice, although some patients may receive other ABO group transfusions with no danger. Determination of compatibility is performed by a test called *antibody-antigen reactions*. Certain maternal tests are performed for expectant mothers to determine if they have Rh or ABO incompatibility between the mother and the fetus, and the mother is monitored throughout her pregnancy in some cases. Some of the tests necessary to determine the safety of a unit of blood may be performed in laboratory sections other than the blood bank.

The blood bank is not highly automated, although new technologies such as **gel technology** in which **antigens** or **antibodies** may be imbedded in a gel reagent are in wide use. Highly skilled technologists and sometimes technicians are involved with measuring and pipetting test reagents and blood in minute volumes. The work is meticulous and records must be extremely accurate. All transfusion reactions observed in the patient must be followed up, even though many of those reactions are of an allergic nature and routine testing will not show any problem areas. Many technologists in the blood bank possess a master's degree in their chosen specialty and perform a great deal of highly specialized testing for unusual antibodies and antigens, which may have a genetic basis. With advances in genetic studies, it is entirely possible that the blood bank will be divided into more than one section, and routine testing for compatibilities of tissues and genetic tests for procedures not currently performed routinely may be offered in this major department.

Clinical Chemistry

Hundreds of chemistry examinations for the blood are performed daily in most chemistry laboratories. It is not cost-effective to perform all of the chemistry procedures that may be ordered, as some are required at such low volumes that it is economically wise to send these to a reference laboratory. Fifty or more tests comprise the majority of procedures performed on a daily basis. Many of these tests are grouped together in *panels* or groups of tests that help to differentiate between various disease states. The large automated instruments used are extremely accurate and specific for many acute and chronic diseases. This department provides more definitive result used in rapid diagnosis than almost any other laboratory section, as the routine tests are available quickly and at any time.

The presence of many different types of organic and biochemical constituents in the blood and other body fluids aids in diagnosing various diseases. For instance, if the kidneys are not properly functioning, there will be an inordinate level of toxic wastes in the liquid portion of the blood, either serum or plasma, indicating that the kidneys are not ridding the body of waste products. And in some cases, malfunction of the kidneys may cause the loss of materials such as minerals and proteins that the body should be reabsorbing and using in its metabolism. When certain tissues are damaged, enzymes peculiar to a particular tissue or organ will cause a rise in certain enzymes as the cells die, giving a clue as to the tissues being damaged. Tests for therapeutic drug levels and drugs of abuse are commonly performed in the clinical chemistry department.

The chemistry department is usually the most automated of all the divisions of the laboratory. In most laboratories, there are one or more large, complex instruments that perform thousands of tests per hour. These instruments are highly accurate, sensitive, and specific, and require that the results be evaluated by the laboratory worker when the values are reported and before they are sent to the physician who will treat the patient. Some large hospital laboratories may have several sections within the chemistry department that perform only certain specific and specialized procedures.

Serology (Immunology)

Serological tests to determine the immune response to an organism are performed in several sections of the laboratory and not in a single department. However, the importance of this variety of procedures requires that they be performed in a unique department. The immune system is the basis of protecting the body from invasions by microorganisms such as bacteria, viruses, rickettsiae (bacterial form of an intracellular parasite, a term that is not often used today), fungi, and parasites such as protozoa. When the body is attacked, the immune system leaps to the body's defense, and its activity in protecting itself gives information that can be used to diagnose the illness.

White cells attack organisms directly, but the liquid portion of the blood will contain proteins called antibodies when an organism is introduced into the body. These antibodies are almost completely specific to a particular organism, with some exceptions, and if the laboratory worker tests for these antibodies, it is an indirect test for infection by specific *antigens* (the organism is the antigen in infections). Allergy tests utilize several mechanisms to determine the products to which a patient may suffer an allergic reaction when coming in contact with the body. This is also a serological test. Other serological tests are available to test for the toxins produced by certain organisms. In some cases, a direct test is done by testing for the actual organism itself (bacterial, viral) rather than by testing for antibodies produced against the organism or for the toxins it produces.

Serological tests are usually performed in batches as most of the work is of a nonemergency nature. Some of these tests may be performed in chemistry or microbiology departments and some automation is available, but there remains a great deal of manual, hands-on work. The serology procedures are evolving rapidly as new technology emerges, and immunologic hormones, lymphokines, and monokines from certain lines of white cells have been isolated and are used to treat diseases that were previously untreatable, such as certain types of cancers. Sophisticated instrumentation is being developed to utilize the increasingly larger numbers of antibodies in increasingly smaller quantities that may be used to fight certain infections and diseases. This department could grow exponentially in coming years with new developments.

Microbiology

Detecting the presence of and identifying pathogenic (disease-causing) microorganisms is the focus of the microbiology laboratory. Microbiological studies represent one of the earliest efforts to detect and treat human diseases in the laboratory. The early development of the microscope by Antonie van Leeuwenhoek (Figure 4-1) in the late 1600s gave a boost to correlating the presence of microorganisms and certain diseases, as the device enabled a visual picture of causative germs.

Clinical microbiology includes the study of bacteria, viruses, fungi, and parasites. In the case of parasitology, protozoa may be visualized and the eggs of many intestinal parasites found in the stool; this facilitates the diagnosis of a parasitic infection. Bacteriology is a major area of most

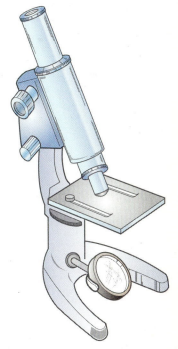

FIGURE 4-1 Drawing of an old microscope.
Source: Delmar/Cengage Learning.

laboratories, and only the larger microbiology departments perform other than routine growing of and identification of bacteria on a nutritive medium from specimens obtained from the patient. Most bacteria can be grown on selective and differential media that are developed to provide materials needed for specific bacteria to grow and reproduce. Not all strains of bacteria have the same nutritive requirements, so a number of types of media are required to grow a wide variety of organisms. Some bacteria, in particular *Treponema pallidum*, which causes syphilis, cannot be cultured on commercial media, so other methods of identification are required.

Detection of and identification of viruses require cell cultures, since these microorganisms can only grow and reproduce in cells (intracellularly), which provide the DNA and in some cases RNA (for a group called **retroviruses**) needed for their growth. The herpes virus and hepatitis viruses are the most prevalent organisms causing diseases, and they are detected directly by sophisticated methods or indirectly by the presence of specific antibodies found in the serum of the blood. Some bacterial organisms, such as the tuberculosis-causing organism, grow extremely slowly on special media, and this process can take weeks to months. Most fungal (mycological) infections are caused by organisms that also grow slowly, but many of the parasites and their eggs are identifiable almost immediately by use of the microscope.

Clinical microbiologists additionally perform an important role in determining the appropriate antibiotic for the physician's use in treating diseases. Injudicious use of antibiotics for viral infections such as colds leads to a greater variety of organisms not susceptible to the medication, and hospitals are often the source of infections in patients who are treated in the facility. Many infectious bacterial organisms are now being identified with new and emerging technology, where the sequence of DNA is specific for identifying various species of microorganisms. But microbiology relies mostly on the skills and intuitive knowledge of the technologist or microbiologist. Many microbiologists earn a master's or doctoral degree, enabling them to perform at a higher level of expertise. Higher levels of certification under the professional certification agencies are available for those who pursue graduate degrees in microbiology.

COMMITTEE FUNCTIONS

Committee functions within the hospital play a vital role in maintaining the quality of services. Many employees, including those from the laboratory, are often called on to serve on a committee where their expertise would be needed. Most accreditation requirements and related issues of health care delivery are handled by committee members who are chosen because of their particular expertise. Some committees are multidisciplinary and have members from several departments within the hospital. Some committees also retain members from outside the facility to gain input from the community. Many committees require multidisciplinary groups that act as experts in some of the areas addressed by the committees. Often these committees are required by accreditation bodies for certain functions, and during a site visit from licensure or accreditation organizations, the site visitors from the professional groups may ask to meet with the committees. Serving on committees is either voluntary or by appointment and is an important function related to hospital accreditation. Committee members provide invaluable service by lending expertise from a number of professions and specialties (Table 4-1). Committee functions are an important facet of providing effective and safe health care for the protection of all patients, workers, and visitors to a clinical facility.

Infection Control Committee and Exposure Control Committee

The **Infection Control Committee or Exposure Control Committee** has the broadest scope of responsibility. This committee touches every department and every aspect of health care. Any department will contain hazards that may be a danger

Table 4-1 Standard Committees in a Health Care Setting, with Interdepartment Representatives

Committee	Purpose	Personnel	Departments
Infection Control Committee or Exposure Control Committee	Protection of patients, workers, and visitors	Custodians Dietitians Educators Laboratory personnel Microbiologists Nurses Pathology personnel Pharmacists Physicians Others	Clinical laboratory Environmental safety Food services Inservice education Medical staff Nursing services Pathology department Pharmacy
Safety Committee	Protection of patients, workers, and visitors	Biomedical technicians Clerical Custodians Electrical technicians Landscapers Nurses Other professionals Physicians Plumbers	Biomedical repair Clinical laboratory Custodial Electrical technicians Grounds and landscaping Medical Nursing services Other Pathology services Plumbing department Receptionists, secretaries Specialty clinics
Tissue Committee	Accuracy in procedures, proper disposal of tissues and generated wastes	Anatomic pathologists Chief of staff Cytologists Histotechnologists Morgue attendants Physician's assistants Surgeons Surgical suite personnel Vital records personnel	Custodians Morgue Operating room suites Pathology department

if a person is exposed or overexposed. Something as innocuous as liquid correction fluid (e.g., Wite-Out) may be dangerous if breathed long enough. Even lubricating oils may be hazardous if they come in prolonged contact with the skin. This committee, which is sometimes separated into both an Infection Control Committee and an Exposure Control Committee, is one of the most important committees within the hospital. It is an interdisciplinary committee with professionals from most of the departments of the institution. This committee includes, but is not limited to, physicians, nurses, laboratory personnel from the various departments within pathological services, and custodial/housekeeping, food service, and pharmacy personnel. Chapter 6, "Introduction to Infection Control," will address specific functions and tasks of these committees.

Safety Committee

The **Safety Committee** works closely with the Infection Control Committee or Exposure Control Committee, and there is often overlap between the duties of the two committees. However, the focus of the Safety Committee involves the entire facility, including the physical plant and all of its systems. Electrical systems, water and sewer systems, and the dangerous conditions within buildings and even on the grounds around the facility are of interest to this committee. Outdoor security (adequate lighting and security personnel) is included in the Safety Committee's responsibilities. Security systems, fire hazards, final disposition of toxic wastes, and the storage and disposal of chemicals and biohazardous materials are often handled by the Safety Committee. Like the Infection Control Committee and Exposure Control Committee, the Safety Committee is involved with protecting visitors, workers, and patients.

Tissue Committee

The **Tissue Committee** likewise often works closely with the Infection Control Committee or Exposure Control Committee. This committee should include surgeons, anatomic pathologists, and other professionals and paraprofessionals such as cytologists and histotechnologists. Statistics are compiled as to the accuracy of diagnosis leading to surgery or from the study of tissues from post-mortem examinations where the patient may have received inadequate treatment. Data for these important functions are reviewed by the chief of staff and accrediting agencies for the facility. Reports from the committee may be of interest to insurance carriers who are providing reimbursement for surgery that may not have been justified.

SUMMARY

Laboratories have not changed much fundamentally in their organization over the past few years. However, the numbers of workers and the types of work performed have changed. Surprisingly, there are fewer hospital beds today to serve a much larger population than in the 1980s, when the number of hospital beds in the United States peaked. Conversely, the number of medical laboratory workers is not as great as in the past, mainly due to automation, with high levels of procedures performed in minutes. However, this decrease in the actual number of workers has been somewhat offset by the larger numbers of tests being performed for diagnosis. Insurance has demanded shorter stays, and treatment is now definitive and quick. Will the organization of the laboratory change in the future? Undoubtedly it will, as the numbers of sophisticated tests available increase and radical treatments for formerly terminal diseases are ratcheted up. In addition, more graduate-level scientists will be required as increasingly sophisticated procedures are developed.

It is possible that more laboratory scientists will be required instead of fewer in the future to perform complex tests that require the critical thinking processes to complete and disseminate the results to physicians and their designees. The next step for technicians and technologists for more definitive and technically demanding work may be just over the horizon. There are new markers discovered on an increasing basis that either predict the risk factors for certain diseases or monitor the treatment of serious diseases. Genetic manipulations and procedures not yet developed may be routine in the next few decades in the hospital laboratory.

REVIEW QUESTIONS

1. Describe how the roles have changed for the CEO of a hospital (formerly known simply as the administrator) now that more hospitals are modeled along the lines of a business.
2. Describe the differences between an anatomic pathologist and a clinical pathologist.
3. The operations of immunohematology (blood banking) and immunology are similar in what way?
4. Describe the difference between a direct test and an indirect test.
5. Name four categories of organisms that may cause an immune response.

CHAPTER 5

LABORATORY SAFETY

LEARNING OBJECTIVES

Upon completion of this chapter, the reader will be able to:

- Describe the personal responsibility of the worker for maintaining a safe environment.

- List a number of physical hazards associated with the workplace.

- List some sources with the potential for transmitting infectious diseases.

- Differentiate between general safety and fire safety.

- Discuss the importance of accident investigations.

KEY TERMS

Acquired immunodeficiency syndrome (AIDS)
Biohazardous materials
Biohazards

Hazardous chemicals
Human immunodeficiency virus (HIV)
Infection Control Committee or Exposure Control Committee

Sharps
Safety Committee

INTRODUCTION

Safety should be foremost in the minds of all employees of a health care facility. Safety is the business of everyone, and prevention is the best cure. However, accidents will continue to occur, and preventive measures (training, documenting steps taken to address dangerous situations) will minimize the impact of injuries on the facility and on a personal basis. Due to the nature of the work, and the persons with whom the workers are in contact, the risks to workers and patients may be amplified. Thus, it is wise to include the issue of visitors to the facility when discussing means of preventing injuries and illnesses. Health care workers should seek to provide good patient care while ensuring that the environment for the patients and the workers is conducive to maintaining physical and emotional health. Safety issues are more than just a responsibility to one's co-workers, oneself, and the patients. They are a volatile legal issue as manifested by suits brought by both patients and workers who have been harmed by injuries and from contracting preventable infections. In the late 1970s, a focus on safety was

Table 5-1 Timeline of Federal Guidelines and Laws Concerning Biological Safety

Year	Issuing Agency/Entity	Guideline/Law
1970	CDC	Published "Isolation Techniques for Use in Hospitals"
1975	CDC	Revised "Isolation Techniques" to include category-specific precautions and prohibition of recapping needles
1983	CDC	Issued nonbinding guidelines for isolation precautions in hospitals, designating seven isolation categories
1985	CDC	Introduced Universal Blood and Body Fluid Precautions (Universal Precautions or UP), primarily in response to HIV/AIDS epidemic
1987	CDC	Issued Body Substance Isolation guidelines
1988	U.S. Congress	Enacted Clinical Laboratory Improvement Amendments of 1988 (CLIA 88)
1991	OSHA	Issued Bloodborne Pathogens (BBP) Standard, which mandated the use of UP
1996	CDC	Issued Standard Precautions, synthesizing UP and Body Substance Isolation
2000	U.S. Congress	Enacted Needlestick Safety and Prevention Act
2001	OSHA	Revised BBP Standard in response to Needlestick Safety and Prevention Act

further spurred by the arrival of the **human immunodeficiency virus (HIV)** that causes the feared **acquired immunodeficiency syndrome (AIDS)**.

Federal and state laws and agencies have been formulated and implemented to protect workers and patients from **biohazardous materials** and toxic and **hazardous chemicals** (Table 5-1). The Occupational Safety and Health Act, adopted by the U.S. Congress in 1970, mandates training for employees by their employers, as a "right to know" that is based on materials a worker is likely to come in contact with in the workplace. OSHA (Occupational Safety and Health Administration) is the federal agency that has the power to force employers to comply with safety issues; in almost all industries, criminal charges may be brought for violation of laws enacted to protect the worker. A rule promulgated by OSHA in 1983 and expanded in 1987 required all employers to provide safety training, to maintain a safe work environment, and to provide protective gear such as gowns, jackets, gloves, boots, etc., when employees work in certain areas. This is especially true in hospitals where the nature of many work areas requires employees be protected from explosive gases, blood and other body fluids and tissues, and electrical hazards, and in any other common sites, where accidents may occur from falls and from being cut by broken glass and other devices.

HAZARDS FOUND IN MEDICAL LABORATORIES

Medical laboratory training programs are required to expend considerable time and effort in educating the student of laboratory science as to the multitude of possibilities for injury and infection. There are several categories of potential hazards in the typical medical laboratory. Biological, chemical, and physical components—in this order of precedence—are all threats to safety in the laboratory environment. The use of toxic chemicals, some of which carry the risk of those exposed developing respiratory problems or even death if inhaled, requires the use of a fume hood (Figure 5-1), the design of which may differ depending on the circumstances of use. Students and workers should be trained on the use of this protective device as well as in the use of respirators when working with both hazardous chemicals and certain organisms that are highly contagious. The biological component of safety known as **biohazards** will be covered separately from the chemical and physical components of safety (see Chapter 6, "Introduction to Infection Control"). Many safety components for physical hazards are mandated by building codes and safety equipment is required by state and local law, which has done a great deal to decrease the number of accidents.

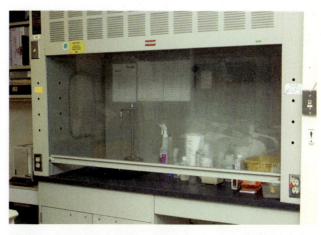

FIGURE 5-1 Fume hood used for toxic hazards found in the laboratory. Source: Delmar/Cengage Learning.

FACILITY SAFETY PLAN

Although the facility's safety plan addresses the entire institution, some of the laboratory accreditation bodies that perform site visits in the medical laboratory will also inspect safety components of the laboratory only for safety hazards. There will be some overlap between agencies that routinely inspect for similar violations of safety rules. Commonly, a medical laboratory safety and exposure plan is adopted with input from a **Safety Committee**, and in the hospital setting, the **Infection Control Committee** or **Exposure Control Committee** will have a great deal of input into the policies and procedures. These committees are highly formal in nature and are an integral part of the administrative team that is involved in fulfilling the regulations imposed by state and federal agencies as well as accrediting organizations. Safety is typically a part of a committee that is separate from the Infection Control Committee, although many of the functions overlap and there is a great deal of cooperation between the two major committees. Both committees monitor activities that are facility-wide, since biohazardous materials are found throughout many areas of the hospital. The Safety Committee monitors occupational risks that extend to patients and visitors as well as risks found on the grounds of the facility. When biohazardous materials or toxic chemicals are stored or used in the facility, the affected areas are required to be clearly identified by the Safety Committee with signs warning of the presence of these materials with the potential to harm those who come in contact with them (Figures 5-2 and 5-3).

The laboratory department is often used as a vital adjunct to the Infection Control Committee or Exposure Control Committee. Environmental sampling may be done on a periodic basis to determine if decontamination and general cleaning of the equipment and the physical building itself are adequate. Environmental surveillance in general, where bacterial cultures were taken from work surfaces,

Safety Alert

Types of Hazards Faced in a Clinical Laboratory

- Bloodborne pathogens
- Airborne pathogens
- Injuries from broken glass and sharp devices
- Toxic chemicals
- Poor physical design of building
- Electrical hazards

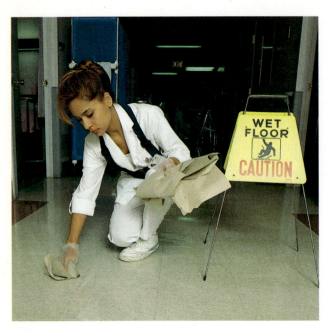

FIGURE 5-2 Examples of symbols and signs warning of potential hazards that may cause injury.
Source: Delmar/Cengage Learning.

drinking fountains, equipment, and other areas, was at one time prevalent but is no longer required by accrediting agencies. However, surveillance is performed on select surfaces and equipment, particularly if there is a dramatic increase in the number of certain bacterial infections, such as those from methicillin-resistant *Staphylococcus aureus* (MRSA), an organism that is prevalent in health care facilities today.

Outbreaks of nosocomial (hospital-acquired) infections are also investigated by the laboratory for the Infection Control Committee. Regarding the appropriateness of antibiotic prescribing, the medical staff, headed by the chief of staff, receives a report of data compiled by the laboratory as to the judicious and effective use of antibiotics. Reports from housekeeping, the dietary department, and other areas pertaining to unsafe or biohazardous conditions are reported to the Infection Control Committee, which often uses the laboratory's expertise in addressing the problems. Most often there is a representative on the Infection Control Committee from the medical laboratory. Infection control, exposure control, and safety are difficult to separate from each other, and demand a cooperative and combined effort from all areas to be effective. But the laboratory is a key component in completing surveillance to determine if indeed a problem exists and in providing a solution to many of the problems related to infection.

PHYSICAL HAZARDS

Physical hazards may be described as ordinary man-made equipment and its surroundings. Many physical hazards exist in the laboratory and include, but are not limited to, open flames from Bunsen burners, electrical equipment, laboratory instruments with moving parts, glassware, and tanks of gases.

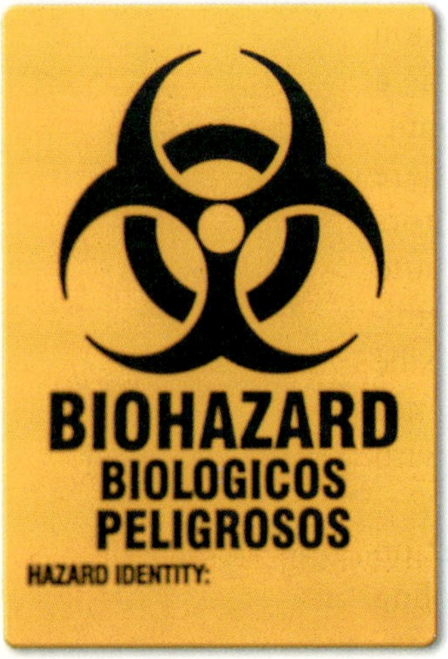

Electricity is a versatile opponent. The electricity itself may provide a fatal shock, or it may cause movement in a piece of equipment or heat some part of an instrument that may cause a severe burn. All electrical equipment should be grounded, and all outlets should be constructed as double-fault outlets that shut off the flow of electricity if a short occurs in the electrical current pathway. This is required in the building codes in many locales in the United States. Frayed cords or any other exposed electrical wire should not be allowed (Figure 5-4). Overloaded circuits may cause equipment failure or even a fire, so careful attention must be paid to having an adequate number of outlets to support the activity in the area. Extension cords should only be for temporary use as they are dangerous in a number of ways, including the possibility of tripping over

FIGURE 5-3 Universal biohazard sign.
Source: Delmar/Cengage Learning.

them if they are on the floor. Heavy-duty and high-quality power strips are acceptable but should be checked by the maintenance department to ensure they can handle the amount of current needed to operate the equipment plugged into them. When work is performed on a piece of electrical equipment, the item should be disconnected before any disassembly begins. If a wire becomes warm to the touch, it is a danger signal.

FIRES

Fires in high-occupancy facilities can be devastating in the number and level of injuries they cause. In past years of laboratory practice, Bunsen burners were commonly used for a number of procedures, particularly in microbiology laboratories. These burners are seldom seen in a modern medical laboratory, so fires have become a relatively minor risk in the laboratory. Open flame devices have largely been replaced by slide warmers. Disposable loops and needles are used more often today, lessening or eliminating the need for bacterial incinerators to sterilize loops and needles, and hotplates and microwaves are used instead of open flames for heating materials. The potential for fires starting in the laboratory have lessened drastically over the past few decades.

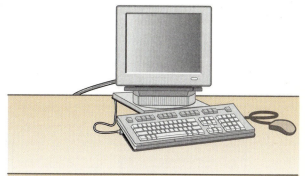
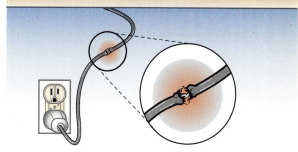

FIGURE 5-4 Frayed power cords create a danger of shock and fire. Source: Delmar/Cengage Learning.

Special cabinets for flammable materials should be properly labeled and should be used to store chemicals away from heat sources. Some chemicals will ignite at relatively low temperatures, so this is a requirement that will draw attention during safety inspections. Even if a fire occurs near the cabinet, the contents will be protected for some time until workers are able to escape.

Fire escape routes and evacuation plans must be conspicuously posted throughout educational and medical buildings (Figure 5-5). Routes of evacuation should be clearly visible, and battery-operated exit signs that remain lighted during emergencies should be present.

Categories of Fires

Fires of various kinds erupt because of and in close proximity to materials that may cause the production of toxic fumes; such fumes may also

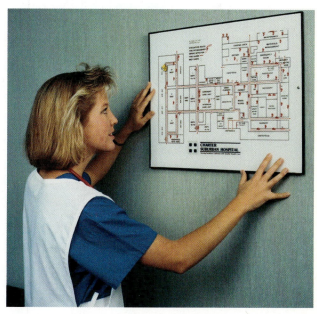

FIGURE 5-5 Escape route for fires and emergency evacuation plans must be conspicuously posted. Source: Delmar/Cengage Learning.

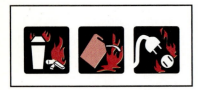

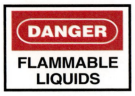

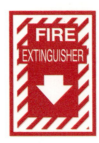

FIGURE 5-6 Common safety signs indicating classes of fire extinguishers and flammable liquids.
Source: Delmar/Cengage Learning.

explode and cause the flames to spread more rapidly. Even adding water to some types of fires may be dangerous or worsen the condition. Figures 5-6 and 5-7 are examples of signs that are seen widely in various types of buildings. These color-coded and explanatory signs should be present anywhere electrical equipment and chemicals are in use. Training in precautions for preventing fires and for combating fires should be provided for all employees.

The National Fire Protection Association provides signs with easy-to-identify threats from fires. Knowledge of the types of threats with which they must contend is essential to firefighters and other responders. These signs are useful to a building's occupants as well as to fire fighters responding to an emergency.

Fire Extinguisher Availability and Location

Fire extinguishers are required to be located conveniently and are to be inspected for proof that they have been regularly tested (Figure 5-8). There are three types of fire extinguishers, labeled A, B, and C. Each type is designed for extinguishing flames from various types of fuel.

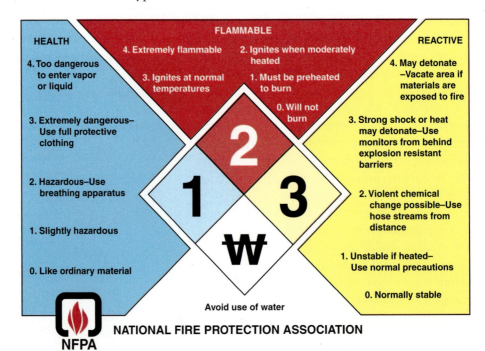

FIGURE 5-7 National Fire Protection Association's (NFPA) color-coded signs warning of chemical hazards, and a means for identifying them.
Source: Delmar/Cengage Learning.

Escape routes should be posted in every area of the building so those seeking to escape a fire will not enter a dead-end hallway or enter an elevator that might stop near the fire.

Personal Safety in Fires

A fire blanket should be available where there is any risk of flames and explosion. If clothing becomes ignited, a fire blanket may be used to extinguish the flames before serious injury occurs. Quick response to extinguish flames on one's clothing and to aid in either putting out flames on one's person or removing toxic chemicals from the skin before serious injury results may be obtained with use of a fire blanket (Figure 5-9) or an emergency shower (Figure 5-10), respectively. Workers should be trained as to the location of the fire extinguishers and in the type to use for various combustible elements, as well as being offered the opportunity to physically hold and operate the extinguisher. Fire drills are required to be held, and escape routes should not have blocked exit doors either from the inside or the outside.

POLICIES FOR DISPOSAL OF MEDICAL WASTES AND TOXIC CHEMICALS

Policies must be instituted for proper disposal of both biohazardous wastes and toxic chemicals. Training of employees is also required to be conducted on a regular basis. All biohazardous wastes must be disposed of according to state, local, and federal regulations. These regulations can vary from one location to another and may change periodically because of research or changing policies by Safety Committees and even government agencies. Most hospitals now procure the services of a commercial waste disposal firm that will provide for safe collection, storage, and pickup of biohazardous wastes for transport to a facility where the materials are incinerated at extremely high temperatures. Since smoke from some of these materials is toxic, the smokestacks sometimes rise to a height of more than 100 feet, and a distillation process

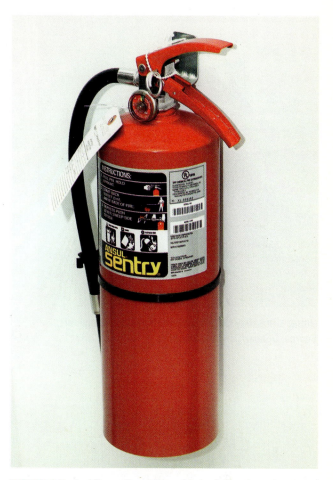

FIGURE 5-8 Typical fire extinguisher with tag indicating when last serviced.
Source: Delmar/Cengage Learning.

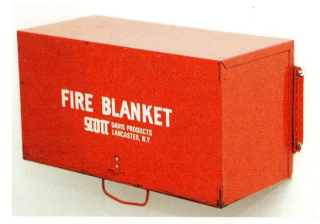

FIGURE 5-9 Fire blanket to extinguish clothing fires.
Source: Delmar/Cengage Learning.

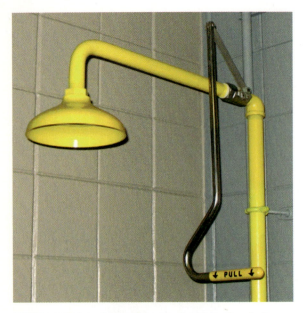

**FIGURE 5-10 Safety shower for removing toxic chemicals.
Source: Delmar/Cengage Learning.**

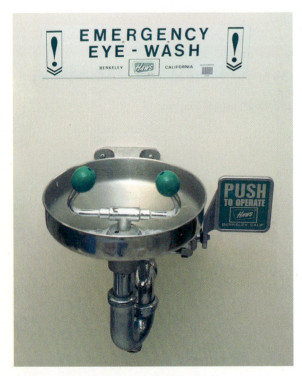

**FIGURE 5-11 Eyewash station for emergency incidents involving biohazards and toxic chemicals.
Source: Delmar/Cengage Learning.**

may also be used to capture and recycle some of the wastes produced by burning the materials. It should be kept in mind that the facility producing the waste materials is responsible for the waste while it is under transport to the disposal facility. This is an aspect of disposal of biohazardous wastes and toxic materials that many do not realize. It is vitally important that both toxic materials and biohazardous spills be taken care of immediately, before widespread exposure occurs, aggravating the situation.

Fortunately, toxic chemicals are not nearly as prevalent in the medical laboratory as they were in years past, when manual procedures were more commonly performed. Regulations for proper disposal of used chemicals or chemicals that should be discarded are to be followed according to policies established by each facility. Some chemicals may be poured into the sewer system if they are highly diluted with water. Others, especially if they contain azides, copper, chromium, or lead and mercury, require special handling by trained toxic waste disposal personnel. Please note that azides should never be poured into the waste water system. In the presence of lead pipes or soldering, an explosion may ensue. Routine training on at least an annual basis is to be provided either through inservice sessions or directly by the laboratory department manager or the instructor in an educational setting. Eyewash stations should be situated in all areas where chemicals or biohazardous materials may splash into the eyes (Figure 5-11). At clinical sites, the orientation of the student to the laboratory will cover disposal of biohazardous wastes and use of potentially hazardous chemicals.

Use of and Disposal of Sharps

Sharp items such as needles, broken glass tubes, scalpels, and other disposable items may cause injury when carelessly handled. If these items are contaminated with patient blood and other body fluids, there is a secondary danger as these instruments are potentially capable of transmitting infectious diseases unless handled with extreme caution to prevent injuries. Used needles should never be recapped by both hands or otherwise manipulated in a manner or technique that involves directing the point of a needle toward any part of the body. Syringes, needles,

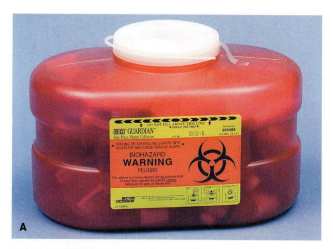
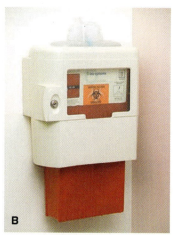

FIGURE 5-12 (A) Rigid container designed for disposal of contaminated sharps. (B) Wall-hung sharps collector.
Source: Delmar/Cengage Learning.

broken glass, and other sharp items should be placed in the appropriate container, which should be strategically located in the work area on a work counter and in any sterilization area. The **sharps** in the container (Figure 5-12) are collected and accumulated in larger waste containers in designated storage areas before being periodically collected by a professional medical waste disposal company. Do not bend or try to break needles before disposal because it is easy to sustain an injury by this act. If a decision is made to recap a needle until it is needed again, use a method called a one-handed scoop technique or the metal needle capping device found in the clinic.

Disposal of Biological and Contaminated Waste Materials

Solid wastes that are contaminated with blood or other body fluids should be placed in a red bag with a red biohazard symbol on it. These bags are strong and impervious to fluid leakage from the contained items. The bag is sealed with a twist tie and placed into a box with a hazardous medical waste sign. Some body wastes such as feces and urine are not considered as potentially infectious materials, but if they contain visible blood, they should be treated as potentially dangerous. Soaked items such as chemical wipes, gauze sponges, and paper towels that blood or other fluids can be squeezed out of or with blood that may flake from the item are considered regulated medical waste. Disposable items that may contain the body fluids of patients but are not subject to medical waste regulations (not soaked with blood or tissue), such as gloves, paper towels, and absorbent paper for use on laboratory counters, should be place in a lined trash receptacle. Red bags should not be used for nonregulated waste. Some containers for biohazardous wastes have a foot-operated lever for opening the lid, protecting the person discarding the wastes by avoiding unnecessary handling (Figure 5-13). To place unregulated wastes, such as gloves that have no blood on them, into a red biohazard bag would involve a great deal of wasteful expense by causing the facility to pay for the disposal of nonbiohazardous wastes.

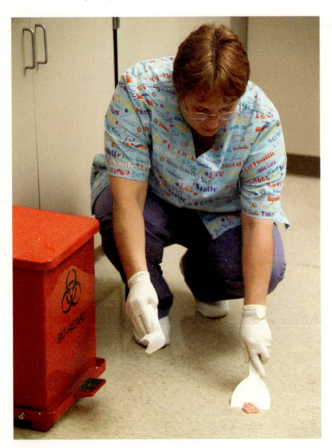

FIGURE 5-13 Wearing of appropriate PPE when cleaning a biological spill.
Source: Delmar/Cengage Learning.

INHERENT SAFETY RISKS IN MEDICAL LABORATORIES

Since laboratories inherently are involved with blood and body fluids that are likely to communicate diseases to others, a formal approach to cleanliness and disposal of sharps and biohazardous materials is practiced in the laboratory. The medical laboratory may also have flammables and compressed gases that pose a safety risk. Tanks of compressed gases must be anchored so they will not fall; this will be regulated by many agencies that perform site visits. A tank of compressed gas (Figure 5-14) that falls with a broken valve may be propelled in the manner of a rocket and has been known to penetrate a reinforced concrete wall.

Because exposure to hazards in the medical laboratory is an ongoing risk, checklists are sometimes maintained in departments of the laboratory, and records are kept of scheduled activities designed to eliminate or reduce occurrences of injury to or infection of the workers. Supervisory observation and check sheets are often used to minimize rates of hospital-acquired infections, provide remedies for areas of increased danger, and prevent the occurrence of injuries.

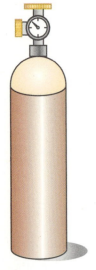

FIGURE 5-14 Compressed gas cylinder.
Source: Delmar/ Cengage Learning.

RESPONSIBILITY FOR SAFETY INFORMATION

Federal laws from the 1970s and 1980s, along with those from many states, have been enacted to protect workers and patients through strict safety codes. Instructors, students, and clinical supervisors have joint responsibility for being aware of, enforcing, and observing these rules and regulations. Documentation of materials covered and of orientation and safety training in the proper procedures to be followed are based on formal regulations. Many of these requirements are monitored and compliance is documented in the workplace by the Safety Committee, which may go by other names in various facilities. Training and educational facilities are also required to provide a safe work environment and to have available the proper tools for practicing safety.

OSHA monitors adherence to its guidelines and its inspectors may appear uninvited and unannounced to survey conditions in a facility and to determine if any violations are obvious. Following an accident or incident, OSHA also investigates the incident and files a report, and administers fines and sanctions against the supervisors and managers of the facility.

Laboratory procedure manuals should have safety practice components built into each procedure. These procedures should be written in a manner that adheres to pertinent laws for disposal of chemicals and biohazardous items. General rules for safety and guidelines for providing and documenting safety training and orientation should be prominently displayed throughout the work-site. The *Federal Register* has a set of OSHA guidelines that should be present in the workplace's library and on its website.

Documentation of Training

Standardized forms are available for providing pertinent safety training. Certain companies also produce and sell complete and comprehensive safety programs along with forms that are periodically updated to comply with changes. On completing training sessions, students and workers sign an agreement that they have received and understand the implications of the safety program and their responsibility to adhere to all regulations. Usually, the law of "right to know" related to the potential for occupational exposure is covered in these training sessions, along with other safety issues that must be addressed.

INFECTION CONTROL CHECKLIST

Various internal committees, such as the Safety Committee or the Infection Control Committee or Exposure Control Committee, will monitor compliance with policies related to safety. Members of these committees and also those from accrediting facilities and government agencies such as OSHA may observe medical workers in the work site. Table 5-2 is an example of a form that would be

Table 5-2 Infection Control and Safety Checklist

Activity	Satisfactory	Acceptable—Needs Some Attention	Unsatisfactory	Not Applicable
1. Utility gloves worn when retrieving items from cabinets				
2. All sharps placed in sharps container				
3. Proper supplies checked and reordered; sufficient inventory				
4. Area kept neat and clean				
5. Cleaning solutions replenished and dated as needed				
6. Lab jackets used appropriately				
7. Contaminated towels and items laundered appropriately				
8. Rubberized aprons used when chemicals or body fluids may be spilled				
9. Chairs and carts properly disinfected				
10. Appropriate plastic covers used				
11. No contaminated items left on counters at end of day				
12. Proper gloves worn at the appropriate time for clean-up				
13. Wash bottles of 10% hypochlorite filled appropriately				
14. Biohazard bags used when indicated				
15. Trash emptied				

used by the Infection Control Committee to document adherence by individuals and departments, but some of these items may also be covered by the Safety Committee. There is a great deal of overlap in some facilities between the Safety Committee and the Infection Control Committee. Sometimes you will hear the term "environmental control" applied to these committees.

PURPOSE AND DUTIES OF SAFETY COMMITTEE

Protection of workers and their patients against the contraction of an infectious disease or exposure to toxic agents is the goal of the Safety Committee, and all of its efforts are devoted to this goal, as well as to protecting visitors to the facility. Although some of this committee's duties include aspects of infection control, the Safety Committee chiefly directs its attention to conditions of the building and whether general maintenance of the facility is adequate (Table 5-3). General safety and fire safety are sometimes handled by one joint committee and in conjunction with the local fire marshal in complying with laws regarding fire safety and prevention.

Fire Safety

This category of risk or hazard is potentially the most dangerous. Fires may block exits and also may ignite chemicals that produce toxic fumes that can

Table 5-3 General Safety Checklist for Building Maintenance, Safe Passageways, and Safety Devices

	Satisfactory	Acceptable—Needs Some Attention	Unsatisfactory	Not Applicable
1. Floors are clean, dry as possible, and free of broken areas containing protrusions and hazards to walking.				
2. Passageways adhere to fire marshal standards, being clear of floor and wall obstructions.				
3. Floors are sealed with wax that is nonskid.				
4. Safety manuals, material safety data sheets (MSDSs), and precautionary documents are found in work areas.				
5. Flammable materials are kept in approved containers and cabinets or store rooms.				
6. Acids and chemicals are kept in approved cabinets on lower shelf.				
7. Safety glasses are available and worn during specified tasks.				
8. Safety hood is used when handling certain materials.				
9. Furniture and equipment have no sharp or broken edges.				
10. Doors are in good working order, including fire doors.				
11. No broken glass is present in windows, cabinet doors, etc.				

render victims unconscious. Clearly marked exits with battery-powered signs in case of electrical outage are required (Table 5-4).

First Aid

First aid supplies should be readily available and adequate numbers of persons available to render first aid. Minor injuries occur with frequency in the laboratory and often do not require emergency treatment. In some facilities, workers are required to complete first aid training and first responder training to be able to react quickly and appropriately if an accidental exposure or injury occurs. Immediate and effective treatment to stabilize the victim of illness or accident often prevents permanent medical problems. In some facilities, the treatment is provided by a team that is ready to respond to emergencies on a moment's notice. Technology has provided equipment for treatment of possible heart attack, and many lives are being saved with a portable defibrillator that is programmed to restore a normal rhythm to the victims of serious heart conditions.

Instructor Responsibilities

The instructor in an educational facility, along with appropriate committees, is responsible for shop, classroom, or laboratory safety instruction in accident

Table 5-4 Exits and Fire Safety Checklist for Unobstructed Movement

		Satisfactory	Acceptable—Needs Some Attention	Unsatisfactory	Not Applicable
1.	Exits are clearly visible and access is indicated, with no obstructions on either side of the exits.				
2.	Exit doors are free of chains or any other device that would prevent the ability to exit building during an emergency.				
3.	Nonexit doors are marked accordingly to avoid confusion in an emergency situation.				
4.	Exit lights are in good working order.				
5.	Evacuation plans are located near the exit door of the lab.				
6.	Fire extinguishers are visibly and conveniently located.				
7.	Fire extinguishers are routinely tested and maintained.				
8.	Training is provided for class A, B, and C fire extinguishers.				
9.	Method exists for reporting unsafe conditions.				
10.	Information is available for obtaining help from both facility and outside personnel for information and emergency help.				

prevention. In the clinical setting where a student may be performing skills practice, the departmental preceptor or instructor has the major responsibility for ensuring the students and other workers are properly oriented and trained in safety matters. The Safety Alert on this page lists the responsibilities of the instructor or the preceptor in the clinical site for a comprehensive accident prevention program in school shops and laboratories.

Student Responsibilities

Students are an integral part of the safety program because they are involved with processes that may expose them to danger if they are uninformed, complacent, or careless. Learning the proper safety procedures prepares them in the proper use of tools and equipment. Safety is an important component of training, and students should be advised on reporting unsafe practices or conditions (see the Safety Alert on the following page), as this responsibility rests on the student worker.

ACCIDENT INVESTIGATION

All accidents should be investigated, and the sooner they are investigated, the more effective the observations will be. Any need for modifications of policies and procedures should be quickly initiated to avoid repeat incidents. Investigators or Safety Committee representatives (and instructors if the incident involves a student) should be prompt and thorough in their investigations. The following steps are intended to assist in investigating accidents. Everyone should be made aware that there is a very real dividend to be earned in safety, not only in the money saved by avoiding costly accidents but also in an improved student morale produced by setting up safety programs. The safety-oriented organization is one that cares about its students' welfare and knows that caring pays off. Obviously, all workplace accidents cannot be eliminated. As long as there are people, accidents will occur. But much can and should be done to train students to work safely and to provide students with safe working conditions. Since some accidents will occur, this section deals with what should be done after an accident occurs. Loss of staff may occur for extended periods of time while recovering from injuries suffered in the workplace. This places an undue financial burden on the institution by requiring that others be required to work overtime, or temporary help may be solicited.

An accident is easily identified and is accurately defined as an unintended occurrence that caused or could have caused personal injury or material damage, such as tripping or slipping and falling on the floor or a transport cart containing equipment or supplies may strike a suddenly opened door. A good example of falls in a hospital occurred when an outside housekeeping and cleaning company received a contract to maintain the floors of a hospital. The company, to save money, used a less expensive floor wax that was not nonskid. Within 1 hour of the application of this new wax, two visitors fell and broke their arms and a phlebotomist rounded a corner and slipped to the floor, breaking all of the blood collection tubes in his tray. The phlebotomist also injured his elbow, which required further medical attention over a considerable period of time. Two lawsuits arose from the condition of the floors in a single day. Needless to say, the type of wax used on the floor was changed immediately.

Four other terms related to safe operations are to be considered:

1. An *injury* is the result of an accident (a nonintentional act) and may be of varying severity and type. Examples of the consequences of an injury would include a cut on the skin of the limbs or other parts of the body, a crushing foot injury, broken bones, or a damaged eye. Most accidents can be avoided, but unfortunately, a string of accidents is often required before preventive action is taken. However, organizations that investigate laboratories for safety violations will often reduce the number of accidents that were historically high in a facility.

2. The *primary cause* is the condition or act that caused the accident. A pool of liquid spilled on the floor or slippery wax may be the cause. Recurring incidents are usually remedied by changing a procedure and requiring additional professional training by the institution of learning or the medical facility. Preventing accidents by safe operations through observation and planning is the responsibility of everyone. Unsafe acts or conditions should be reported and acted on quickly.

3. *Secondary causes* are other acts or conditions that contributed to the accident. These include the reasons a spill on the floor had not been cleaned up. Additionally, the spill may have been caused by a leaking plumbing system or a leaking roof or window. Often it is difficult to separate the primary from the secondary cause. But this should not hinder an accident investigation, because all causes should be listed. The important thing is to detect and correct all of the defects or unsafe conditions by determining what department or what individual is responsible for monitoring the area, and adjusting schedules or possibly hiring additional personnel to ensure the important tasks are being performed in a timely manner.

Safety Alert

Student Safety Responsibility

Students of clinical laboratory programs have an equal responsibility for contributing to and observing safety requirements to protect themselves and others.

- Practice good safety habits and attitudes through actual training and practice in the clinical facility and the laboratory classroom.

- Develop a sense of responsibility for your own safety and the safety of others.

- Observe and evaluate potential hazards in educational work that will be required in future careers, and learn to practice the appropriate prevention measures.

- Do not let your guard down, and never forget to follow the safety rules and regulations.

- Report hazards that may exist in the classroom, laboratory, or clinical site to the proper authority.

- Report any defective supplies, services, or equipment to the instructor or training preceptor.

- Only perform hazardous procedures after receiving instructions on how to safely and properly perform the work.

- Wear the appropriate personal protective equipment wherever there is potential danger or hazards in the classroom lab or work environment.

- Always report all accidents to the instructor regardless of nature or severity.

- Demonstrate knowledge and understanding of the safety rules and regulations of the school and the instructional program.

- Participate in training programs in the clinical site pertinent to the performance of procedures.

4. *Other causes* are conditions that could result in accidents but had no effect on the specific accident currently being investigated. Many times when an investigation is ongoing, additional risks are identified quite by chance and are handled along with the original management of the dangerous condition.

Why Should an Accident Investigation Be Initiated?

An investigation is performed mainly to prevent a recurrence of the accident. Nearly all accidents offer the possibility of preventing another accident at some time in the future. Thus, it is important to examine each accident as soon as possible, to find the cause and to remedy the situation. Even under heavy workloads and time constraints, workers are required to work within practical limits. Even under ideal circumstances, the work situation is not going to be perfect. It is necessary to maintain schedules and account for adequate staffing, absenteeism, or sickness while maintaining or even increasing the quality of service and increasing the speed at which work must be completed. Not all job hazards can be eliminated, but student, worker, and patient welfare require the elimination of all identified job hazards. Practical measures can be taken to eliminate many of the dangers associated with students' jobs. Injury prevention and accident prevention are often confused. For example, when students are required to wear safety shoes or safety glasses, the possibility of some injuries is reduced, but not the possibility of an accident. Nevertheless, when it is not possible to eliminate the accident potential, there must be concentration on preventing the injury. In some situations, a simple solution may be available where both the injury and the accident are preventable, but most situations do not limit themselves to such a simple solution. The first consideration should be to prevent the accident. If this is not possible, then action must be taken to prevent the injury that may occur as a result of the accident.

Responsibility for Safety Investigations

Again, Safety Committees are an integral part of a medical facility as well as of educational institutions. There are no set rules dealing with how a Safety Committee must be set up. Each organization must tailor its staff and equip its workers and students for its own needs, regardless of size. In educational institutions, the instructor is in contact with the students and is responsible for all operations within the class, including safety. This person may be the classroom and laboratory instructor in the college or function as a preceptor for students in clinical settings, but both categories of instructor are usually the best qualified to investigate an accident in the area he or she knows best. Instructors who work with the students are aware from experience of the students' attitudes, the work they will be performing, and the hazards involved. This does not mean that the instructors share all of this responsibility. But ultimately everyone should be involved. The student and administrative staff share the responsibility with the instructor for students' safety.

Timeframe for Investigation

Again, safety violations and incidents should be investigated as soon as possible following an accident or a potential for an accident, where conditions exist for a possible accident. The accident investigation should begin immediately on learning that an accident has occurred. Just as in a crime scene, signs left by the accident and physical evidence quickly begin to disappear, such as in a spill or a biohazardous spill. Clean-up crews will move things and erase important details. Other shifts come on the job and soon many of the clues are gone. Witnesses may leave the scene. While impractical in some instances, photographs of the accident can save time in gathering accurate information. The use of a digital camera to take pertinent pictures of the accident scene would greatly bolster the evidence for procedural, if not policy, changes. If considerable injury has occurred, interviews including questioning of the victim(s) may be done later but certainly before the memory has faded in those injured. The critical point is to start the investigation while all the facts are present and fresh in the minds of those involved.

Information Collection Following an Accident

For obvious reasons, for a successful accident investigation it is necessary to determine the cause of the accident. Investigators must be trained in the sort of things to look for in the area and be able to recognize this evidence. Documentation of each step of the accident or incident will enable the committee to more easily change policies and procedures, if necessary.

Accidents may be broken down into two basic categories. Some causes are readily observable, but some require intensive effort before the real cause of an accident can be found. Patterns of similar accidents are often the easiest to analyze and to arrive at the root cause or causes. When related to the initial cause(s), the two categories are:

- Unsafe conditions (mechanical failure or physical causes)
- Unsafe acts (human failure)

In most cases, an accident investigator or Safety Committee will have three sources of information. Equipment can be tested and visually checked for malfunctions or improper use. Materials or supplies may be defective or used for a purpose for which they were not intended. Although people, the third source of information, will have psychological components of their estimates of the cause, especially if serious injury has occurred, equipment and material and the conditions of each of these will be fairly reliable if still present. They are not affected by any psychological overlays or by memory or subjectivity. The key to inspecting objects is to know what to look for. Which came first? In some cases a piece of equipment causes damage to a building, which later causes another accident. The equipment would be the cause and not the damage to the building, such as a hole in the floor. Was the machinery in good condition with no defective parts and was it being operated properly? A "yes" answer to any of these questions helps to narrow the investigation.

People, on the other hand, can be more difficult to handle because the method of approach to them will often determine the amount of information to be received. An impartial and impersonal attitude must be taken. Trying to fix blame or find someone to "blame it on" (or giving this impression) can be counterproductive in gathering meaningful information. Laboratory workers along with members of the health care team from other departments are often called on to be a member of the Safety Committee, to provide expertise from a number of viewpoints as needed. Many companies and facilities have become so savvy as to accident prevention that they will openly advertise that there have been no accidents during the past posted number of weeks or during the past number of thousands of man hours worked.

GENERAL PREVENTIVE EQUIPMENT MAINTENANCE SCHEDULE AND RELATED SAFETY ISSUES

General preventive maintenance on a routine basis not only keeps equipment in good operating order but also is a means to prevent accidents, such as those that may result from damaged electrical components. Laboratory professionals and students of laboratory medicine should follow the manufacturer's directions for providing preventive maintenance both to prevent accidents and to avoid breakdowns. An accident might result in an injury to the worker as well as cause downtime due to damage to equipment. Sometimes the accident investigation causes a work stoppage or slowdown while the investigation is ongoing. And lawsuits may arise because of conditions that led to the accident or incident. Following directions and being mindful of the potential hazards associated with one's work help to avoid a slowdown in work production, which in the health care facility translates into delays in treatment and efficiency of the facility. All major pieces of equipment in a medical laboratory will have a posted list of measures to be taken in cleaning and maintaining the machinery so it does not fail at critical times and to ensure it produces quality results.

LABORATORY SPECIFIC SURVEYS

Certain areas of the laboratory are inspected by any of a number of internal committees, a local fire marshal, or any accreditation body performing a site visit. These inspections include, but are not limited to, a survey of safety equipment (Table 5-5), equipment and supplies for safety of the laboratory personnel (Table 5-6), and a sharps injury log (Table 5-7). The latter requires a follow-up for those injured by needle sticks and cuts from glass and equipment, etc.

Documentation of Departmental Surveys and Follow-up

Committees and external agencies will look for certain pieces of safety equipment and protective clothing when surveying a clinical laboratory. The Infection Control Committee and Exposure Control Committee will routinely perform an inventory of available engineered control devices and work practices in the department. Table 5-5 contains some essential items that will be accounted for on a routine and recurring basis by perhaps several groups, including institutional committees and external accrediting agencies.

Table 5-5 Safety Equipment and Supplies Available in the Medical Laboratory

		Yes	No
1.	Adequate sinks with handwashing solutions for effective cleaning of hands		
2.	Eyewash stations at each sink		
3.	Fire blanket on wall near entrance		
4.	Safety shower near entrance		
5.	Safety storage cabinets for storage of stains, bases, and acids		
6.	Fume hood available for performing exams with certain pathogens		
7.	Spill kit located on safety storage cabinets		
8.	Barrier shield for opening tubes of blood		
9.	Adequate gloves in all sizes		
10.	Impermeable aprons for use with certain liquids, as indicated		
11.	Disposable gowns for use in laboratory		
12.	Disposal containers for sharps and potentially infectious materials		

Table 5-6 Sharps Injury Log for Incidents Involving Sharp Implements

Date of Injury	Facility Where Occurred	Brief Description	Follow-up Necessary (Y/N)	Prophylactic Immunizations Documented	Notes

Safety Equipment and Supplies in the Medical/Clinical Lab

The department will be organized so as to contain the proper stockage levels of chemicals, protective equipment, and engineered controls for maintaining safety (Table 5-5). Wastes will be discarded on a regular basis, in proper containers, and disposed of according to institutional policy.

Table 5-7 Required and Essential Safety Equipment Survey

This is a sample form for relating complete safety information to the student.

1. Be familiar with the location of the nearest fire extinguisher.
2. Know the location of the nearest fire alarm.
3. Explain use of the ABC fire extinguisher located in the MLT laboratory.
4. Learn the muster point outside the building if an evacuation order is given.
5. Relate location of the designated safe area in case of dangerous weather warning.
6. Indicate the location of the first aid kit.
7. Understand who should render first aid in the medical laboratory area.
8. Relate awareness of how the institution is notified if an accident has occurred in the clinical site.
9. Locate the MSDSs and the emergency plan location.
10. Understand responsibilities for safe operations in the medical laboratory.
11. Describe use of eyewash stations after demonstration.
12. Point out fire blanket and relate use of it.

Sharps Injury Logs

It is not uncommon for sharps sticks and cuts to occur on a regular basis. When this type of accident occurs, policies and procedures dictate that certain practices are followed. A log is maintained to document that the incident was reported properly (Table 5-6) and the victim was treated in accordance with policies of the health care facility. Proper orientation, regular inservice education and a willingness to observe safety measures will help to eliminate many injuries.

Most institutions, including educational facilities, require a log of all injuries by needles and other sharps (Table 5-6). Medical follow-up must be documented and filed for a prescribed period of time. A designated health care provider will complete the medical examination to include the information in Table 5-6. Proper follow-up will be the responsibility of the initial health care provider.

Essential Safety Equipment Survey

Whether a student is in a clinical site or the educational facility, he or she should be oriented to and become familiar with the location of safety items, evacuation routes, and safe places for weather emergencies (Table 5-7). Students and workers should be periodically updated on safety practices for their facility.

Other Areas Requiring Safety Measures

Fires and natural events such as weather are areas that require safety measures for patients, visitors, and health care workers. These events would require preparation by the staff of educational and health care institutions and include drills that ensure everyone knows the proper action to take in the event of such an event. These are generic instructions similar to those that will be posted in all college buildings and health care facilities for each department or division. As previously mentioned, periodic drills for these activities will be conducted on an institutional

Table 5-8 Fire, Inclement Weather, and Terrorist Threat Response Procedures

Threat	Description
FIRE EVACUATION *In the event of a fire:*	A continuous pulsing ring of the fire alarm system will indicate a fire emergency. Immediately evacuate work areas or the health care facility by prearranged exits. Evacuation routes are posted, and a rally at a predetermined point outside the building will be established when orienting new employees. A verbal command from an administrator to the faculty and staff will indicate the *all clear* signal.
TORNADO EVACUATION *In the event of a tornado:*	A verbal warning will indicate a tornado evacuation emergency. Proceed to an inner hallway of the designated building, away from exterior doors and windows. A verbal command from the administration to the administrative, designated professional, or support staff will indicate an *all clear* signal when the danger is past.
MEDICAL EMERGENCY *In the event of a medical emergency:*	If a life-threatening accident or event occurs to any person that would require first aid, immediately dial 9 for an outside line if necessary and then "911" on any telephone readily available. Render assistance to the injured person and keep him from endangering himself further. Stay with the injured person until help arrives. Notify the administrative, designated professional, or support staff, or clinical preceptor of an incident immediately.
HAZARDOUS CHEMICAL EMERGENCY *In the event of a hazardous chemical emergency:*	Notify the administrative, designated professional, or support staff, or the instructor that you are using a chemical for your lab exercise. Consult the appropriate MSDS prior to using any chemicals, except when an instructor has oriented the entire class as to the dangers of and precautions for a given chemical. If a spill occurs, notify the administrative, designated professional, or support staff, or your instructor, or clinical preceptor immediately. Keep all personnel away from spill until it has been addressed by the appropriate personnel such as housekeeping. A spill kit is available in the medical laboratory to absorb and neutralize possible hazardous materials. Obtain an MSDS for the chemical spilled and ensure proper action has been taken. Evacuation may be required at the discretion of the administrator or instructor. Handling chemicals is usually included as a part of continuing education and staff development and must be documented in the students' and medical workers' files.
TERRORIST THREATS *In the event of a terrorist threat:*	Help from the local police and fire departments and Homeland Security and FEMA personnel will arrive quickly. Identification of organisms or toxins, or the disposal of bombs by a specially trained team with dogs to sniff out hidden threats, will likely occur. There will still be a need for medical personnel to treat victims of such an attack while maintaining personal safety.

or facility-wide basis as a requirement of various accreditation agencies as well as local fire departments and emergency management planning. Exits and fire safety documents will be completed by survey of the facilities (see Table 5-4).

Emergency situations involving fire, severe weather alerts and warnings, release of toxic chemicals, and mass casualties require prior training and preparation for an actual event. The headings and instructions in Table 5-8 provide examples of actions to take in an actual emergency. Policies at various educational and health care facilities differ slightly but all generally address the same basic topics. And with the potential for terrorist activities, many facilities also have plans for bomb threats and actual explosions that occur, which might release biohazardous organisms or biochemical toxins.

SUMMARY

Safety is the business of everyone, not only in a health care facility but also in one's personal life and one's occupation. The various safety considerations for a health care facility include biohazardous and toxic hazards and apply to employees, patients, and even visitors. There are legal ramifications that may impact a facility where injuries occur due to negligence and to commonplace occurrences that are not a result of carelessness or neglect by the employees of the health care facility but are accidents. Therefore, policies and procedures must be adopted and carried out to avoid as many of these occurrences as possible.

In addition to policies and procedures for each facility, there are local, state, and federal laws where certain practices are mandated, in an effort to circumvent injuries and deaths due to conditions where specific policies and procedures will prevent many accidents. Safety Committees and Exposure Control Committees (including Infection Control Committees) are organized to initiate and implement policies and procedures designed to protect the health of all categories of personnel who might be associated with the health care facility.

Physical hazards must be addressed by identifying them and, in some cases, by containing them in specially designed cabinets or areas where little or no harm may be present. Engineered controls to be used to prevent fire and the release of chemicals or pathogens are two important components of a safety program. In addition, a "right to know" law makes available Material Safety Data Sheets (MSDSs) for employees to consult to know how to avoid danger or how to treat oneself in a case of exposure. Appropriate signs for escape routes, and warning signs for flammable and toxic chemicals and for electrical hazards should be used.

Disposal of broken glass and sharp items must be done in a proper and safe manner. Specially trained personnel should have the knowledge to safely handle these materials. Biohazardous materials must be properly collected, isolated from patients, employees, and visitors, and properly packaged for pick-up and transport to a commercial waste disposal operation by trained personnel. Training is mandatory based on the tasks performed by each health care employee and is done on at least an annual basis and when job duties change. Documentation of this training is maintained for a lengthy period of time for those who have undergone the training.

REVIEW QUESTIONS

1. What is the purpose of a Safety Committee?
2. Who is responsible for safety and for reporting hazards?
3. What is the main purpose for reporting and following up on accidents, including injuries and exposure to toxic and biohazardous materials?
4. When should safety training be provided for employees, and who is responsible for providing this training?
5. In your own thinking, what is the number one reason that accidents occur?

CHAPTER 6

INTRODUCTION TO INFECTION CONTROL

LEARNING OBJECTIVES

Upon completion of this chapter, the reader will be able to:

- Understand the role of the medical facility in protecting medical workers, patients, and visitors.

- List examples of work practice controls.

- List examples of engineered controls in the typical medical care facility.

- Discuss methods to interrupt pathways for infection into the body.

- Provide information relating to the three categories of medical care workers regarding potential exposure.

- Relate an exposure incident and give the immediate steps to take following exposure.

- List preexposure procedures, including education and training components.

- Discuss processes involved in postexposure activities.

- Relate steps for the donning of personal protective equipment.

- Give the methods of transmission for the major bloodborne and airborne organisms: HIV, hepatitis B virus, and tuberculosis.

KEY TERMS

Bacillus Calmette-Guérin (BCG)
Bloodborne and airborne pathogens
Centers for Disease Control and Prevention (CDC)
Decontamination
Engineered controls
Exposure incidents
Gamma globulin
Hepatitis B virus (HBV)
High efficiency particulate air (HEPA) filter masks

Human immunodeficiency virus (HIV)
Human T-lymphotropic virus 1 and 2 (HTLV-1 and HTLV-2)
Iatrogenic
Infection Control Committee or Exposure Control Committee
Malaria
Nosocomial
Other potentially infectious materials (OPIM)

Personal protective equipment (PPE)
PPD (tuberculin) skin test
Safety Committee
Severe acute respiratory syndrome (SARS)
Standard Precautions
Tuberculosis (TB)
Universal Precautions
Work practice controls

INTRODUCTION

Infection control is an all-encompassing program that is headed up by a committee responsible for making policy and providing ongoing surveillance of all aspects of hospital operations, with a goal of protecting both workers and patients against hospital-acquired infections. Federal regulations address some bloodborne and airborne organisms, called "covered organisms," and require that training be provided by the employer for these important organisms. These include **human immunodeficiency virus (HIV**, the acquired immunodeficiency syndrome [AIDS]–causing virus), **hepatitis B virus (HBV)**, and **tuberculosis (TB)**. However, there are countless other pathogenic organisms to which the health care worker may be exposed and should be made aware of. Additional common and important organisms, of necessity, must be included in infection control programs. There are inherent risks in the hospital from which patients, visitors, and workers must be protected. All health care workers must be aware of their responsibility for avoiding infection or creating situations apt to cause infectious disease, while protecting their patients and sometimes visitors.

What is infection control and why is it important? In other chapters of this book, some of the basics for bloodborne and airborne infections are specifically discussed. The bloodborne and airborne pathogens section in this chapter is focused mainly toward the individual. Infection control programs, however, focus on the institution, for the protection of the individual worker as well as the patient. *Infection* is defined as the invasion and multiplication of any organism that has the potential to harm the body of a human or other organism. Infection control for a medical facility where patients may contract an infection while hospitalized is one of the most important facets of the holistic approach to delivery of health care. Most diseases in humans either are or were the result of an infectious process where pathogenic organisms invaded and set up residence in the human body. In some disease states, an infection may have subsided or have been overcome, but the damage done causes lasting problems for the victim, leaving him or her with permanent problems that may shorten or limit the enjoyment of life. The focus in this chapter is to acquaint the medical worker or student with the methods used by most health care institutions to protect their workers and patients from infection.

Covered Bloodborne and Airborne Pathogens

Only a few organisms that may cause serious diseases or death are classified as "covered pathogens." These are deemed by the **Centers for Disease Control and Prevention (CDC)** as having sufficient impact on the medical community that they require special training and responses to the infections they cause. They are termed **bloodborne and airborne pathogens** and include HIV, HBV, and TB organisms. These organisms are given special status in the orientation and training of new health care workers. These are not the only diseases that are of great import for the medical laboratory worker, but following guidelines for prevention of these three diseases will provide protection against most other potentially serious infections.

History of Infection Control

Several centuries ago, scientists learned that many diseases were caused by very small living organisms called *germs*. In the 19th century, a French chemist and bacteriologist named Louis Pasteur contributed to the founding of the modern science of microbiology. His greatest endeavors were related to the fields of bacteriology and immunology, a study of the body's reaction to disease. One of his most important discoveries was that disease organisms could be killed by "pasteurization," a process that applies high temperatures of approximately 140°F (60°C) for 30 minutes. Milk is rid of harmful bacteria by this process without damaging the nutrients found in it. Everyone, regardless of where he or she works, may be daily exposed to numerous organisms and toxic chemicals and, without good health, the body is often unable to combat the onslaught from these environmental dangers. Changing procedures to avoid or minimize contact with pathogens and toxins is the most effective way to prevent exposure incidents.

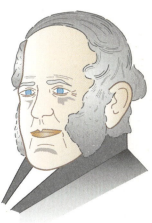

FIGURE 6-1 Sir Joseph Lister. **Source: Delmar/Cengage Learning.**

Another contributor to the field of bacteriology is Joseph Lister, a British surgeon (Figure 6-1). Lister determined that germs (bacteria only) could be killed with carbolic acid (also known as phenol). At the time, many deaths in hospitals were related to the unclean conditions of the health care facilities. Lister demanded that surgical wounds be kept clean and that the air in operating rooms be kept clean and circulating. The number of deaths related to complications from surgical procedures diminished dramatically when his changes were instituted. These practices eventually found their way to the battlefield, and wounded soldiers needing amputations greatly benefited from this advance.

During the U.S. Civil War, many deaths were caused by infection rather than the severity of the wound. Practices developed during the war were later adapted for civilian use in medicine. This included practices such as transportation of the wounded by ambulance for treatment behind the lines and setting up of treatment facilities, which may be in a house or other building or a tent. The model for this treatment persisted into World War I and, from this modest beginning, evolved into rapid treatment in sanitary facilities for the wounded soldier.

MODERN-DAY INFECTION CONTROL

Human Immunodeficiency Virus (HIV) and Its Effect on Infection Prevention

Most people have a healthy fear of contracting HIV, and the implications of becoming infected require that specific training for prevention of infection be provided to the medial laboratory worker, along with all those in other medical professions with possible contact with blood and body fluids. HIV causes a disease called AIDS (acquired immunodeficiency syndrome). A syndrome is a group or collection of symptoms and signs associated with a particular disease. The original source of the virus is in disagreement among many medical specialists. Two theories have been proposed as to its origin. Some postulate that the organism originated with the hunting and eating of the green monkey of Africa, and others believe that the disease originated with the administration of polio vaccine made from the kidneys of rhesus monkeys. Neither theory has been proved to date. Manifestations and symptoms of the disease and are well documented and predictable. With proper precautions, the health care worker is at no more risk of contracting HIV than the average layperson.

Several strains of HIV (the AIDS virus) exist, and some are similar to those found in animals. For instance, feline leukemia is thought to be caused by a strain of virus that is almost identical to that of HIV; to date, humans are considered naturally immune to this strain of the virus. In addition, other significant blood-borne viruses pose threats to human life and to blood supplies. In some parts of the world, epidemics of both **human T-lymphotropic virus 1 and 2 (HTLV-1 and HTLV-2)** have occurred. This poses such a risk to the blood supplies of the United States that testing of each unit of blood for HTLV-1 and HTLV-2 is performed. Such was the case in the 1991 Persian Gulf conflict, during which massive quantities of blood were collected and tested for the presence of these two bloodborne viruses. Symptoms associated with AIDS are caused by the presence of a virus that commonly attacks the immune system, leaving the victim susceptible to a number of opportunistic infections. Symptoms will depend on the site of infection and the organism involved. Initial symptoms may be insidious or mild, with nonspecific symptoms such as those associated with a flu-like illness. Signs and symptoms may include lymphadenopathy (enlargement or tenderness of the lymph nodes), anorexia, chronic diarrhea, weight loss, fever, and fatigue. Later stage symptoms include Kaposi's sarcoma, manifested by red-brown to purple lesions of the skin and mucous membranes.

AIDS has been found worldwide. It was first identified in the United States in 1981, but may have been present for some years before sufficient occurrences, diagnostic technology, and documentation existed to investigate it as an important malady. Some reports indicate that tests performed on the blood serum saved from an adolescent who died with an undiagnosed and wasting disease in the late 1960s indicate that there may have been antibodies developed against HIV at that time. The disease is now raging in a number of areas of the world, and efforts to eradicate it have not been effective to date, often because of political views by heads of states in some developing countries.

Humans are now recognized as reservoirs of HIV. A reservoir may be an environmental habitat such as water or soil, or a living organism such as humans. The transmission or passing of the AIDS virus from one person to another has been found to occur chiefly with blood, semen, saliva, tissue fluids, and vaginal fluids. Urine, tears, perspiration, vomitus, and feces may also contain the virus (Table 6-1). However, to date, there have been no documented cases of transmission from contact with fluids other than blood, semen, and vaginal secretions. In

Table 6-1 Substances Recognized by the CDC as Having the Potential to Transmit Pathogens

Blood	Synovial fluid
Blood products	Vaginal secretions
Semen	Pleural fluid
Peritoneal fluid	Pericardial fluid
Amniotic fluid	Unfixed tissue specimens
Cerebrospinal fluid	Breast milk
Urine	Sweat
Organs	Saliva in dental settings where bleeding occurs

adults, the virus is most often spread through sexual contact or by the sharing of needles, although early in the history of the disease, before testing for the virus or antibodies was performed on blood donor samples, transfusions resulted in a large number of infections. Most infected children acquire the virus in utero from infected mothers. Some cases have occurred as the result of transfusions of blood or blood products, such as the blood factors necessary to treat patients with hemophilia. HIV may be spread through the blood from an infected person getting into broken skin, open cut, or abrasion, or into the mouth or eyes.

Infection Control and Its Relationship to Health Care Facilities

All personnel employed in the health care environment are required to have a basic knowledge and understanding of disease and disease transmission. This knowledge is focused on the protection of both the patient and the health care worker. A number of issues related to infection control are common to all categories of health care workers to accomplish the goal of preventing workers and their assigned patients from becoming infected through exposure to pathogens. The issues of protecting patients and medical workers from contracting a serious infection is of such importance that federal legislation has been implemented to prevent or at least minimize the number of these incidences. Certain minor practices in the workplace will provide a means for preventing potentially tragic occurrences.

According to a report in *The Chicago Tribune* in July 2002, a number of startling charges were made related to infection control in hospitals. Infection control is designed to protect both patients and workers, but even in this day with increased availability of products and services designed to do just this, there are many breaches of established policies in many hospitals. This article states that approximately 75,000 patients needlessly die each year due to dirty hospitals and that the most effective and simple way of preventing the spread of pathogens, handwashing, is practiced by only about 50% of physicians and nurses as they go from patient to patient. The most helpless of patients, those who are infants, neonates (babies just born), the elderly, and immunocompromised or weakened, are at the greatest risk for the development of a hospital-acquired infection.

More than a century ago, pioneers such as Hungarian physician Ignaz Phillip Semmelweis recognized the importance of handwashing. He showed that simple handwashing could dramatically lower the infection rate. This practice is still not being conscientiously practiced, even with a requirement for documentation of the use of both work practice and **engineered controls**. These two terms refer basically to manufactured items for protection (*engineered controls*), and what one personally does for self-protection (*work practice controls*).

Many people can be observed going into the restroom and then leaving without ever washing their hands. In numerous cases, workers, including restaurant employees, will prepare food or eat their food and shake hands with others immediately afterward, with never a thought as to the organisms on their hands. It has been observed that conscientious handwashing will also reduce the incidence of colds since these infections are most often passed by the hands coming in contact with dirty surfaces and then with the mucous membranes of the eyes, nose, and mouth.

Official Agencies Responsible for Policies Related to Infection Control

Many federal agencies work with state and local governments to foster effective infection control in medical care, agricultural processes, and manufacture of products that may release organic or toxic chemicals. There is no doubt that these organizations are achieving great strides in protecting the health of the public, as evidenced by an expanding life span in the United States and other developed countries. Biohazardous materials containing blood and other body fluids or tissues are the major sources of the spread of infectious diseases. Some facilities have both an **Infection Control Committee** and an **Exposure Control Committee**, but in many facilities, the two are combined. Therefore, many facilities will also rank exposure to toxic chemicals as being comparable in seriousness to exposure to infectious materials, and will call the committee by the term "Exposure Control," rather than separating the two entities.

Organizations that work to prevent unnecessary disease due to contact with infectious materials include, but are not limited to, the National Institutes of Health (NIH), CDC, U.S. Department of Health and Human Services (HHS), Environmental Protection Agency (EPA), Food and Drug Administration (FDA), Occupational Health and Safety Administration (OSHA), and a host of state and local agencies that are often funded in part by the larger federal agencies. The Federal Emergency Management Agency (FEMA), to a lesser extent, works to provide safe water and sewage disposal during natural and man-made disasters, and to contribute to the good health of and prevent epidemics among the population of the United States. Most often, government offices and a number of national and international organizations, such as the American Red Cross and the Salvation Army, work together during disasters. They help to provide healthful living conditions for those displaced from their homes or those whose homes have been damaged so as to cause unsafe living conditions.

Since the bubonic plague (Black Death) devastated Europe in the mid-1300s, civilized nations have done a great deal to control the spread of infectious diseases. Basic sanitation can go a long way toward preventing many diseases on both a personal and a global basis.

Hazard Communication

OSHA provides guidelines for employers in its Standard 1910.1200, which spells out the obligations of the employer when there is a potential exposure to hazardous chemicals. This information must be provided to the employees in health care facilities through inservice education and training on an annual basis. The training for hazard communications is usually combined with required training for categories of health care workers who are at risk of contracting infectious diseases from patients or from equipment and supplies used in the treatment of the patients. Information required in the training includes a comprehensive hazard communication program regarding container labeling, warning signs, and symbols as well as material safety data sheets (MSDSs). Specific information is available on the Internet for setting up such a program and implementing it.

Information concerning the hazards of materials that one may come in contact with in the workplace must be periodically updated and changes in job responsibilities may require additional training for affected workers. Even very simple materials normally found in the workplace may, if proper care is not exercised, pose a threat to the health of the user of the materials. Information concerning the risk and the first-aid procedures to follow when exposed to a chemical agent is required to be available through MSDSs that are located in the departmental area where the exposure is likely to occur. Any changes in materials that may pose different or additional risks to the patient or worker will require updates. The Exposure Control Plan, usually a part of infection control, should be reviewed at least annually, usually at the beginning of each fiscal year, for effectiveness and updating. The annual update will include a review of the general employee instruction sheet containing elements of Universal Precautions, as outlined previously. Any updated information from any regulatory agency or by facility policy changes will be prepared for dissemination to the employees at this time.

BLOODBORNE AND AIRBORNE PATHOGENS

As described previously, three organisms are associated with the majority of infections by bloodborne and airborne pathogens. Infection control is not limited to these three pathogens, but includes all organisms—bacterial, viral, protozoal, and fungal—that may invade the human body and cause infectious processes. However, the major pathogens that are considered "covered organisms" by federal agencies receive the most attention in infection control and exposure control documents. While protecting the medical worker against bloodborne and airborne pathogens, the work practice and engineered controls protect the worker and the patient against many other organisms.

Patients undergoing invasive procedures may be at risk for contracting infections both by pathogens and by the transfer of "normal flora." Normal flora include a large variety of bacteria that naturally occur in certain parts of the human body. Normal flora are in large part found in the mouth and the intestine but may be transplanted to another anatomical site, producing an infection. Any organism from the body that may be normal in one area may not be normal in another area. Normal flora are helpful bacteria that aid in preventing other bacteria, yeasts, and various microorganisms from growing in certain tissues, such as the mucous membranes of the mouth, nose, eyes, anus, and urogenital tract. But when they are introduced to another part of the body, the organisms become a problem that may lead to serious consequences. These types of infections often occur through careless practices and failure to disinfect work areas and equipment. Inordinate numbers of these types of incidents in a department of the health care facility would warrant an investigation by the Infection Control Committee to determine the cause and prevention of the incidents, possibly leading to procedural changes to prevent future occurrences.

Major Organisms Requiring Precautions

Prevention is the best way for the medical worker to avoid contracting an infection, and certain requirements contained in policies and procedures for the medical worker are discussed in this section. The medical laboratory, by the nature of the work that is performed there, will pose more risks than, for instance, the medical billing office. Many of the diseases that require hospitalization are a result of infections by a considerable range of species of microorganisms. This places the patient at risk for acquiring these diseases from other patients and workers who have been in contact with ill patients.

Examples of diseases that have caused much suffering abound in medical history. The world has a history of widespread infectious diseases since the beginning of recorded history, with a number of notable examples. Bubonic plague in Europe several centuries ago and, more recently, smallpox in this country, which devastated the Native American population, exacted a heavy toll and could have been prevented by simple processes. However, during these two periods, the general population and even the health care professionals of that day knew little about microorganisms and their roles in infection.

Today, much medical progress has been made in identifying organisms, which has led to prevention or treatment of diseases. This success has virtually eliminated large-scale epidemics or pandemics to date. But the progress we have made could quickly be undone if precautions are not understood and practiced by everyone to prevent the spread of infectious agents. A number of surveillance organizations, from state health departments to the federal CDC, are constantly making efforts through research and regulations to prevent much of this unnecessary suffering from infectious diseases. In addition, the World Health Organization (WHO) uses workers from every country to track, immunize against, and treat outbreaks of infectious diseases in the underdeveloped parts of the world. Were it not for these agencies, the world would undoubtedly have experienced an outbreak of biblical proportions that might have eclipsed anything experienced previously, including that of bubonic plague in the 15th century.

Most larger hospitals have comprehensive microbiology departments that are able to identify and provide information for the initiation of adequate treatments for a number of virulent pathogens. The five basic categories of microorganisms are bacterial, viral, parasitic, rickettsial (a specialized bacterium of increasing prevalence), and fungal organisms. There are a few others, including subviral particles called prions, (the source of the well-publicized "mad cow disease"). In the case of rickettsial infections, the causative organism is usually transmitted by a tick vector or carrier. Newer and less well-defined organisms other than these five categories will doubtless be discovered.

The administration of antibiotics that are specific for only certain bacteria is of little value in treating many bacterial organisms. Some broad-spectrum antibiotics will indiscriminately destroy most bacterial strains, including normal flora. This presents an opportunity for potentially harmful organisms to take the place of the normal flora. Also, most respiratory infections such as the common cold are caused by viruses against which antibiotics will do nothing or may even exacerbate the growth of the virus. The wholesale prescribing of antibiotics without identifying the presence of a pathogen has led to the rise of many bacteria that are resistant to almost every antibiotic currently in use. Many infections that are difficult to treat arise in patients who are hospitalized and have contracted an antibiotic-resistant organisms while in the facility. Major sources of hospital-acquired infections (termed **nosocomial** infections and **iatrogenic** infections) are caused by organisms that gain entry into and colonize the body through the introduction of medical devices used for various treatments.

With the proliferation of new medical procedures, some of an elective nature, the rise in infections by resistant strains may cause a local epidemic within a health care facility. In a number of cases, the Infection Control Committee will trace certain strains of bacteria to a single physician, to instruments, or to other health care workers. Protecting oneself against these dangerous organisms is paramount, and most disease prevention efforts are focused toward teaching the health care worker protection against a whole host of organisms. Infection by bloodborne and airborne pathogens other than HIV, HBV, and TB, as well as by environmental organisms, must be prevented through the use of precautions designed to protect both the worker and the patient. Economy and efficiency dictate that effective and conscientious efforts be pursued to avoid either the health care professional, the student, or a patient from being infected. These efforts will pay dividends in lowering our health care costs as a nation, as well as preventing needless suffering and inconvenience.

To protect workers and employees against infection by HIV, HBV, or TB, the infection control program of each medical facility and each educational institution classifies job positions by potential for exposure. These levels of potential risk range from Category I through Category III, with Category I including workers at most risk, and Category III representing health care workers with little risk of exposure. Although literally thousands of organisms are capable of causing serious infections in humans, only two major organisms associated with the majority of infections by bloodborne pathogens are given a status that requires specific training for health care personnel. It bears repeating that while the emphasis is on only two bloodborne organisms—HIV and HBV—focusing attention on other pathogenic (disease-causing) organisms among humans cannot be neglected. Hepatitis A virus, which is chiefly transmitted through water and food, is an important pathogen that can now be prevented through immunization, and the hepatitis C virus, which is bloodborne or sexually transmitted in most cases, is becoming increasingly important (sometimes dual immunization occurs for both hepatitis B and hepatitis C during a single immunization).

At this time, hepatitis A and C are not treated in OSHA guidelines as "covered organisms" requiring periodic training of the health care worker. Exposure to biohazards is inherent in some tasks and in those who perform them. Not only health care professionals but also other personnel who may come in contact with bloodborne pathogens or other body fluids may contract and spread organisms by virtue of their professions. Table 6-2 contains a list of most professionals who are at risk.

Blood is an extremely good bacterial medium, and viruses are intracellular organisms, meaning that they may grow well inside blood cells. Another organism that grows in blood cells is the **malaria** organism, of which there are four major strains capable of infecting humans. The strains of malaria organisms, called protozoa, that infect humans are not prevalent in North America currently but are rampant in other parts of the world. There are strains of malaria in the United States that infect birds, but humans fortunately have natural immunity against these strains.

This immunity of humans to certain animal pathogens seems to have been breached recently with certain organisms previously unknown to have infected humans. An example seen in outbreaks in Asia is **severe acute respiratory syndrome (SARS)** caused by organisms normally found only in chickens, turkeys, ducks, and migratory fowl. Exposure to the blood of animals is currently a topic for research, as diseases harbored by mammals and birds to which humans are currently immune may eventually find an avenue to directly infect humans.

Table 6-2 Workers Who May Be at Risk for Exposure to Bloodborne Pathogens*

Physicians	Dentists and other dental workers
Nurses	Laboratory and blood bank technologists
Pathologists	Medical technologists
Phlebotomists	Research laboratory scientists
Dialysis personnel	Emergency medical technicians
Some laundry workers	Morticians
Medical examiners	Some maintenance personnel
Paramedics	Some housekeeping personnel

* Exclusion of a job category here does not denote lack of risk.

CATEGORIZATION OF MEDICAL CARE WORKERS, FACULTY, AND ALLIED HEALTH STUDENTS

Educational institution faculty members and students in programs or course areas requiring direct contact with patients, with their body wastes, and with the wastes associated with their care are considered as Category I (high risk). Occupational exposure to HIV, HBV, and TB in certain health care professions is considered to fall under federal guidelines. Specific tasks are assigned to workers in these occupational areas, such as those related to nursing care, but are not limited to nurses and include other professionals and custodial types who may perform duties with certain risks involved. The process of categorizing tasks for Categories I, II, and III relates to the potential for contracting covered infectious diseases relative to the specific tasks these workers perform. The Infection Control Committee normally categorizes occupational tasks for medical workers on an ongoing basis due to the changes in duties and evolution of technology.

Three general groups of workers in health care facilities have been identified, and training for them has been directed toward specific tasks with a level of risk. Appropriate training is provided for all the various levels of health care workers categorized into the three groups. These levels of workers are placed into categories based on their potential for being exposed to blood, respiratory secretions, and other body fluids in the course of their treatment of patients and in handling of infectious wastes. In general, the three types of workers are as follows: Category I personnel have the greatest risk of exposure to infectious materials, Category II personnel handle materials that might have come in contact with infectious materials, and Category III personnel have the least risk of becoming infected in the workplace. Infection control/exposure control manuals often break down tasks with instructions for methods to be used to protect oneself depending on the category to which one is assigned as a result of job duties.

Category I

Nurses, emergency responders, and certain physicians, along with medical laboratory workers, including those working in histopathology laboratories and morgues, are at one of the highest risk levels due to the potential for contact with human blood. Medical laboratory workers are listed as Category I health care workers since the majority of the work performed by this group involves blood specimens and other body fluids and tissues. In addition, some medical laboratory workers perform procedures directly with infectious agents, such as those workers employed in the microbiology laboratory. Blood and certain other body fluids carry the highest risk of transmitting an infection to the unwary health care employee who comes in contact with them. Engineering controls, or equipment designed to protect the worker, must be used when testing blood and **other potentially infectious materials (OPIM)**. When protective equipment and supplies are used where there is potential for contact with body fluids, the possibility of becoming infected is greatly minimized (Figure 6-2).

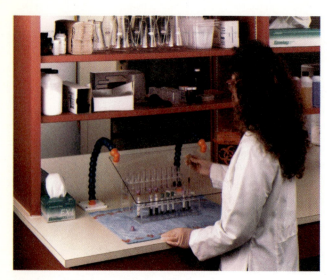

FIGURE 6-2 A laboratory worker wearing gloves and laboratory jacket while handling blood.
Source: Delmar/Cengage Learning.

All health care employees with potential contact with blood and OPIM are classified as Category I, even when barrier devices and **personal protective equipment (PPE)** are used. Especially for Category I employees, regular training is required at least annually and when job requirements change and increase the potential exposure to blood and OPIM increases. Health care employees other than medical laboratory personnel who are listed as Category I are those who work with hospitalized patients in a direct care manner, such as patient care assistants, radiology workers, patient transport personnel, teams that provide infusion services (IV), and surgical workers. In a large and complex medical facility, there could also be any number of other specialty areas where employees may be involved with direct patient care.

The basic components of PPE are tailored specifically to the likelihood of exposure during various procedures. In the medical laboratory, the needs are quite different, for instance, from those of nurses working with patients with contagious diseases and from those of surgical and other technicians and surgeons who work in areas where invasive procedures are performed, such as in operating room suites (Figure 6-3).

Category II

Custodians and laundry workers are classified as Category II employees since many of their tasks include procedures where there is a definite possibility that they will handle blood, blood products, and body fluids during the disposal of such materials. Although barrier equipment should be worn, there is a potential for accidental exposure through needle sticks for those removing trash from treatment areas and because laundry workers routinely handle linens soiled with body fluids and wastes. Several decades ago, medical wastes were simply thrown into ordinary trash bins and dumpsters or autoclaved (sterilized) and then discarded in ordinary trash. These wastes are now required to have special handling due to local, state, and federal regulations that mandate how this potentially infectious material is to be disposed. Commercial providers supply collection containers and collect the contaminated material on a regular basis for disposal, usually by burning.

Transportation of these infectious wastes is strictly regulated from the collection point to certification that the wastes have arrived at the disposal facility and have been properly disposed. Disposal facilities are specially designed to provide for safe and effective disposal of waste products that may transmit infections if a person comes into contact with the material. Medical and other biohazardous wastes generated by the health care facility are the responsibility of the generating facility until disposal, including the travel to the disposal facility.

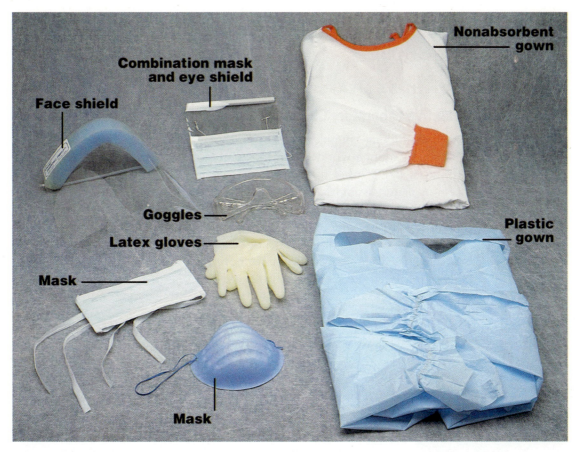

FIGURE 6-3 Personal protective equipment used to protect the medical worker against biohazardous materials.
Source: Delmar/Cengage Learning.

If a shipment is lost, the health care facility and not the waste transport company may be responsible for ensuring that the wastes are recovered and are properly disposed of according to local, state, and federal laws.

Category III

Clerical jobs and dining room tasks pose little likelihood of the worker coming in contact with blood and body fluids. However, this category of worker is often in contact with the patient for information gathering, interviews for admission processes, and perhaps dietetic consultations, so TB has the potential for being transmitted to Category III workers if the patient is coughing forcefully. In some facilities, clerical personnel may be required to accompany the patient and to obtain a history from emergency patients in treatment areas, where they may come in contact with the patient in question or with other patients. In this event, the clerical worker would be treated the same as a worker providing direct patient

Infection Control Alert

Categories of Health Care Workers

Category I Workers
Subject to the highest potential for exposure to infectious and toxic materials

Category II Workers
Incidental to the nature of their job duties, these workers may be exposed

Category III Workers
Seldom or ever subject to exposure; clerical personnel may unwittingly be exposed to patient with TB, however, when taking patient history and admitting patients

care if a patient were found to be contagious, and should wear a mask if the person being interviewed is listed as one requiring respiratory precautions.

PROTECTIVE MEASURES FOR HEALTH CARE WORKERS

Protective Laboratory Clothing

Protective clothing suitable for the job being performed is provided by the employer. In routine work, a uniform is usually required, such as scrubs and lab jackets. PPE is used in both the classroom laboratories when potentially infectious materials and hazardous chemicals are being used, and in the clinical sites. When there is a danger of spillage and splatter, a laboratory jacket should be worn at a minimum. Although it is a common practice, laboratory overgarments such as lab jackets should not be worn outside the workplace. Some facilities even have employees remove their scrubs and don street clothing before leaving the building. Gloves are worn at all times when blood and other body fluids, and solid waste such as feces are handled. Aprons that are plasticized or rubberized are necessary where there is a danger of spilling strong acids and alkalis while working. Latex gloves used for simple procedures are not adequate for handling strong chemicals. Reusable gloves should be available for use when strong chemicals are being handled. A splash shield may also be used when opening vials of blood or other body fluids. Goggles and face shields (Figure 6-4) are necessary when there is a danger of splatter or aerosolization of fluids.

The wearing of long dangling earrings, necklaces, and bracelets may be dangerous for the medical laboratory worker. Long hair, hair extensions, and dangling braids may dip into the materials being tested or used in testing and may contaminate certain items and persons in the laboratory. An additional risk related to long hair lies in its potential to catch in moving parts of equipment, posing a risk of injury to the laboratory worker. A potential hazard from wearing dangling jewelry is that electrical shocks have occurred when jewelry made of metal has come in contact with and conducted electricity to the technical worker, resulting in serious injury. Shoes should have closed toes for protection from hazardous materials and from items falling onto the feet. They should be comfortable and stable for standing for long periods, as is often required when working in a medical laboratory.

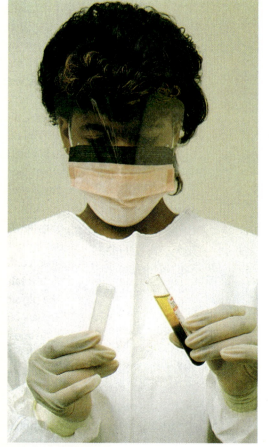

FIGURE 6-4 Personal protective equipment includes eye goggles or shield.
Source: Delmar/Cengage Learning.

Required Personal Protective Equipment

The clinical facility or the educational institution must provide PPE as appropriate in sufficient numbers and types to enable health care employees, students, or instructors to protect themselves from exposure to contagious diseases or toxic materials. Training will be provided in classroom activities and during orientation to clinical facilities for both employees and students. The costs incurred for the required training and the necessary PPE to perform tasks in the safest manner possible are the responsibility of the medical facility. Department supervisors of the various facility areas are responsible for maintaining sufficient supplies of each protective item needed. However, individual workers are also required to inform supervisors of shortages of items and to maintain the equipment and supplies assigned to them.

While laboratory workers other than phlebotomists seldom come in direct contact with patients, collection of blood or other body fluids may be required of the technician or technologist under some circumstances. Isolation rooms are provided for patients with extremely contagious diseases as well as those in reverse isolation, used where the patient's immunity is low. It is necessary to fully protect oneself or the patients in these circumstances. When entering the room of a patient in an isolation rooms (Figure 6-5), PPE is donned on entering the room and discarded as the worker leaves the room.

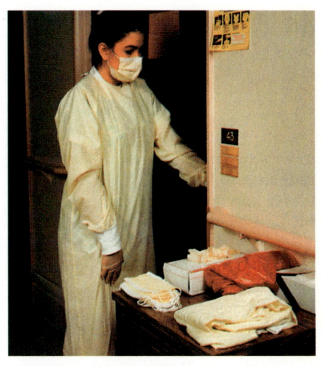

FIGURE 6-5 Laboratory employee wearing gown, gloves, and mask on entering a patient's room where transmission-based precautions are in effect.
Source: Delmar/Cengage Learning.

Gowns and Other Overgarments as Barriers against Contamination

Gowns are used to protect caregivers from becoming infected while they provide prolonged procedures for the patient. Gowns may be sterile or nonsterile, as determined by the procedure being performed. Normally, sterile gowns are worn to protect the patient from contamination when an invasive procedure is being performed. Moisture-resistant gowns may be used if there is a danger of splatter of infectious materials from the patient. These gowns must be removed before leaving the patient's room when they have been used for performing procedures involving body fluids. Gowns that have been used in the performance of medical procedures are considered contaminated materials and should not be worn in general areas of the health care facility.

All overgarments such as protective gowns and overshoes are to be removed before leaving the facility and are not to be worn in public areas. Gloves, masks, and gowns are worn at any time when there is a possible risk of being contaminated with blood or body fluids or with respiratory secretions from a patient suffering from TB. Goggles and face shields may be necessary when performing certain procedures. This information will be provided to the student by the section supervisor or the preceptor training the medical laboratory worker. Certain minimal risk tasks require only gloves (along with suitable clothing), while others may require a mask, a face shield, or all three. Generally, only gloves are worn (as protective equipment) for the following tasks:

1. When there is a likelihood of contact with patient's blood or other body fluids, except for perspiration
2. When collecting or transporting a specimen
3. When cleaning up spills of body fluids
4. When transporting or handling soiled bed linens or towels
5. When the student or worker has open cuts or sores on, or chafing of, the hands and arms

Transparent shields are used in the laboratory for opening tubes of blood from which spatters of blood or aerosols may be generated.

EXPOSURE POTENTIAL AND PREVENTION

All medical workers have a responsibility to themselves and the institution to be safety conscious at all times. Using preventive practices enables workers to avoid making mistakes that will cause them to come in direct contact with blood and body fluids. It is best to avoid **exposure incidents** by following the policies and guidelines of the institution and by obtaining good information and training. By conscientiously following these measures, there is very little likelihood of contracting AIDS, hepatitis, or TB in the course of the performance of the medical worker's tasks.

Prevention and Treatment for Bloodborne and Airborne Pathogens

There is currently no cure for HIV infection or AIDS. HBV infections run their natural course, and approximately 90% of those infected recover and show no evidence of the disease after the condition is resolved. However, 10% of those contracting HBV become chronically infected and are known as "carriers." Carriers are difficult to identify just from appearance, as the infected person may appear quite healthy.

TB is the most prevalent airborne disease and may be cured in the early stages of the disease by the administration of specific antibiotics in most cases, except for those cases arising from resistant strains of organisms. However, the emphasis should be on prevention rather than cure for both bloodborne and airborne pathogens.

What Is Meant by *Potential Exposure*?

Potential exposure occurs when a health care employee may be exposed to blood or body fluids or to a patient with a respiratory illness in the course of duties being performed. The terms "exposure" and "exposure incident" are used somewhat interchangeably when there is an actual exposure to a hazardous condition, such as working with a patient who later is determined to have active TB, or if the hands or clothing are soiled with blood from a patient with an infectious disease. An exposure incident more accurately occurs when there is an unexpected situation where a release of blood or toxins occurs accidentally and persons are exposed. A physician makes the determination regarding an actual exposure. If damaged skin comes in contact with body fluids or if the employees receives an accidental needle stick from a contaminated needle or a cut from contaminated instruments, an exposure incident has occurred. An exposure to airborne pathogens most often occurs when an employee is exposed to a patient who is later diagnosed as having active TB.

An exposure may involve a number of products, but primarily either biohazardous materials or toxic chemicals for the purposes of this section. Any time a layperson or medical worker comes in direct contact with body fluids or provides treatment to a patient later found to have an infectious disease, the status of the person exposed should be assessed. Any other worker who was possibly exposed to the infected patient should also undergo a health assessment, especially if contact with blood and body fluids may have occurred. This assessment might require only counseling but may include preventive immunization or the collection of a blood sample to determine baseline laboratory values. Prophylactic treatment is sometimes initiated where a high likelihood of exposure has occurred. Postexposure prophylaxis (PEP) may be initiated in which treatment is begun to prevent replication of viruses such as HIV, or gamma globulin–containing antibodies against an organism such as HBV are administered.

Usually at 2 weeks following an exposure incident, a second blood sample may be collected to determine if any changes have occurred. The first sample, drawn immediately following the incident, is called the *baseline sample* or the *acute sample*. Blood is drawn aseptically and is separated into blood cells and plasma or serum (liquid portion of the blood). The acute specimen should be negative for antibodies against the suspected organism if the blood sample is drawn almost immediately after exposure and the person has had no prior exposure or immunization to the particular disease organism. The sample collected 2 weeks after the acute sample is called the *convalescent sample*. If the particular antibody is negative in both samples, no infection was contracted. If the first sample is negative, and the second positive, more than likely an exposure has occurred that has led to infection. Positive results from these samples will confirm an exposure and subsequent contraction of a disease.

Exposure through Spills of Biohazardous and Toxic Materials

When biohazardous materials or toxic chemicals are spilled, it is important to observe the following procedures to protect others who may enter the area. Warning signs should be placed as necessary in areas where foot traffic occurs, before beginning the clean-up process described below.

1. An absorbent material or a specially designed gel should be used to cover the entire spill. The custodial staff will be responsible for the proper removal of the spills and will provide thorough cleaning of the area. Wastes should be removed to an area for storage until disposed of properly.

2. Spill kits may be designed for both biological and hazardous materials cleanup, as well as for neutralizing toxic chemicals, and are to be provided and used as required. Either type of kit is designed to absorb or contain biohazardous materials for disposal.

3. Following the absorption process, disinfectants are to be used to thoroughly clean the area of any residual material.

How to Assess a Potential Exposure

When confronted with a situation with a high potential for exposure to blood, body fluids, or hazardous materials, or when such exposure has already occurred, an individual should ask the following three questions:

1. *Assess the situation; is it serious enough to determine that medical help is needed?* If the victim is bleeding profusely, or has any broken bones, there is a potential for exposing the person providing aid to the victim. Serious injury would necessitate calling 911. (Note that in some areas a 911 number is not available, so you should post the proper number to call in the case of an emergency in the work area. Many health care facilities will have already done this as a function of the infection control personnel or in some cases, a **Safety Committee**, and the numbers will often be posted conspicuously near each work area, including maintenance and mechanical shops where traumatic injuries may occur. All individuals should be familiar with the proper procedure for reporting an emergency situation.) Primary treatment would focus on keeping the victim comfortable and avoiding further injury by preventing the victim from moving about, until emergency personnel arrive.

2. *Can the situation be managed with simple first aid and removal of the hazard without professional help?* If the helper/rescuer has only come into contact with a body fluid and has no breaks or cuts in the skin, washing of the affected area(s) with soap and water is sufficient. In case of doubt, or if questions arise, contact the infection control coordinator or seek medical attention in the absence of the infection control officer. It is best to seek the advice of a medical professional as early as possible following an actual or a potential exposure to infectious body materials. A baseline set of diagnostic tests and a review of the immunization records are always good ideas. A delay in treatment is not advantageous to the exposed person, as early treatment enables a better outcome if the person has been infected.

3. *In case of doubt, should treatment be sought?* It is better to err on the side of caution. Making a proper assessment and, if necessary, instituting treatment quickly, may prevent substantial harm. In the case of exposure to a known substance, it is possible to ask for consultation with a professional who may give valuable information regarding the possibility of the need for further treatment. Even though the health care industry is chiefly concerned with exposure to bloodborne and airborne pathogens, it is possible that exposure may occur with materials that are chemical in nature and that are equally as dangerous to the health of the worker as are disease-causing organisms. Engineered and **work practice controls** (Figure 6-6) are essential

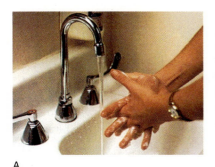
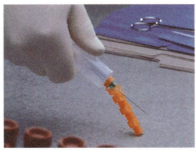
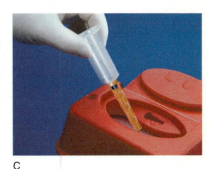

A   B   C

FIGURE 6-6 (A–C) Work practice controls.
Source: Delmar/Cengage Learning.

to the prevention of unnecessary contraction of disease or exposure to toxic materials that may harm the health care worker, the patient, or coworkers.

EXPOSURE TRAINING AND IMMUNIZATION FOR PREVENTION OF INFECTION

The sequence of events to prevent or minimize exposure, prevent or treat the effects of exposure, and treat following exposure, is categorized using three different labels. The three types of activities are preexposure, actual exposure, and postexposure treatment and actions. To be exposed to toxins and biohazards does not absolutely indicate that the person exposed will suffer any ill effects from the incident. There are many exposures daily in health care facilities, but only a small fraction of these persons are affected adversely because of a number of factors that play a role in protecting the individual. A healthy lifestyle leading to a healthy and disease-free body, preventive medicine, and intact skin help substantially in preventing any harm from most types of exposures. It is easier and safer to use work practice and engineering controls along with common-sense precautions to prevent contraction of an infectious disease, rather than later having to treat a medical condition. Repetitive training and practice should cause the health care professional to always practice safety, as eventually this awareness of the need for practicing self-protection will become a part of the affective domain and will be done without thinking.

Preexposure

Immunization, when vaccine exists to protect against certain organisms, along with training to enable health care workers to avoid becoming infected, are the most effective ways to avoid becoming infected. In a number of institutional and government policies, this type of training is mandatory on a regular basis. Safety Committee and Infection Control Committee activities to prevent infection can also be lumped under the preexposure category. The cliché, "Prevention is the best cure," is the best way in which to approach any kind of infection.

Human Immunodeficiency Virus

To date, there has been no effective vaccine developed to provide immunity against HIV. Several strains of HIV exist, some of which are similar to those found in animals. For instance, feline leukemia is thought to be a viral strain almost identical to that of the HIV strain that infects humans. In some parts of the world, epidemics of both HTLV-1 and HTLV-2 have also occurred. This poses such a risk to our blood supplies that testing of each unit of blood for HTLV-1 and HTLV-2 is performed.

Hepatitis B Virus Vaccination

An HBV vaccination is offered to all medical care workers and students. The risk of contracting HBV is minimal if proper precautions are followed, but close contact with blood and other body fluids, as well as with patients with the disease, puts clinical laboratory workers at higher risk than those in the general population.

1. Category I and II employees having occupational exposure or potential exposure to blood or other infectious materials are offered the HBV vaccination at no charge to the employee. The vaccination is made available within 10 working days of initial work assignment unless the employee has previously received the complete HBV vaccination series and declines immunization (see item 2) or antibody testing reveals the employee is immune or the vaccine is contraindicated for medical reasons.

2. Students in occupational areas with potential or likely exposure to blood-borne and airborne pathogens are required to receive the HBV immunizations or to sign a declination form indicating that the student is aware of the risks of not being immunized. By signing a declination form, the student agrees to hold the clinical facility and the educational institute blameless if an exposure results in the disease. The student is required to pay for his or her immunizations and the series of three injections are usually provided for the student at cost. Students should receive the first vaccine dose before any patient/client contact and before performing any tasks, procedures, or activities that involve exposure potential.

3. An antibody titer is a prescreening test that may be offered but is not required before receiving an HBV vaccination. An antibody titer determines the presence of already existing antibodies against HBV, and is also offered at no charge to the employee and at cost to the student. Each employee and student who tests positive for the antibodies has the right to refuse vaccination by completing a declination form. Those who later decide to be immunized against HBV will be offered the immunization at no cost to the employee and at cost for the student.

4. A repeat vaccination is also offered as a postexposure follow-up for all instructors, medical employees, or students with an occupational exposure incident [skin, eye, mucous membrane, or parenteral (intravenous, subcutaneous, intramuscular, or mucosal) contact with blood or OPIM]. A simple repeat vaccination or administration of protective antibodies is a small price

to pay for the assurance that protection from a potentially dangerous infection is in effect.

5. Documentation of the immunization status should be kept in each individual faculty member's personnel record as well as in a master vaccination file. Documentation of student vaccination is to be maintained in the student's record file and master training file. Any faculty member or student declining vaccination will be counseled on the benefits and safety of the vaccine and will sign a statement to that effect.

Preexposure Records Storage and Maintenance

Preexposure documentation of training and baseline testing of the employee or student for preexisting conditions is important. When a health care worker is exposed to an infectious agent, procedures called *baseline determinations* that were performed before the incident are compared with those obtained immediately following exposure. This documents the presence or absence of a preexisting condition. Medical records are maintained as required in the Blood Borne Pathogens Standard implemented by OSHA. Student medical records shall be retained for a period of 1 year after graduation, completion, termination, or leaving the educational facility. Faculty medical records as well as those for medical workers and other employees of the medical facility are retained for a period of 30 years after the date employment ends for each employee. These records are often accompanied by documentation of training for the employees.

Immediate Action after Possible Exposure

If soiled clothing or broken skin is present following a possible exposure, immediate action may be necessary. First, the amount of blood present is assessed. A small amount less than the size of a 50-cent piece that cannot be squeezed from the clothing would not necessitate removal of one's clothing. Extremely bloody clothing should be removed and NEVER worn home. Those exposed should clean themselves carefully and place soiled clothing in a plastic bag. Clean clothing should be available for wearing during travel home.

Second, bloody clothing must be handled with precautions in mind. Bloody clothing with a considerable amount of blood on it should be secured in a closed and intact plastic bag to prevent contamination of others in the vicinity who may be assisting with or providing aid. Extremely bloody clothing should NOT be washed in commercial washers. It should be soaked in a dilute bleach solution before it is placed in a washing machine or sink. Very little danger exists from dried blood, but it is important to be very careful. It has been documented that HBV may survive 10 to 14 days in dried blood. Fortunately, HIV survives for only a short time in dried blood.

Skin breaks, rashes, or cuts and abrasions provide a direct portal of entry into the body for infectious microorganisms, including both bacteria and viruses. If skin breaks are present, one should seek medical attention if exposed to blood. If the infection control officer is not present and broken skin or mucous membranes are involved, one should go either to a physician in the emergency department or to his or her private physician. The educational institution or medical facility is responsible for charges incurred when exposure occurs during duties related to the medical program in which a student is enrolled. Incident reports are initiated at the clinical site and must be supervised by a physician.

Postexposure Treatment for Exposure to Blood or OPIM

Follow-up actions with a physical evaluation and counseling should be immediately initiated. When an exposure is determined by investigation to have occurred, an exposure incident evaluation and follow-up report form should be completed. These forms should be available in all departments, and additional forms may be obtained from the infection control officer. Counseling should be scheduled for those who have been exposed to infectious materials to determine the status of the individual and the reasons for the exposure. The infection control representative should make a report for discussion with the entire committee to determine if any policies were violated or if there was actually a policy that could have prevented the incident. An incident may precipitate the implementation of new policies or revisions of existing policies.

An accidental exposure to the blood of a suspected or confirmed case of hepatitis B should be followed by administration of **gamma globulin** within a few hours of the incident if possible. Gamma globulin is the portion of blood called serum that contains specific antibodies against certain organisms. If gamma-globulin is administered no later than 7 days following exposure, it is often effective in preventing infection from occurring. This is also true for a number of other organisms. Therefore, if an exposure to any potentially hazardous organism occurs, it is prudent to seek medical advice so quick treatment may be provided when indicated.

The health care employee, faculty member, or student is deemed to have experienced an exposure to possible harmful pathogens if there is a skin break, a dirty needle stick, a cut or puncture by contaminated glass or a broken object, or a splash into mucous membranes such as the eye, nasal mucosa, or mouth. A cutaneous (skin) exposure due to chapped, abraded, or other nonintact skin should also be reported as an exposure incident to the medical facility departmental supervisor and the educational institution's infection control officer or coordinator.

DOCUMENTATION OF EXPOSURE INCIDENT

Following the report of an occupational exposure incident, the medical worker, faculty member, or student is required to complete an accident/incident report, available from the infection control coordinator. The forms to be completed are organized in such a way that a supervisory employee will be able to complete all steps necessary immediately following the exposure if the incident occurs during the evening, night, or weekend hours when the infection control coordinator or a designee is not on site. The records related to preexisting conditions and any immunizations, as well as immune status, will be gathered from the exposed person's records on file as required. This will ensure that all appropriate steps are performed for any employee at any time. Remember, except in limited situations, the patient has the right to refuse to have his or her blood tested, so it is important that a person with a potential exposure make a rational decision. The potentially exposed employee will be offered a confidential medical evaluation and follow-up, which will include the information below.

Essential Steps for Documentation of an Exposure Incident

1. Documentation of the route(s) of exposure, previous HBV and HIV antibody status of the source patient(s) (if known), and the circumstances under which the exposure incident occurred.

2. If the source patient can be identified and it is feasible, with the patient's permission, collection and testing of the patient's blood should be conducted to determine the presence of HIV and/or HBV infections.

3. If the patient does not consent to furnishing a specimen, the employer shall establish that legally required consent cannot be obtained. If the source individual's consent is not required by law, as is covered by applicable laws in some states, his or her blood, if available, will be tested and the results documented. If the source patient is already known to be HIV or HBV positive, repeat testing is not required.

4. Results of the source individual's testing should be made available to the medical worker, faculty member, or student, and the affected persons should be informed of the applicable laws and regulations concerning disclosure of the identity and infectious status of the source individual.

5. The exposed health care employee or student's blood should be collected as soon as feasible and tested after consent is obtained from the person exposed to HBV or HIV.

6. If the medical facility employee, instructor, or student consents to baseline blood collections but does not give consent at that time for HIV serologic testing, the sample is preserved for at least 90 days. If, within a 90-day period of the exposure incident, the individual elects to have the baseline sample tested, testing will be done as soon as feasible.

7. The educational facility and the medical facility shall ensure that the health care professional responsible for the medical worker's, instructor's, or student's hepatitis B vaccination is provided a copy of the regulation for "Occupational Exposure to Bloodborne Pathogens."

8. The educational institution shall ensure that the health care professional evaluating an employee after an exposure incident is provided with the information in the "Infection Control Alert" box on the next page.

9. The facility shall obtain and provide the employee with a copy of the consulting health care professional's written opinion within 15 days of the completion of the evaluation. The health care professional's written opinion for HBV vaccination shall be limited as to whether the vaccination is indicated and if the medical worker, instructor, or student received such vaccination. NOTE: An employee who declined HBV immunization and is subsequently exposed may be immunized within a few days of the incident. This will usually provide protection to the employee, as will administration of gamma-globulin–containing antibodies against the virus.

Infection Control Alert

Obligations of the Health Care or Educational Facility Following Exposure Incident

- A copy of the regulation for "Exposure to Bloodborne Pathogens" is provided for the individual to ensure that he or she understands the risks involved and that the treatment is adequate.

- A description of the duties for a medical worker, instructor, or student as they relate to the exposure incident will be available to determine if the employee was performing a procedure outside the scope of his or her training and the incident could have been avoided.

- Documentation of circumstances leading to the exposure incident, including the route of exposure, will be provided. Statistical evidence indicating more than one occurrence under the same conditions would possibly lead to modification of employee training.

- Results of the source individual's blood testing, if available, are to be provided with the source individual's consent. The source individual may only be be asked but is not legally required to provide a blood or body fluid sample, and he or she is allowed to refuse to do so in some states.

- All medical records relevant to the appropriate treatment of the employee, including vaccination status, are the responsibility of the facilities to maintain and should be available to the counselor who is performing preliminary processes to document the exposure incident and to determine the risk to the employee.

10. The health care professional's written opinion for post-exposure evaluation and follow-up is limited to the following information:

A. Medical facility employee, faculty member or student is to be informed of the results of the evaluation.

B. The faculty member, medical worker, or student is to be told about any medical conditions resulting from being exposed to blood or other infectious materials that require further evaluation and treatment if clinically indicated.

NOTE: All other clinical findings are confidential and are not included in the written report to be provided to the exposed medical worker.

LIMITING THE SPREAD OF HIV

It should be reassuring to the health care employee that AIDS is not known to be spread by coughing, sneezing, hugging, or contact with eating utensils, faucets, or toilet seats. It is possible, however, that AIDS may be spread through kissing, if a person infected with the virus has oral-to-oral contact with someone who has vigorously brushed his or her teeth and has minute bleeding of the gums. AIDS may be transmitted in a similar manner as HBV, so learning about the spread of one of these organisms will enable the health care provider to protect himself or herself against both, as the precautions are similar. In addition to sweat, tears, urine, and vomitus, NO transmission is known to have yet occurred through vectors such as mosquitoes, fleas, ticks, or other insects or animals. The possibility of transmission through animal and arthropod vectors is remote but is periodically investigated on the chance that this may eventually occur.

The incubation period is the time required for the virus to grow and to reproduce to a level where symptoms and signs appear. The incubation period for HIV is unknown and therefore may be variable. Asymptomatic persons are known to have harbored the virus for more than 10 to 15 years. Some who have been diagnosed and who have been successfully treated for a number of years are living somewhat normal lives due to advanced and improved treatment that has developed over the intervening years since the first cases of AIDS were documented. In transfusion-related cases, the incubation period has most often been about 2 years or less. Fortunately, with routine testing of blood supplies, the number of transfusion-related cases has practically disappeared.

The stage or period of time following the infection of a person before the HIV organism may be transmitted to another person is unknown. It is believed that the disease may be transmitted before the appearance of symptoms and that it persists even after successful treatment has alleviated the initial symptoms. It should be noted that a person who has been successfully treated may appear normal while continuing treatment but may be able to infect others. Therefore, preventive measures in relation to sexual practices and performance of medical procedures should always be taken.

Prevention and control of HIV infection go hand in hand. Because most cases are transmitted sexually or by shared using of drug paraphernalia, these practices must be modified or curtailed by those who are positive for HIV. Good rules to follow are to avoid indiscriminate sexual contact with new partners, particularly those whose background is unknown and to avoid the use of IV drugs and the sharing of IV drug items. In the health care facilities and when treating patients at the sites of accidents, scrupulously careful cleaning and disinfection of blood and body fluid spills are necessary to avoid the spread of the virus. Cleaning practices should include protection for the person responsible for cleaning contaminated area such as those where medical procedures have been performed that generate blood or other body fluids and tissues. Protective aprons or other clothing impervious to liquids, such as safety aprons, should be worn over the clothing normally worn for work, along with reusable gloves that are in good condition and that are cleaned between uses.

Medical laboratory technical personnel are encouraged to clean their work surfaces and equipment frequently with a fresh 10% bleach (Clorox or sodium hypochlorite) solution. This is the most effective disinfectant that is readily available and should be made fresh on a daily basis. Surfaces and objects contaminated with blood or body fluids that may contain blood (e.g., vomitus or urine) must be cleaned with detergent and water and disinfected immediately. The disinfecting solution of household bleach and water at a 1:10 ratio is extremely effective against HIV and almost all other viruses and bacteria.

For effective cleaning of work surfaces, a procedure should be followed in which fresh 10% bleach solution is used to generously saturate the area and then the surface is allowed to air dry. DO NOT RINSE. The solution loses its potency within a few hours so it should be prepared fresh daily. Some medical facilities use materials other than bleach and use additional procedures for disinfecting all surfaces within the clinical areas. Policies for disinfecting areas are published in a facility's policy and procedure manual and will be documented as being effective by the Infection Control Committee before the procedure is adopted.

HIV may be found in conjunction with other infectious organisms, because of the immunocompromised condition of the patient seeking treatment, which gives other microorganisms the opportunity to grow. It is important to test accident victims following treatment where a number of medical responders may have been exposed to the victim's blood.

HIV and other potentially dangerous organisms may be found in body fluids even when there are no symptoms to suggest infection is present. Some HIV-infected persons are diagnosed during routine testing, and show no signs or symptoms of infection. A person with an HIV infection ultimately develops a weakened immune status and thus is also vulnerable to a host of opportunistic infections with organism not normally found as human pathogens. These patients may require reverse isolation to protect them from exposure to others, including health care providers who may transmit organisms to them. Laboratory workers should always wear disposable gloves when handling blood and other body fluids, secretions, and excretions. However, only blood, semen, vaginal fluids, and bloody body fluids are known to enable transmission of the HIV organism. Note that sweat is the only fluid not included in Standard Precautions guidelines issued by the CDC. Tears and urine may also contain the viruses, but no transmission has been made through these body fluids to date.

After contact with any body fluid, the hands should be washed as soon as possible. There is no substitute for ordinary hand soap, warm water, and friction in washing all parts of the hands, including the cuticles. Although disposable latex gloves are necessary to prevent contamination when performing ordinary laboratory work, reusable gloves that are sturdier and more impenetrable should be used for cleaning spills of body fluids and sharp objects such as broken glass. The work practice control of washing the hands is the easiest method for preventing contamination of oneself as well as others with whom the medical worker comes in contact. Even if gloves have been worn, the hands should be washed thoroughly and vigorously with running water and soap for at least 30 seconds after removing the gloves, ensuring that the webbing between the fingers is scrubbed. Remove rings and other jewelry to do a more thorough job of washing of the hands and arms. Particular care should be taken to wash around the cuticles of the nails, with vigorous rubbing together of the hands to produce friction.

Remember, handwashing (Figure 6-7) is indicated before donning gloves and after removing them. The area where procedures are performed should be cleaned before removing one's gloves.

LIMITING THE SPREAD OF HEPATITIS B VIRUS

Hepatitis B is the second important bloodborne pathogen that is considered a "covered" disease. The causative organism is HBV, which is spread much in the same manner as HIV, through sexual practices and exchanges of body fluids. However, unlike HIV, immunization is available for this organism and it is required in many health care facilities unless the worker declines vaccination. Although 10% of those who contract an infection with HBV become *chronically infected* and can still transmit the disease even when asymptomatic, the remaining 90% recover spontaneously after varying periods of time.

The symptoms for HBV are similar to those of HIV with the exception, in part, of nausea and jaundice (yellowing chiefly of the skin and eyes). Anorexia (loss of appetite), tiredness, nausea, and vomiting, often accompanied by arthralgia (joint pain), and sometimes a rash are often but not always present. Jaundice is most often present in adults but is ordinarily not found in young children. Symptoms will vary widely from person to person, with some patients having almost no symptoms at all, while others become seriously ill. Again, a person with HBV may exhibit almost no signs, yet be capable of infecting another via the exchange of body fluids through sexual activities and the sharing of needles and contaminated blood products.

HBV is found throughout the world, and the disease is rampant in many areas where medical care and immunization are not readily available. The only

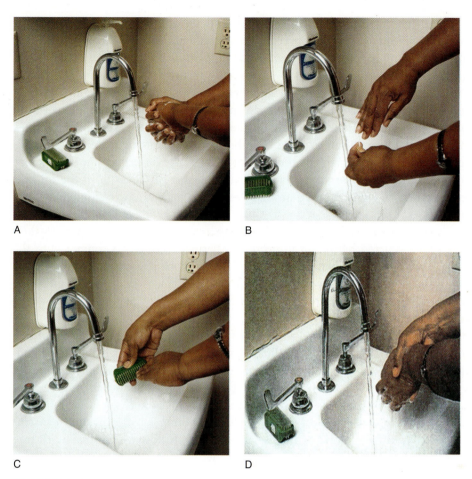

FIGURE 6-7 (A–D) Work practice of washing hands before and after a procedure.
Source: Delmar/Cengage Learning.

known reservoir for HBV is the human body but, unlike HIV, HBV may persist in dried body fluids for as long as 10 to 14 days. Careful cleaning and **decontamination** of work surfaces and equipment would prevent most cases in which this disease is contracted by contact in the workplace. Transmission of the disease has occurred through a number of routes or portals of entry into the body.

A laboratory test for HBsAg (hepatitis B surface antigen) tests for the actual viral particles and provides a direct test for the organism, unlike other tests in which the antibody response to the virus is measured. Although HBV has been found in infected persons in virtually all body fluids, from tissue secretions to wound excretions, only blood and blood products, semen, and vaginal fluids, as in HIV, have been found to be the source for transmitting the disease. As in HIV, HBV can also be spread person-to-person from a person's blood by finding its way into open skin cuts or abrasions. Splashing of blood and other body fluids into the eyes of another person may cause contraction of the disease, as will sexual contact. Transmission from a mother to her baby is common when the mother is HBsAg positive.

Accidental inoculation through needle sticks or shared razors and tooth-brushes has been documented on rare occasions. Fecal-oral transmission has not been demonstrated for either hepatitis B or HIV, but is associated with hepatitis A, another important disease that is more easily spread than hepatitis B but does not have the important medical ramifications that HBV infections do. The incubation period for HBV is about 45 to 180 days, with an average of 60- to 90-days elapsing from the exposure incident to the onset of signs and symptoms. The amount of inoculum or dose (number of organisms or materials containing the organisms entering the body) accounts for the differences in time before symptoms appear, as larger doses of inoculum most often result in the quicker manifestation of signs and symptoms. Preventive measures are similar to those for HIV.

Procedures for cleaning and disinfecting areas where blood and body fluid spills have occurred before an unprotected person comes into contact with the material are most effective in preventing spread of the organism. After properly disposing of biohazardous wastes (Figure 6-8), surfaces and objects contaminated by blood, blood products, or body fluids must first be cleaned with detergent and water and then disinfected.

Proper cleaning of work areas is of paramount importance. Disposable gloves are mandatory when handling blood or injuries accompanied by bleeding, or bloody and body fluid–contaminated items, as well as when cleaning or disinfecting work surfaces or clothing. Open cuts, rashes, or sores on the hands require special precautions when removing the gloves and when washing the hands. Extreme care should be taken when handling needles or sharp instruments and supplies. Hand washing immediately following contact with any body fluids is required even when gloves are worn. It is possible that the outside of the gloves may come into contact with portions of the hands when removing the gloves. Wash hands thoroughly and vigorously with soap and running water for a minimum of 30 seconds. Also, please note that hands should be washed BOTH before donning gloves and after removing them following completion of disinfection of work surfaces or treatment of a patient with injuries or illness of an unknown etiology.

Postinfection treatment for hepatitis B is not currently available, so prevention is of the essence. Therefore, avoiding infection through preventive measures is the best protection against this disease. Prophylaxis is the most effective manner of preventing spread of any infectious disease, along with conscientious cleaning and use of aseptic techniques in the treatment of patients. The word *prophylaxis* means "to prevent disease" from occurring. Immediately following a probable exposure to a biohazardous material or an infectious patient, hepatitis B immune globulin (HBIG), which contains antibodies against

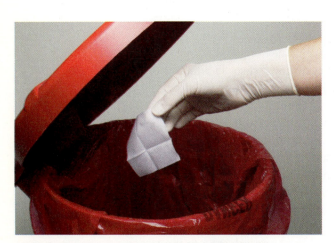

FIGURE 6-8 Engineering controls, where a biohazardous container is used for disposal of nonsharp objects. Source: Delmar/Cengage Learning.

the organism, should be available for postexposure treatment. If HBIG is to be used, it should be given as soon as possible and always within 7 days following an exposure incident. An exposure through a needle stick injury would be of the most concern and would provide the greatest potential for transmitting the organism from a patient to the health care worker. Blood splashes to the eyes or blood or other body fluids that contaminate cuts, rashes, and abrasions on the hands would also give cause for concern.

Situations where contact with blood or other potentially infectious materials occur should be carefully evaluated. The source patient should be considered for testing if available to determine if blood came from an infected patient. Remember, a source patient does not have to agree to have his or her blood collected and tested.

Prevention of hepatitis has been readily available for more than 20 years. HBV vaccine is provided by the employer in health care facilities and other agencies where a high likelihood exists for coming in contact with the virus. Although a worker may decline the immunization, it is highly recommended for persons considered to be at high risk for contracting this illness, particularly for health care workers. Immunization for HBV leaves few side effects and is the most effective and specific way to avoid contracting the illness.

Prehospital health care personnel, such as emergency treatment personnel, are considered to be in the high-risk category. These emergency responders are required to either undergo the three-dose immunization or to sign a declination form stating that the risks are known but that the worker does not wish to be immunized. HBV infections are often accompanied by hepatitis C viral infections. Although only approximately 10% of hepatitis B–infected persons become chronically infected, hepatitis C has more long-term effects. One serious long-term effect of hepatitis C is the statistical increase in liver cancer among those who were infected even decades earlier. Often, the contraction of hepatitis B and hepatitis C occurs simultaneously, along with several other lesser-known viruses known to cause hepatitis (most common are the delta and echo varieties).

TUBERCULOSIS IN THE HEALTH CARE SETTING

By virtue of working with patients who are ill, and those particularly who have some sort of compromising condition of the immune system, such as HIV infections, health care providers are at particular risk for contracting tuberculosis (TB). Therefore, education and training on a regular basis are required for persons with direct patient contact and those who handle items that may have become contaminated by patients.

Introduction to Tuberculosis

A number of airborne pathogens exist, and the medical worker or student is exposed to many organisms that may be transmitted through the respiratory tract. TB, however, is the only disease currently included in federal guidelines for airborne pathogens requiring specific training as protection against the organism. *Mycobacterium tuberculosis* is the organism that causes TB. (As a point of interest, certain parts of the world have colonies of persons infected with a similar organism that causes the disease of leprosy. That organism is called *Mycobacterium leprae*, and it has been infecting persons at least since biblical times.) TB was thought to have become almost completely eradicated in the developed and modern world, but in the past few years, large pockets of the disease have broken out, dispelling the belief that there was no longer a danger from this disease. Drug-resistant cases are being discovered almost daily, and cases of atypical TB are on the rise. Atypical TB may include diseases similar to TB but fostered by a different causative organism than *M. tuberculosis*.

Before the development of antibiotics effective against the TB organism, treatment consisted of isolation in a sanitarium. The focus of treatment was to help the patient become as healthy as possible through adequate nutrition and the provision of fresh air. Patients stayed until their sputum no longer carried the organism. This sometimes occurred when areas of the lungs became calcified and effectively walled off colonies of the TB organism. Isolation or quarantining was the only treatment available and often patients were kept in sanitariums for years before they were released to live among the uninfected population. When relapses occurred, as they almost invariably did, patients were readmitted to a sanitarium.

TB is caused by a bacillus (rod-shaped bacterium) that is more difficult to treat than many bacterial organisms. Different strains to which humans are also susceptible occur in both birds and cattle. The diagnosis is made by performing a skin test to determine if the patient has developed a reaction against this particular organism. If the skin test is positive, a chest radiograph is obtained to determine if the person is in an active stage of the disease.

Routine tuberculin skin tests to determine if an unknown exposure has occurred are required before entering a clinical facility for both students and medical workers. This is routinely done as part of the physical examination on health care students and new employees in medical facilities. OSHA regulations require testing twice per year to determine if a medical worker or student has been exposed to the *M. tuberculosis* organism. Medical facilities will not allow anyone to work in direct contact with patients unless the worker has been tested for the disease or for recent exposure. Both actual infection and recent exposure will yield positive results on the **PPD (tuberculin) skin test** (Figure 6-9). The PPD skin test is an intradermal injection that will cause a positive reaction for those who have ever been exposed to the TB organism.

Although antibiotics are effective except in the more resistant strains of *M. tuberculosis*, the administration of antibiotics for treating uncomplicated cases of TB requires daily doses of the antibiotics isoniazid and rifampin for 2 months, followed by 4 months of additional self-administration of these antibiotics. There is an 80% mortality rate for those with the multidrug–resistant strains of the organism.

Symptoms and signs of the disease include fatigue, fever, and weight loss. These signs and symptoms may occur early in the illness. During the advanced states of the disease, cough, chest pain, hemoptysis (spitting up of blood), and hoarseness may be prevalent. The disease is found worldwide but most often occurs in crowded areas of cities and in facilities where persons are housed in close proximity to each other. The disease most commonly infects the respiratory system but may become systemic in the blood and is capable of affecting any of the organs of the body. For example, the disease may also affect the gastrointestinal and genitourinary systems, as well as the bones, joints, nervous system, lymph nodes, and skin.

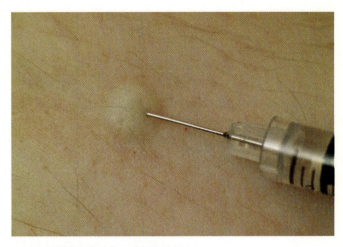

FIGURE 6-9 Administering of PPD skin test. Source: Delmar/Cengage Learning.

The main reservoir for TB is humans. Next in importance, in some instances, are cows, through their milk, and sometimes birds who live in close proximity to humans. A number of similar organisms thought to be harmless have recently been implicated in cases of pulmonary fibrosis mimicking TB that have produced lesions. Cleanliness and sanitation of public facilities, inspection of cattle by government agencies, and control of birds roosting and nesting in buildings may help alleviate some of the conditions that give rise to larger and more prevalent reservoirs for the organisms. Secluding those suffering from TB while symptoms are acute and treatment is ongoing is the most effective process for avoiding the spread of the organism.

Transmission of the disease is primarily through airborne droplets from sputum of persons with infectious TB (Figure 6-10). Repeated and close exposure to an infectious case often leads to the infection of close contacts, including family members. When a family member is diagnosed with TB, other family members should be tested and given prophylactic treatment if necessary. Often a person is infected but lives among the general population for a considerable period of time before signs and symptoms become noticeable. The organism may incubate for a period ranging from 4 to 12 weeks before the victim is alerted by symptoms to seek medical treatment; by then, a number of persons who have come in close contact with the infected individual may be at risk for contracting the disease.

A person who is infected by the TB bacterium may transmit the disease for as long as he or she is harboring the organism. This may occur when an asymptomatic patient is hospitalized for another ailment and TB is then diagnosed. As a general rule, the person is considered to be able to communicate the disease to others as long as the bacterium can be isolated from the person's sputum. Improvement of sanitary conditions and wearing of PPE are the best methods for preventing and controlling the spread of TB. Those who have come in close contact with a person who later develops symptoms of the disease require surveillance, diagnosis, and possibly early treatment.

Good work practices such as effective hand washing, provision of filtered ventilation if available, and good housekeeping practices should be maintained as provided for in the infection control manual. Organisms found in sputum may survive for days on inanimate objects, necessitating the practice of good

AIRBORNE PRECAUTIONS
In Addition to Standard Precautions

Visitors - Report to Nurses' Station Before Entering Room

BEFORE CARE	DURING CARE	AFTER CARE

BEFORE CARE

1. Private room and closed door with monitored negative air pressure, frequent air exchanges, and high-efficiency filtration.

2. Wash hands.

3. Wear respiratory protection appropriate for disease.

DURING CARE

1. Limit transport of patient/resident to essential purposes only. Patient/resident must wear mask appropriate for disease.

2. Limit use of noncritical care equipment to a single patient/resident.

AFTER CARE

1. Bag linen to prevent contamination of self, environment, or outside of bag.

2. Discard infectious trash to prevent contamination of self, environment, or outside of bag.

3. Wash hands.

FIGURE 6-10 Airborne precautions in addition to Standard Precautions.
Source: Delmar/Cengage Learning.

and regular cleaning of surfaces and objects used in patient care. The medical worker should wear a mask when a patient may cough or sneeze in the face of the medical worker or student. This practice is extremely effective in avoiding TB. All health care workers and students in the health professions are to be fit-tested and provided with **high efficiency particulate air (HEPA) filter masks** (Figure 6-11) when treating patients who are under Respiratory Precautions status as well as those having symptoms of respiratory diseases. Patients who are under Respiratory Precautions must wear a mask when being transported about the facility, as their sputum may harbor the organism for several days and infect the unprotected worker and any others who may have come in contact.

Protective Equipment

Both engineered (based on supplies and equipment available) and work practice (what the worker does, such as washing the hands) controls will be provided during training in the educational facility and during clinical practice

FIGURE 6-11 Health care provider wearing N95 respirator.
Source: Delmar/Cengage Learning.

at a clinic or hospital. It is the responsibility of the student to observe all precautions to which he or she has been introduced. The level of protective gear is based on the risk posed by the job being performed.

HEPA Mask Fit Test Kit

Workers who may be required to perform direct patient care should be fit-tested for a HEPA mask. Differing facial sizes and shapes require that a person be tested for proper fit as one size does not fit all. Facial hair such as beards, mustaches, or heavy and extensive sideburns that encroach on the face may impede a fit design that will protect the worker.

Types of Workplaces Covered by These Guidelines

Persons are more susceptible to TB when living in unsanitary conditions. Those groups confined to crowded areas with poor ventilation are at greater risk of contracting TB than are others in less-cramped and better-maintained facilities or homes. The workplaces listed in the sidebar on the next page have been identified as being likely to house inhabitants with active TB. They are considered as workplaces with an inherent potential for exposure to TB.

What Comprises Exposure Potential to Tuberculosis?

An exposure potential is defined as an exposure to the inhaled or exhaled air of a person suspected of TB disease or confirmed to be infected by a skin test and radiograph. The medical laboratory worker who is responsible for collecting blood from a patient would be at some risk if the patient coughed while in close proximity to the face of the worker. Masks are worn when a patient is under "Respiratory Precautions" or has been confirmed as being infected with the TB bacillus. Besides being coughed on by a patient with TB, the worker who handles contaminated items in the patient's room or sputum specimens without conscientious hand washing can contract the disease.

Certain procedures performed on an individual with suspected or confirmed TB disease also have an extremely high potential for producing infectious airborne organisms through respiratory secretions. Specific procedures that place the medical worker at greatest risk are those involving aerosolized medication treatments and assisting in or performing bronchoscopies, sputum inductions, intubations, suctioning procedures, and autopsies. While performing these procedures, the workers should wear PPE, including a face shield with mask if droplets and aerosols may be produced. Often after diagnosis, a hospitalized person will be in a room designed to isolate the patient from other patients and visitors. Only those who are performing direct care of specimen collections will enter the

Infection Control Alert

The CDC Requirements for Training, Education, and Use of PPE

The CDC's "Guidelines for Preventing the Transmission of Tuberculosis in Health Care Settings (with Special Focus on HIV-Related Issues)" provides for postexposure reporting and follow-up guidelines for TB exposure in a medical area where there is a potential for exposure to patients with TB. The requirements for HEPA respirator training and education and the use of PPE are addressed in this document. These guidelines are to be in effect until the Occupational Exposure to Tuberculosis; Proposed Rule 29 CFR 1910.1035 is acted on by OSHA. Changes may be required at that time.

Infection Control Alert

Workplaces with Potential for Exposure to TB

CDC's "Guidelines for Preventing the Transmission of Tuberculosis in Health Care Settings, With Special Focus on HIV-Related Issues" are expanded to cover other high-density population facilities:

1. Health care facilities, such as hospitals and clinics

2. Rehabilitation facilities for posthospitalization, etc.

3. Correctional facilities

4. Homeless shelters and battered-spouse facilities

5. Long-term health facilities such as nursing homes

6. Drug treatment centers

7. Any other facility where groups of people are congregated in close contact with each other. Travelers to parts of the world where TB is endemic often contract the disease if proper precautions are not observed.

8. Areas where large numbers of refugees and immigrants from lesser-developed countries have resulted in increases in the rate of TB, including cases caused by drug-resistant TB organisms

room, and full protective gear will be worn. Removal of wastes from the room requires special handling.

Workers Most at Risk for Occupational Exposure

One of the greatest and most unexpected risks of contracting TB occurs when both clerical and medical personnel are performing admitting procedures. When the patient has not yet been diagnosed with TB nor is even suspected of having TB, the clerical worker takes no precautions for personal protection. All medical workers or persons with both direct or indirect patient care and even those with responsibilities not directly related to medical procedures but who perform activities that merely place the person in close proximity to an infected person are considered to be at risk for contracting TB. As patients from all walks of life and with various ailments come into health care facilities, any possible contagious infection will eventually present itself.

A number of categories of health care workers, including physicians, nurses, physician's assistants, respiratory therapists, radiography technologists, laboratory workers, morgue workers, emergency medical services personnel, corrections personnel, students, and medical course instructors, are most at risk (CDC, 1993, 2005). A physical examination of students entering medical laboratory science programs is required, and the student will be tested for a previous exposure or disease conditions as a pre-exposure requirement. If the worker, student, or faculty member previously showed a positive reaction to the TB organism, determination must be made by radiograph that the person is no longer contagious and likely to transmit the organism to patients or coworkers. The person with a positive PPD skin test must have completed adequate therapy before assuming duties in a medical treatment facility and must provide appropriate documentation of having met these requirements. Some countries vaccinate their citizens with a **Bacillus Calmette-Guérin (BCG)** organism that supposedly provides protection against TB, although there is some doubt that this mode of immunization is effective. Those who have been "immunized" in some countries against TB by BCG will always show a positive result for the PPD; this is not a true positive, since the immunization itself leads to a positive result, and not contraction of the organism causing TB. It may be determined that a chest radiograph is also necessary at this time.

First-Time Positive Reaction to PPD (TB Skin Test)

A covered medical worker, faculty member, or student who shows a first-time positive reaction to the skin test must receive medical clearance by a physician before further contact with patients or coworkers. This clearance must be in writing and filed appropriately as required by the medical facility or educational institution. Personnel found to have active TB disease should also be offered HIV antibody testing, as TB frequently occurs in immunocompromised persons such as those with HIV infections or those on immunosuppressive medications. Covered faculty members and students with a documented history of a positive PPD skin test or adequate treatment of latent or active disease are not required to obtain further testing unless signs and symptoms of active TB disease develop. Often, persons in this category must be routinely screened periodically to determine if the disease has returned to an active status. Initial and follow-up tuberculin skin tests should be administered and interpreted according to current CDC guidelines. A copy of infection control manuals and/or other manuals and documents should be available to inform employees of potential risks and actions to follow when potentially exposed to a pathogen. These manuals and associated documents are available to all employees and will include protocol required for further testing or treatment when a positive PPD occurs.

Postexposure Treatment and Follow-up for Tuberculosis

Immediately after an instructor, student, or worker in an occupational area covered by guidelines is exposed to a clinically confirmed case of TB, the following procedures are to be followed. All workers, instructors, and students who have had close contact with the infected person will be advised to have a PPD skin test. A negative result must be obtained before reentering the clinical area. As described previously, the person must be medically cleared before further participation in the clinical area or attendance in the classroom. A person who is exposed to TB and who has a documented history of positive PPD skin tests and radiographic findings must obtain a current chest radiograph to assess his or her infectious status before further participation in educational or clinical activities.

Repeat testing of PPD-negative medical workers, faculty members, and students should be conducted periodically to identify persons whose skin tests convert to a positive reading. The frequency of repeat testing is risk dependent. Routinely, the schedule for persons performing high-risk procedures is every 6 months, as required by OSHA. Initial and periodic tuberculin skin tests are offered to covered faculty members at no cost to the employee. However, students are responsible for the cost of their skin tests, even after a potential exposure.

Documentation of any exposure incident should be performed within 24 hours of its occurrence if possible. A baseline determination of immune status as soon as feasible, indicating an earlier exposure or lack thereof, is of the utmost importance. Exposure to TB is determined to have occurred when any worker is exposed to a patient or client who exhibits symptoms of active disease or who tests positive for the disease. There are those who do harbor the organism and exhibit no symptoms. Some individuals who test positive for TB may have been exposed years earlier and now have colonies of the organism that are calcified and walled off in the lungs. This category of person may be a health care worker or a patient, either of whom may be unaware of the fact that he or she can be a danger to others.

Infection Control Alert

Workers Most at Risk for Exposure to Tuberculosis

- Physicians (includes pathologists)
- Nurses
- Physician's assistants
- Respiratory therapists
- Radiography technologists
- Laboratory workers (specimen and patient contact)
- Morgue workers
- EMS personnel (EMTs and paramedics)
- Corrections personnel
- Students in various health care programs
- Medical course instructors

Education and Training Required for Faculty and Students

Education and training for faculty and students are required to enable them to protect themselves in a medical environment where highly contagious patients may be treated. This education and training are to be relevant to the areas in which these persons will be working. Students may be required to purchase some supplies and equipment. Supplies and equipment will be furnished to instructors at the expense of the educational institution and will be specified in program outlines.

1. Each medical worker, instructor, and student is to receive education and training relative to TB as part of the bloodborne and airborne pathogens section of instruction, as required by law. Medical workers should receive training and education during their orientation to medical facilities as well as through annual updates. Instructors should receive annual refresher training throughout their tenure. The educational facility's infection control coordinator is responsible for monitoring and evaluating effectiveness of the education and training process, ensuring that appropriate documentation has been achieved.

2. Training should be documented as specified in the institute's exposure control plan. This plan is written to include guidelines from OSHA, the National Institute for Occupational Safety and Health (NIOSH), and the CDC, as well as any other state or federal governmental entity that has input into the process. Each student will have the appropriate documentation relative to compliance with the training needs as outlined by the institutional committees, accreditation officials, or statutory bodies.

Training and Education Elements

Training to prevent contracting TB requires that certain standards be met. This is accomplished most practically with a formal class, in which both didactic presentations and laboratory exercises are included, which emphasizes the need for information and practical application of measures designed to prevent the contraction of TB. Minimum educational requirements designed for effective training and education of the health care worker for bloodborne and airborne pathogens will include the diagnostic information shown in Table 6-3.

Table 6-3 Characteristics of Tuberculosis

Modes of transmission	The mode is the method by which a disease is passed on to another. The mode may be mechanical through equipment or person-to-person.
Pathogenesis	This term refers to where and how the development of a disease progressed from its inception.
Diagnosis and assessment of TB	Skin tests (tuberculin) should be read after 48 hours. The body reacts to the antigen (organism) causing the disease by forming a raised and discolored lump at the site of injection. This reaction indicates that the body has been exposed to and has made antibodies against the TB organism (remember that BCG may give false-positive results). Positive PPD tests require a radiograph of the chest to determine the condition of the patient.

PROTECTION AGAINST AND PREVENTION OF INFECTION BY BLOODBORNE AND AIRBORNE PATHOGENS

Medical laboratory workers and other prospective medical care providers by law must be provided with information on specific bloodborne and airborne diseases. This is necessary to enable the medical laboratory employee and the student assigned to the laboratory to make informed decisions regarding self-protection to prevent contracting disease on the job in the course of treating patients. Students and health care professionals who practice the precautions outlined in this section will face little possibility of becoming accidentally infected.

Practices and Precautions for the Medical Laboratory Worker

The two most effective means for protecting the laboratory worker as well as other professionals providing health care are personal protection and appropriate and effective immunization. Not all pathogens have effective immunizations designed for them (e.g., HIV). But HBV has been greatly minimized as a disease among health care workers due to effective immunization, now required for all health care workers unless they exercise their right to decline the procedure.

Personal Protection

- Protective Equipment: This principally entails the wearing of appropriate protective garments, masks, and respirators while providing care to patients who are known to be or are potentially infectious. The wearing of appropriate protective clothing and devices protects both the patients and the workers or students who have had contact with other contagious patients and who might transmit the infection from one patient to another.
- Work Practice Controls and Engineered Controls
  - *Work practice controls* relate to the practices of the medical care worker to minimize risk of contamination. It is related to what the worker does rather than what he or she uses in the way of devices. One example of a work practice control is washing of the hands before donning gloves and after removing the gloves following the performance of a procedure.
  - *Engineered controls* refer to controls that include manufactured items such as sharps disposal containers, self-sheathing needles, safer medical devices such as sharps with engineered sharps injury protections and needleless systems, and hand washing and eyewashing facilities. These equipment or supplies serve to isolate or remove a bloodborne pathogen hazard from the workplace.

Immunizations

An *immunization* is the most specific way of protecting oneself. There are no immunizations to date for certain infectious diseases. While great strides have been made in the past few decades to rid the world of certain epidemics, there are no vaccines against certain organisms such as HIV or the TB bacterium.

Even when immunizations are available to prevent infection by certain organisms, the medical employee must continue to practice self-protective measures. While immunization is specific against specific infectious organisms, there are numerous organisms other than the three major bloodborne and airborne pathogens. The bacterial strain that causes *tetanus* has a long history of effective immunization and immunization shortly after exposure can provide immunity against this potentially fatal disease. This is one of only a few bacterial organisms for which an immunization that lasts for a substantial period of time is available. Generally, immunization against viruses is much more effective than that for bacteria, often giving virtually lifetime immunity unless the strain mutates sufficiently to become an organism no longer recognized by the antibodies previously produced.

Minimizing Exposure to Infectious Organisms

To eliminate or at least minimize incidents where a medical worker is exposed to infectious patients or materials that may be contaminated by infectious organisms, certain precautions are provided. Training of medical workers and students should be geared toward following procedures designed to protect the medial laboratory worker as well as other health care providers. Exposure incidents are usually the result of a failure to follow proper procedures while performing medical procedures, exposure to a patient who is newly admitted and who may have no symptoms, or exposure to materials contaminated while performing a medical procedure.

Universal Precautions and Standard Precautions

Is there a difference between Universal Precautions and Standard Precautions? Sometimes these terms are used synonymously but they are really focused on protecting different groups. Standard Precautions were designed primarily to protect the patient from becoming infected while in the medical facility. Universal Precautions are aimed at protecting the health care worker who is handling blood and bloody materials. Protective practices for each type of medical procedure require precautions to protect oneself and were issued in 1996 by the CDC (Figure 6-12).

Standard Precautions

These guidelines were recommended by the CDC to reduce the risk of the spread of infection in the health care facility. These precautions include hand washing and the use of gloves, masks, eye protection, and gowns, and they apply to blood, all body fluids, secretions, excretions (except sweat), nonintact skin, and mucous membranes of all patients. They are the primary strategy for successful prevention of nosocomial infections. Nosocomial infections are those that the patient did not contract outside the hospital but were acquired during a visit or

STANDARD PRECAUTIONS

FOR INFECTION CONTROL

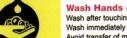

Wash Hands (Plain soap)
Wash after touching **blood**, **body fluids**, **secretions**, **excretions**, and **contaminated items**.
Wash immediately **after gloves are removed** and **between patient contacts**.
Avoid transfer of microorganisms to other patients or environments.

Wear Gloves
Wear when touching **blood**, **body fluids**, **secretions**, **excretions**, and **contaminated items**.
Put on **clean** gloves just **before touching mucous membranes** and **nonintact skin**.
Change gloves between tasks and procedures on the same patient after contact with material that may contain high concentrations of microorganisms. Remove gloves promptly after use, before touching noncontaminated items and environmental surfaces, and before going to another patient, and wash hands immediately to avoid transfer of microorganisms to other patients or environments.

Wear Mask and Eye Protection or Face Shield
Protect mucous membranes of the eyes, nose, and mouth during procedures and patient–care activities that are likely to generate **splashes** or **sprays** of **blood**, **body fluids**, **secretions**, or **excretions**.

Wear Gown
Protect skin and prevent soiling of clothing during procedures that are likely to generate **splashes** or **sprays** of **blood**, **body fluids**, **secretions**, or **excretions**. Remove a soiled gown as promptly as possible and wash hands to avoid transfer of microorganisms to other patients or environments.

Patient-Care Equipment
Handle used patient–care equipment soiled with **blood**, **body fluids**, **secretions**, or **excretions** in a manner that prevents skin and mucous membrane exposures, contamination of clothing, and transfer of microorganisms to other patients and environments. Ensure that reusable equipment is not used for the care of another patient until it has been appropriately cleaned and reprocessed and single use items are discarded.

Environmental Control
Follow hospital procedures for routine care, cleaning, and disinfection of environmental surfaces, beds, bedrails, bedside equipment and other frequently touched surfaces.

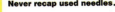

Linen
Handle, transport, and process used linen soiled with **blood**, **body fluids**, **secretions**, or **excretions** in a manner that prevents exposures and contamination of clothing, and avoids transfer of microorganisms to other patients and environments.

Occupational Health and Bloodborne Pathogens
Prevent injuries when using needles, scalpels, and other sharp instruments or devices; when handling sharp instruments after procedures; when cleaning used instruments; and when disposing of used needles.

Never recap used needles.

Do not remove used needles from disposable syringes by hand, and do not bend, break, or otherwise manipulate used needles by hand. Place used disposable syringes and needles, scalpel blades, and other sharp items in puncture–resistant sharps containers located as close as practical to the area in which the items were used, and place reusable syringes and needles in a puncture–resistant container for transport to the reprocessing area.

Use **resuscitation devices** as an alternative to mouth–to–mouth resuscitation.

Patient Placement
Use a **private room** for a patient who contaminates the environment or who does not (or cannot be expected to) assist in maintaining appropriate hygiene or environmental control. Consult Infection Control if a private room is not available.

The information on this sign is abbreviated from the HICPAC Recommendations for Isolation Precautions in Hospitals.

Form No. **SPR** BREVIS CORP., 3310 S 2700 E, SLC, UT 84109 © 1996 Brevis Corp.

FIGURE 6-12 Guide to Standard Precautions for infection control.
Source: Delmar/Cengage Learning.

a stay in the hospital. Essentially, Standard Precautions is a term that refers to those procedures that prevent the spread of organisms to the patient, and in so doing serves to protect both the worker and the patient.

Universal Precautions

Guidelines established for protecting workers with occupational exposure to bloodborne pathogens are called Universal Precautions. These "universal blood and body fluid precautions" require the use of gloves, masks, and gowns, as recommended by the CDC in 1985. They were mandated by the OSHA Bloodborne Pathogens Standard in 1991 for workers in all U.S. health care settings.

Preexposure Precautions

Work practice controls and engineered controls are important methods by which to combat infection of workers and cross-contamination of other patients in multiple patient cases.

Personal Protective Equipment and Work Practice Controls

The first line of defense includes proper washing of the hands routinely before donning and after removing gloves following a procedure. Disposable gloves are used for medical tasks, and strong, reusable gloves that require cleaning between tasks are used for cleaning purposes. When airborne precautions are necessary, disposable surgical face masks are used one time and then discarded. When a mask becomes wet, it is removed as it is no longer effective as a preventive measure. Goggles or face shields are required when splashing of blood and body fluids is likely in tasks such as cauterizing, suctioning, and creating aerosols of any type. Special clothing, including impermeable aprons, is worn to prevent saturation or contamination of clothing by either chemicals or biohazardous materials.

Immunization and Vaccination

Immunization and vaccination are extremely effective to protect against certain pathogenic organisms or to determine if exposure has occurred. Unimmunized persons will react to immunization or to actual exposure in the same way, with antibodies formed in both categories of persons. The PPD skin test determines if exposure to the organism has occurred and if antibodies have been formed. However, this test does not prevent TB but merely demonstrates exposure to TB. If a chest radiograph is used to diagnose active TB, antibiotics may cure the disease in its early stages.

HBV vaccine is now required of all who work directly with patients and their body fluids, unless the worker elects to sign a declination form indicating that he or she understands the risks and does not wish to be vaccinated. Immunity is long term, but occasionally booster vaccines are administered to increase one's level of protection. MMR immunization is required of everyone, but those entering health care professions are required to show proof of immunization. This vaccination gives immunity for varying periods against the childhood diseases mumps, measles, and rubella. Programs for immunizing the majority of the population have made these diseases somewhat rare in the United States. Tetanus toxoid vaccinations give up to 10 years of immunity and are usually administered routinely every 8 to 10 years, and again if a traumatic injury occurs.

Multiple Patient Situations

"Multiple patient situations" is a term used to indicate the responsibility of the health care industry to protect patients from exposure and transmission of disease when using instruments and supplies that have been used for treating other patients. Immunosuppressed patients are those whose immunity is compromised by other conditions. This may be related to age, as both the very young and the very old have less immunity against biohazards than other age groups. Some disease conditions also weaken the immune system, resulting in a higher rate of infection among individuals with a particular condition. Some medications are also responsible for causing changes in elements of the immune system, putting the person at greater risk than those not under treatment.

Exposure-Prevention Education

Guidelines for preventing exposure to infectious patients, supplies, and body fluids are usually provided by the Infection Control Committee and Exposure Control Committee. Guidelines should be in place for workers to follow, dictating measures to prevent possible exposure to infectious diseases for the following situations when functioning as a medical laboratory worker.

- During classroom lectures and lab practice in educational facilities, there is some minimal risk for an exposure to a potentially infectious material. Using appropriate supplies and equipment is the first step toward avoiding illness related to exposure as engineered controls. Clinical applications such as those found in hospital laboratories would be appropriate for the practice of procedures in the classroom labs. Lecture and then rehearsing pertinent case studies and relating the appropriate activities and responses would be effective.
- During clinical rotations, most of which would occur in a hospital laboratory for a medical laboratory technician or technologist, monitoring would be required for safety consciousness while working with preceptors. These preceptors or clinical instructors should constantly alert the student as to the risks of contracting bloodborne and airborne pathogens during clinical practice.

Postexposure Considerations

Even if the worker has been immunized, there are certain procedures to follow after determining that a potentially infectious incident has occurred. Answering the question of whether an incident has occurred is primary. A situation in which a worker has been spattered with blood or OPIM that might have entered mucous membranes such as the eyes, mouth, and nose would constitute an exposure. A worker with chapped or abraded skin and torn nail cuticles whose hands become contaminated with blood would be deemed an exposure. Needle sticks from used needles and cuts by glass with blood or other body fluids on the glass would also constitute a definite exposure. A worker who performed procedures on or even interviewed a patient who was later found to have active TB would be classified as having experienced an exposure.

Postexposure considerations should be attended to as quickly as possible. A medical laboratory student or worker should first contact his or her clinical preceptor or supervisor. In the classroom, the student would inform the instructor of a possible exposure. Steps to be taken are contained in policies in either the medical facility or in the educational facility manuals. In most facilities, the worker or student is interviewed by a medical professional and often by a representative from the Infection Control Committee. An airborne pathogen exposure would require, at a minimum, a PPD skin test. Another test would be performed at a later date, and if either test is positive, a chest radiograph would follow and appropriate antibiotic therapy would be initiated for an active case. Students and workers who are found to have contracted TB are assigned other duties until the case is resolved and a physician clears the person for return to previous duties.

In the case of a blood exposure, the results of the source patient's testing are considered, if available. The source patient cannot normally be required to undergo testing except in states where nonvoluntary testing is mandatory following an exposure incident. The worker or student will have the medical records on file from prior physical examinations, if such tests were performed. These results are then compared with repeat testing. A worker who was previously negative for HIV or HBV infection and who later shows a positive result will have most likely been exposed and at the time of exposure have contracted the disease. Laboratory tests may be performed if in the opinion of the medical professional there was a possibility of exposure to a disease. Records of these interviews, laboratory tests, skin tests, and medical examinations are kept in a confidential file, usually for 30 years following the end of the worker's or student's affiliation with the facility.

GUIDELINES FOR INFECTIOUS EXPOSURE

Guidelines should be in place to follow for precautions for possible exposure to infectious diseases in any situation that a medical worker or student may experience. There is a potential for exposure when a student or worker comes in contact with infectious patients, wastes, and body fluids. Specimens from hospital patients are often used in classroom and college laboratory practice sessions. Instructors should monitor a student's work, ensuring the use of proper protective equipment and safe practices. Clinical rotations for medical laboratory students afford the most potential for exposure. Students should be taught at the beginning of education and training to practice safety, report exposure incidents, and receive treatment for affected patients and workers.

Disposal and Decontamination

Decontamination of work areas, nondisposable equipment, and supplies should be practiced on a daily basis. Students should be taught to properly and effectively decontaminate work areas daily, as well as how to properly dispose of biohazardous wastes and chemical hazards according to policies. Disposal of these items must also be performed in a manner to protect sanitation workers and other employees. Disposable equipment should be cleaned before disposal, and contaminated waste materials should be properly stored and identified by marking them before disposal. Needles and other sharps that may have come in contact with blood are disposed of in rigid sharps containers. Needles should never be recapped, bent, or broken before disposal as these activities often result in an accidental needle stick or a cut from sharp objects, including glass. The clipping or breaking of needles may also create aerosols or splatter, creating an additional reason to not mechanically destroy needles. Even bed linen is handled while wearing gloves and is transported in a linen cart that is closed and has a protective cover that is impermeable to liquids.

SUMMARY

Diseases that are caused by various organisms and that are transmitted from person to person and from inanimate object to a person have been the scourge of humanity throughout humans' inhabitation of the earth. More people have died of infection than by any other illness or injury, even including the millions killed in wars. Organisms such as HBV and HIV (as well as hepatitis C virus) are mainly transmitted through blood and other body fluids. TB, which is the chief disease transmitted through airborne means, is of vital and growing importance. All of these disease organisms are virulent and are sufficiently contagious that they have specific government regulations requiring training, the offering of immunization where possible, and preventive practices designed to minimize the occurrences of infection by these organisms. Of no less importance is the possibility of contracting other types of disabling conditions through exposure to chemicals. Such exposure may have severe health consequences.

A significant number of people working in scientific fields have contributed to advances in protecting the entire populace from being unwittingly exposed to dangerous pathogens and chemicals. Agencies of the federal government and some state agencies have been organized to determine causes of disease outbreaks and to provide research into the prevention of these diseases. Visitors from foreign countries where immunization is not routinely performed may require immunization for a number of diseases before they enter the country.

Local health departments are found in every state, and a chief focus is to immunize or to facilitate the immunization of the entire population against diseases that have a vaccine available. We now have immunization against HBV and hepatitis A virus, but as of yet no effective vaccine exists for the AIDS virus (HIV). Work practices and engineered practices are required to prevent the contraction of a number of diseases and to protect health care workers, patients, and visitors. The morbidity and mortality from infectious diseases and exposures can be minimized through conscientious work practices and research.

REVIEW QUESTIONS

1. What is the purpose of the Infection Control Committee and the Exposure Control Committee?
2. What organisms are called "covered organisms" by the federal government and why are they considered most important?
3. How are biohazardous wastes disposed of in a health care facility?
4. What should occur if a laboratory worker suffers an exposure to biohazardous materials?
5. Who is responsible for treatment of an exposed worker?

CHAPTER 7

MEDICAL ECONOMICS AND LABORATORY EQUIPMENT

LEARNING OBJECTIVES

Upon completion of this chapter, the reader will be able to:

- Describe the hierarchy of administration of a modern health care institution.
- Identify the medical consumer and how he or she pays for medical care.
- List some lifestyle factors that contribute to poor health.
- Explain how a wholesome lifestyle might help alleviate the nation's health care crisis.
- Discuss the reason for and the importance of reference laboratories.
- List the key factors in producing test results in the laboratory.

- List the measures taken by laboratories and entire health care units for controlling costs.
- Describe point-of-care testing (POCT).
- List the major departments within the medical laboratory and their basic functions.
- List the equipment and basic instrumentation of a hospital laboratory.
- Describe the reasons that a hospital laboratory would refer a procedure to a reference laboratory.
- List the importance of cost-effectiveness and the

sending of samples to a reference laboratory.
- Compare and contrast the factors involved in evaluating whether laboratory procedures should be performed on an automated system versus using a manual procedure.
- Describe situations when automation would be advantageous.
- Relate the importance for laboratory workers of understanding the manual methodology of routine procedures.
- Discuss factors that would be important in choosing automated systems.

KEY TERMS

Anticoagulated specimens
Assignment of health care benefits
Autoanalyzers
Biological safety cabinet
Breakeven point
Centrifuges
Cost centers
Financial management

Fume hood
Health care providers
Health care savings accounts (HSA)
Immunohematology
Lease-purchase
Lifestyle costs
Medicare and Medicaid
Point-of-care testing (POCT)

Preferred provider option (PPO)
Preceptor
Proficiency testing programs
Reference laboratories
Reimbursement
Rotor
Screening tests
Spectrophotometer

INTRODUCTION

Historically, most hospital administrators were physicians. Although physicians were singularly suited to treating the ills of the public and to dealing with other physicians, they were most often poorly equipped to handle the complex finances of the modern health care facility. As the financial complexities burgeoned, it was obvious that a more businesslike approach to handling and controlling cash flow was needed. Business office managers and resident accountant positions were created for compiling the intricacies of costs and income. It should be noted that medical centers and hospitals are theoretically nonprofit but must maintain a cash reservoir for handling unexpected expenses of updating, facility repairs, loss of cash flow for various reasons, and, in some cases, expansion. Many hospitals have evolved from a general or community hospital to a "medical center" or a "health care system," increasing the size and complexity of the organization and the structure of the management team. The sometimes far-flung specialty clinics and full-size hospitals of health care systems create a need for using an established business model, similar to that of large industries, for maintaining fiscal soundness.

Complex systems such as those found in the health care industry are growing. Budgets have expanded, as services rendered to patients are increasing in number and the advanced technology used for these services are more expensive. The medical industry is an ever-evolving industry, with funds for services generated from a variety of sources, including government agencies, private insurance, and, in increasingly rare cases, through direct payment from the consumer. **Assignment of health care benefits** from insurance companies has helped to fund increasing levels of medical care, particularly during the past few decades.

Another concept, that of **cost centers**, has arisen in health care facilities in the past few decades. The term is somewhat of a misnomer, as these centers or departments often generate revenue in some cases, although others lose money. The clinical laboratory and the pharmacy typically generate a great deal of revenue, while costs for patient rooms and operation of the emergency department traditionally exceed revenue generated for these areas. To cover certain operating costs, most often the laboratory is assigned a portion of the overhead or perhaps other types of operational costs, paying with revenues generated, to help in balancing the budget for the entire health care institution. The mechanism for this type of system is complex, but in simple terms is essentially as presented here.

In the last half of the 20th century, most hospitals were increasingly headed by a business type of officer or "administrator." This official worked directly with the medical board through the chief of staff and with the various department heads. Administrators are now called CEOs (chief executive officers), just as they are identified in large businesses, a category in which medical centers now belong. Most often these CEOs have no background in medicine as any sort of medical practitioner, as was the case in the past. Departments in larger facilities are now typically handled by assistant administrators, who report directly to the CEO. Thus, most large hospitals and certainly the large health systems or corporate hospital systems have a distinct division between the business aspects of operation and the actual provision of care to the patients.

Medical departments where patient care is rendered are usually managed by specialists from various departments in the health care facilities.

Medical care consumes a large portion of our national gross domestic product (GDP) annually. The medical industry is now larger than the federal Department of Defense. The costs of medical care have risen from a modest 5% of the GDP in 1960, to 14% in 1998, and to an estimated 16% currently! Blame has been laid at the doorstep of many offices within the medical care system. It has been popular for many years to blame the physician for the rise in health care costs. But the rise in health care costs cannot be blamed on any individual or group of individuals, but possibly on the mismanagement of resources and the lack of a prudent use of available technology. Perhaps George Bernard Shaw, Irish dramatist, literary critic, and socialist spokesman, was attempting to focus on preventive medicine in a backhanded manner, when he defended physicians as follows:

> It is not the fault of our doctors that the medical service of the community, as presently provided for, is murderously absurd ... to give a surgeon a pecuniary interest in cutting off your leg, is enough to make one despair of political humanity ... and the more appalling the mutilation, the more the mutilator is paid. He who corrects the ingrown toe-nail receives a few shillings; he who cuts your inside out receives hundreds of guineas, except when he does it to a poor person for practice.
>
> George Bernard Shaw (1856–1950)

The Medical Consumer

In the beginning, the services of physicians were mostly directed toward the more affluent in communities. Those with less money and influence relied on folk remedies and subjective diagnoses by members of the community who often had self-appointed curative abilities. Most of the ill had to get well on their own without the benefit of the medical profession, or to suffer the alternative fate of death. Delivering babies was left to the skills of either midwives or female relatives who had the practical experience of having their own babies and then assisting with others. "Native healers" such as Native American medicine men or priests provided some medical care, and religious orders sometimes built hospitals as part of their mission to their parishioners and the poor. Surgery was sometimes performed by barbers and most anyone could set a broken bone, no doubt leading to a great number of bone deformities.

Medicine gradually and all-too-slowly evolved into what it is today. But still, many common ailments such as the common cold and other viral infections have resulted in few advances in the arsenal of the physician for effective treatment. However, medical care for a variety of conditions has greatly improved, and some advanced procedures fall just short of the miraculous. Treatments of illnesses associated with aging and techniques to deal with injury and infectious diseases have advanced so much that the physician of the past bears little resemblance to the physician of the present. Today, medical care is considered by most to be a right of everyone, and if a patient has no money or insurance, care is often provided at the expense of those who do pay for their services, through increased costs for service. Some insurance, funded by taxpayers through federal government programs such as Medicare and Medicaid, pays reimbursement to hospitals and physicians at a somewhat lower rate than the actual costs of providing the service.

Health Care Providers and Insurance

Early in the history of the United States, the physician was paid directly by the patient. Often the amount charged was related to the financial status of the patient. A rich person was charged much more for a physician's service than a poor one. The country doctor often accepted his payment in produce, eggs, or chickens, and sometimes labor. Where teaching hospitals were found in the major cities, indigent patients were treated free of charge to provide experience and training for medical students and their comparably well-paid professors of medicine. Medical school professors were on salary but typically had time to treat private patients for pay to supplement their salaries, a practice that is still common today in a number of medical schools.

As our nation became more industrialized, moving from a largely agrarian economy to an urban one, reimbursement for medical services began to change. Particularly at the end of World War II, changes occurred precipitously as many then had the means with which to pay for medical care, because many families were becoming more prosperous in a postwar economy. This gave rise to group insurance plans that gave an economical manner in which to pay for medical services. The familiar Blue Cross-Blue Shield system of medical insurance was initiated at this time and was often called "the doctor's plan" because it was originally organized by and for physicians. A large insurance program, the Kaiser-Permanente Medical Care Program, was put in place in 1945 by industrialist Henry J. Kaiser. It was probably the first nonprofit HMO (health maintenance organization). It provided first-rate medical care at a lower cost than the fee-for-service Blue Cross. Physicians were salaried and worked an 8-hour day if they decided to accept employment by this organization, which was desirable for many who had previously worked long hours in private practice. Although physicians were not as well compensated as those in private practice, a normal and regular family life often overrode the reduced compensation. It also became obvious that Kaiser's physicians, who were salaried, tended to order fewer unnecessary procedures and less surgery than did those who were paid for these procedures. In other words, the profit motive has a profound effect on how medicine is practiced. Although HMOs are still prevalent in some regions, they have been significantly replaced by PPOs and other plans. The executives of many insurance plans are often paid handsomely, in most cases, rivaling industrial standards for CEOs and administrative assistants.

The Medicare system, a government-run entity, was begun in 1965, and provided medical insurance for people 65 years of age and older. Medicaid was also passed at that time. An unintended result of these programs to provide adequate care to many resulted in skyrocketing numbers of persons seeking health care. HMO facilities were designed specifically to control costs but were no more successful in doing so than were Medicare and Medicaid insurance. Certain services have diminished over the years, such as the old familiar house calls, which will most likely never return.

In summary, health care insurance and plans designed to provide optimum medical care for the majority of the population have fallen short of providing this care on a more economical basis.

Direct and Indirect Pay

When the consumer pays for his or her own care, it is called *direct pay*, and includes the required co-pay at the time of service. When the insurance company pays for the medical care by collecting insurance premiums, it is called *indirect* pay. In the opinion of many citizens, there should be a balancing between insurance and direct responsibility by shifting the cost burden to the consumer of medical care. Consumers of health care may have a choice in the type of insurance they choose. Lower premiums are available if the consumer chooses to pay a high-deductible amount of the first few thousand dollars for care. This forces the consumer into a direct pay mode, until a certain level is reached, at which time the insurance plan begins to pay for at least a portion of the services. Others may choose health care insurance that covers the majority of the costs, from the beginning, with a low or no deductible provision. This type of insurance often requires the paying of higher premiums for the luxury of having coverage immediately. The plan where direct pay is required for the first few thousand dollars of care tends to encourage the consumer to avoid medical visits except when absolutely necessary.

Another option lies in the funding of a universal type of health care that is paid at least in part by the taxpayers. Some political activists seek to require taxes to pay for the care of everyone. There is a possibility that medical care would then be rationed and limited to all except those who can afford to pay their entire medical costs.

A system along a business model in which everyone contributes and which allocates costs, risks, and contributions in an equitable manner would be the optimum solution. Lifestyle choices usually are often responsible for either health or lack of health, and in the minds of some, those who practice risky behavior and lifestyles should be required to pay more for their care.

Insurance and Reimbursement

No current insurance plan for health care reimburses the consumer or pays for the entire cost of medical procedures, and laboratory services are no exception. Most often, the consumer is asked to pay a co-pay of a set amount for any service provided, including charges for prescription drugs. There is also a hefty deductible in most insurance plans that must be met before any payments are made by the insurance provider. Some HMO plans allow a certain number of visits per year, and a certain level of services without a co-pay, to discourage overuse of the services. There are also lifetime limits imposed by most insurance plans, and when these funds are exhausted, the insurance will no longer cover the consumer. In some cases, the limit is $1 million per lifetime; some companies have recently raised this amount to $2 million. This sounds as though it would be sufficient, but some major surgeries with the attendant expenses may cost in excess of $500,000 for one hospital stay! Some states have laws regarding catastrophic coverage and will subsidize treatment for some chronic illnesses. For those using Medicare and Medicaid, there is also a requirement to pay at least some fees out of the patients' pockets.

Acceptance of Assignment

Some insurance companies have made contractual arrangements with certain providers, including physicians, hospitals, and clinics. These arrangements provide for a certain level of care at no additional cost to the consumer. Hospitals and some physicians will accept assignment for patients covered by Medicare. Those who have both Medicare and Medicaid are not usually liable for any of the charges for medical services. In the case of a system called preferred provider option (PPO), the health care provider often accepts assignment when the institution provides medical care to all employees of a certain company at a contractual cost. This plan shows that competition could work to the advantage of the consumer, but this system must be carefully monitored to ensure that all patients receive appropriate care.

Attempts to Aid the Consumer

Better-informed and educated consumers would lead to better health and better provision of medical care throughout the world. Through use of the Internet, and given the availability of information regarding laboratory testing and medical procedures, many patients are able to determine the course they wish to follow as to diagnosis and treatment. However, this can cause problems where patients question physicians regarding a medical condition if the patient is only partially aware of the impact of a disease and the reasons for embarking on a particular course of treatment. A new company, Carol.com, is one of the beginning efforts to aid the patient in gauging the cost of treatment in an online medical marketplace. It is probable that this is just the beginning of efforts to inform consumers and to answer their questions about their health. Such availability of information is timely in that it is said that the health care system is "broken" in this country and that the nation's health care crisis shows both acute and chronic problems that must be addressed personally and politically.

Will putting more choices in the consumers' hands drive down spiraling health care costs? A valid fear is that the vast array of choices may be too complex for the average person to make informed selections. In some companies, the previously expected health care insurance as part of the employee benefits package is rapidly disappearing. It has been replaced by health care savings accounts, sanctioned by the government, that include a tax benefit. In addition to health care changes, pensions have been replaced by 401(k) investment plans in place of a retirement plan managed by the company. As an advantage, employees are now able to change jobs and take their retirement accounts and their health care accounts with them if allowed.

Some employers, such as General Motors, have given the health care insurance responsibilities to the union representatives, due to the large expenses of providing insurance for both current and retired workers. So after a struggle of many years where the employer shouldered at least a portion of the medical costs, many employers are pushing for a 401(k)-style setup for health care. Over the past several decades, the costs of medical care have increased at a greater rate than inflation. In a 401(k)-style health care package, the employers may contribute money to a plan, but employees are responsible for spending their money wisely by investing in healthy behavior. These health care savings accounts may be cumulative and often have an incentive for the employee and his family to spend wisely, as the amount that can be spent can easily be exhausted by frivolous visits to the physician for such minor ailments as colds that can be treated at home in a palliative manner.

A consumer-driven attempt in controlling medical expenses to the customer is the demand for information on prices, services, procedures, physicians, and hospitals. Hospitals and clinics may pursue groups of patients with certain ailments by bundling related tests, services, and procedures for a set price, with consumers and not insurers in mind. This would allow a comparison of what is being offered at a number of health care facilities, particularly in larger cities where choices may be possible as a competitive advantage, perhaps lowering prices.

Previously, insurance companies contracted for negotiated prices for groups of employees, but many believe that the emphasis should be placed on the consumer, and proponents of this effort say that open competition will drive down costs and raise quality. The Center for Studying Health System Change in Washington, DC, stresses the continuation of placing the focus on individual responsibility and open competition for both the improvement of health care access and holding down costs. Current attempts by elected officials to provide government-subsidized health insurance runs counter to the capitalistic method of competition as a means of controlling prices and quality of health care. Heated and emotional debates are growing increasingly vitriolic in 2010 among taxpayers who may be responsible for substantially increased costs and political figures who believe that one of the federal government's responsibilities is to provide health care for all. It is a certainty that some changes to the current system of reimbursement for provision of medical care will be the result.

FACTORS AFFECTING THE COST OF MEDICAL SERVICES

Lifestyle Costs—Should They Be Passed on to the Consumer?

An area that is getting greater scrutiny relates to whether the increased lifestyle costs of those with risky lifestyles should be passed on to all of those who are insured. A great deal of information is now available that shows unequivocally that certain lifestyles contribute to conditions that require greater levels of health care than do more prudent lifestyles, especially in the latter decades of life. A prudent lifestyle is one in which risk factors that can be avoided are, and those that cannot be changed are dealt with by proper diet, rest, and reduction of stress, to name a few. Obesity and smoking are the root cause of many illnesses that could be prevented by changing the diet and by exercising. Is it fair for those who abuse their bodies to cause insurance premiums to increase by double-digits percentagewise on an annual basis? Many taxpayers and health care consumers emphatically voice a "No!" response to this question.

Some companies are hiring only nonsmokers in return for lower health insurance premiums that are offered by companies who have a pool of employees who practice a health-conscious lifestyle. It is legal for companies to hire only nonsmokers and refuse to pay for medical treatment for smoking-related illnesses, or to fire workers who have signed a pledge that they do not smoke but then begin smoking.

Given the rapidly rising health costs for which employers share at least part of the burden of coverage, it is probable that more companies will place restrictions on those who work for them. Most causes of type 2 diabetes can be actually reversed or cured by weight loss. Hypertension may be caused by smoking and, along with obesity, contributes greatly to heart disease and to an increased risk of cancer. Some employers are supplying workout areas in their companies as well as restricting vending machines to low-fat foods that have little or no processed sugars or white flour in them, both of which are culpable in weight gains leading to obesity. Some insurers now charge a surcharge for employees who smoke and for those who refuse to adopt a healthier lifestyle. So far there has been no legal decision that would prevent such practices by the insurance companies and employers.

Laboratory-Specific Economics

In a similar manner to that of the **health care providers** who have either chosen or have been pressured to be cost conscious, the laboratory has been pushed to control costs. Many insurance companies, as well as Medicare and Medicaid, reimburse for laboratory services at a much lower rate than the costs associated with performing the tests. As in the hospital, low levels of reimbursement lead to higher costs for other tests to make up the difference. Contractual arrangements are also made by laboratories to garner a large amount of procedures that can be performed in bulk at a much lower cost than if only lower volumes of individual tests are ordered. This is the idea behind "panels" of tests, which began in the 1960s. Panels for high levels of fats in the blood, kidney disease, heart disease, anemia, endocrine problems, and many others were developed to cover a wide array of tests that led to a quick and definitive diagnosis of specific ailments in most cases. These panels are much cheaper than running each test individually. They provide multiple test results where one test may confirm the results of another or may indicate that additional tests may be necessary for confirming a diagnosis.

The basic role of the laboratory is to provide diagnostic test results to aid in the evaluation of patients for both diagnosis and prognosis. But to hospital administrators (CEOs and assistants), the laboratory may also be viewed as a "cost center" along with radiography, pharmaceutical services, respiratory therapy, and certain other departments—providing critical sources of funding for the entire hospital. Laboratory revenues may be used to cover the costs of operation of the laboratory, such as overhead, employees and benefits, costs of equipment and supplies, and licensure and accreditation fees. In addition, the laboratory, along with the aforementioned departments, may also be assigned a portion of the cost of the overall operation of the hospital, to cover the areas where costs exceed revenue.

An example of a department that requires funds other than the amounts it generates is the emergency department, where many patients are uninsured and unable to pay for their care. Room rate income for hospitalized patients, although it appears exorbitant, does not cover the costs associated with staffing the floors and providing for supplies and equipment on a 24-hour basis, 7 days per week. Service areas such as custodial and maintenance workers, dietary personnel, grounds workers, and clerical personnel do not generate revenue, so they must also be compensated from revenue generated by cost centers that provide services for which charges are incurred.

Included in laboratory revenue are the decentralized laboratories found in some larger facilities. Satellite laboratories that perform testing with quick turnaround in areas where the demand is high for certain tests are economically operated for a limited number of tests that are essential in the area in which they are located. These laboratories do not require large quantities of specialized equipment except for the limited tests they offer, so efficiency and economy are possible. For instance, there is sometimes a "stat" laboratory located in the emergency department. This laboratory would typically be able to perform only tests routinely needed in the emergency department, such as complete blood counts, urinalyses, blood glucose, drug screening, electrolytes, and a number of quick screens for infectious diseases. More time-consuming tests and those requiring large and sophisticated equipment would still be performed in the main laboratory, by collecting the blood or other samples from the patient and transporting them to the larger laboratory.

Reference Laboratories

Early laboratories performed almost 100% of the laboratory procedures requested "in house" by a single hospital laboratory. However, low volumes of certain tests made it economically unfeasible for these tests to be performed "in house," because quality control measures, personnel, and expensive equipment for only a few tests per week or month required that the test bear a high cost for performance. Of course, the insurance companies would not reimburse one laboratory for an expensive procedure that another laboratory would be able to perform for a fraction of the cost. This led to the birth and somewhat explosive growth of reference laboratories.

The availability of rapid transport of laboratory samples, sometimes via air to a distant laboratory, and the ability to transmit results instantaneously have resulted in decisions by hospital laboratories and physician's office laboratories to use reference laboratories more freely. These reference laboratories are also able to justify the cost of extremely expensive and sophisticated equipment as they receive large numbers of samples from the entire country, which are shipped to them via air if necessary. Reference laboratories have formed mergers over the years, and hundreds of small, independent reference laboratories were bought by the large corporate giants. Some of these reference laboratories even have contractual arrangements with each other whereby they share the costs of expensive tests that have a low volume of use. This enables them to avoid duplicating the purchase of expensive equipment and supplies where specialized tests for rare conditions are seldom requested. In this way, they can gain even more of a competitive edge by performing thousands of sophisticated tests at greatly reduced costs. Performing large numbers of laboratory tests is much more efficient and cost-effective than running small numbers of seldom-performed tests. An added advantage lies in the fact that the ranges for quality control results will become "tighter" by compiling statistics from larger numbers of analyses (see Chapter 10, Quality Assurance).

Physicians' office use of reference laboratories is prevalent, as a number of tests collected are not performed in the physicians' office laboratories (POLs) because of Clinical Laboratory Improvement Amendment (CLIA) regulations. POLs are allowed to perform more than a relatively small number of "waived" tests that require little or no training of the person performing the tests. However, some of these offices take advantage of the system and collect the blood or other samples for even simple tests, which they send to reference laboratories for testing at low prices. They may then charge the patient a substantially higher price for the test, justifying this practice as the cost of collecting the sample and handling the results. Some offices may make tens of thousands of dollars per year by merely collecting the samples and having them picked up by a courier, while the reference laboratory most often provides even the phlebotomy equipment and supplies for collecting the samples. This is an area that is getting increased scrutiny by insurance companies as well as government insurance programs such as Medicare and Medicaid, as they are billed for the tests at a much higher rate than was charged to the POL by the reference laboratory.

Mechanization of the Laboratory

Laboratory testing is becoming increasingly more sophisticated. The number of tests that may be performed has increased and the newer procedures are in the realm of nanotechnology and molecular biology. Genetic testing should be commonplace in the clinical laboratory only a few short years in the future, if research that is published in professional journals almost daily is to be believed. Many of these tests do not have a manual procedure that can be performed without the use of expensive and technologically advanced equipment.

While many of these new-generation tests will be performed in reference laboratories, the more common ones will no doubt be performed in most medium-size to large laboratories, where the volume of tests will justify the practice. But routine tests and panels of tests that are performed on virtually all patients on admission or during their stay in the hospital will still comprise the bulk of the procedures performed in a routine laboratory. Tests that are performed on a daily basis and in large numbers are normally performed on expensive machines that have a through-put (number of tests per time unit) of hundreds or even thousands of individual tests per hour.

Space-age technology of the past few decades has led to machines that are computer driven, increasingly smaller, and more efficient. This technology has revolutionized the clinical laboratory. It would appear that fewer technicians and technologists are now needed to perform the great array of testing required by the modern hospital. However, the volume, due to a greater array of available procedures, some of which are quite sophisticated, has increased sufficiently to offset the need for fewer technical personnel, resulting in an increased need for laboratory professionals in some laboratories.

Automated instruments can provide accuracy and efficiency with small volumes of both sample and reagent that cannot be duplicated by manual methodology. These instruments are also safer to use, and the reagents are not as toxic as they once were, as some of the old reagents were notoriously carcinogenic. Even the tissue and cellular pathology department has been invaded by sophisticated technology. Instruments with templates for normal cells can match patient samples and determine the presence of cancer or other pathological conditions more rapidly than manual methods. An example of this type of equipment is a system capable of screening Pap smears in large numbers in a short period of time; originally, these had to be screened microscopically by cytotechnologists and pathologists at a much slower rate.

Elements Involved in Calculating the Costs of Performing Tests

A great number of variables must be considered when establishing the cost of a laboratory procedure, to determine the price that should be charged for this procedure. In the *Medical Laboratory Observer,* March 2007, Daniel M. Baer stated that the major facets of determining cost and subsequent charges for the procedures must include certain basic requirements that must be considered before affixing a price to the procedure. To determine the true cost of performing a given test, the numbers obtained by the manager doing the calculations are paramount. Technicians and technologists are often called on to evaluate new tests or new methodology to replace a test already being performed. These technical personnel look for accuracy, specificity, and labor involved in terms of time along with other factors. The manager may provide other points of consideration to be used in determining a price for an analysis under review for revision or change in methodology.

Basic calculations would include the following information. There are two separate costs that are important to establish. There is a *cost per reportable test* and a *cost per billable test.* What is the difference between these two? One must accurately count the number of tests performed in a specific time period, such as a 1-year or a 6-month timeframe. For accuracy in the realm of reportable test volume, counts should include patient samples, proficiency tests, controls (including control verifications), calibrators, and a percentage of repeat tests that are necessary because of random system errors or errors by the technical personnel. For billable tests only, the analysis will count those tests that were actually reimbursed. Once the technician or technologist has accurate test volumes, the costs to run that volume of tests should be added together. Essential costs would include direct costs such as reagents and consumables, as well as indirect costs such as regulatory fees and proficiency testing costs. It is extremely important to include the overhead for the laboratory only and not for the entire facility. Allocation of a portion of the laboratory revenue for the facility overhead is determined separately after the costs per reportable and billable tests are calculated.

In calculating these costs, one must ensure that accurate costs for equipment purchase, lease, or other manufacturer's arrangements for procuring use of a piece of equipment are included. Expenses such as equipment maintenance and all personnel costs, including phlebotomists and clerical personnel and the cost of benefits, should be added. Overhead expenses will be a difficult cost factor to determine. Information should be sought from the office manager or administrator to determine what is appropriate for the purpose of determining the costs of providing laboratory services. Again, remember that a portion of the overall overhead of the entire facility must be added as a percentage of the overhead for which a laboratory is responsible. Professional associations are often helpful as a resource for information on cost analysis. The sum of all costs for a particular test divided by the correct volumes of tests performed yields the costs per reportable test and costs per billable test. Determining all the costs by going through contracts and invoices is a time-consuming process, but it is important to reconcile invoices with contracts to ensure the lab does not pay more than its contracts with outside vendors of equipment and supplies state. This often happens!

Screening Tests

For some medical laboratory tests, it is possible to perform a cheaper and easier procedure before becoming involved with the increased work and expense to the patient of a more extensive procedure. As a general explanation, it is possible to determine if a condition exists in a patient, such as that for general inflammation, before performing more costly and time-consuming tests, many of which might yield a negative clinical finding. In some routine tests, initial test results might need to be confirmed by another test before a more advanced procedure is needlessly performed. A good example of this is found in the simple urinalysis where a dipstick with chemically reactive pads is dipped into the urine specimen. A positive protein would be significant but would sometimes require the collection of a 24-hour urine specimen, which requires refrigeration and would be an inconvenience for the patient, as well as an expense. A simple test using a precipitating acid to confirm the presence of protein rather than some innocuous substance that by use of the dipstick would give a falsely positive result will save a great deal of money and will avoid providing the physician with erroneous results. This will be explained in chapter 12, Procedures for Urinalysis and Body Fluid.

Although it is not the same as performing a **screening test** before performing a more advanced test, some agencies find it necessary to screen large populations for early evidence of disease. Screening tests are inexpensive methods that may be used to screen out the healthy members of the population from those who will require further testing for positive results. This process is often performed at health fairs and is particularly true for government agencies that provide health care to segments of the country's population as well as to those in less-developed countries. The screening procedures selected must be adequate for screening large populations for certain prevalent diseases.

These screening tests must have the specificity (sometimes called validity) for "picking up" diagnostic findings on patients who are either diseased or at risk for becoming so. *Specificity* is defined as a test measuring what it is intended to measure, with little or no interference from other materials, and providing a true or specific value. Optimally, a test must be specific enough that it does not yield a positive result for other materials in the body (cross-reactive) but possesses the sensitivity to pick up low levels of constituents for which the test is being used. Sensitivity should not be so high that normal patients will show erroneous positive results. Sensitivity of diagnostic testing indicates that the test is designed to detect clinically significant levels of a constituent of the blood, as an example, by its ability to pick up positives on minute amounts if necessary. But it should not be too sensitive in that some tests will give a false positive in patients with values for constituents of the blood or other body fluids that are normally found at low levels in the body.

Contracts for Services, Equipment, and Supplies

Contracts in general are promulgated for the convenience and advantage of both the provider and the consumer. It is to the advantage of the manufacturer to capture a large account from which the institution will order all of its reagents and control specimens for calibrating and operating its equipment. Another large category included in many contracts is that of consumable supplies that are used in large quantities. Bids may be sought by entire government agencies such as the Veterans' Administration for its hospitals, or by large health care systems that may include a number of hospitals or clinics.

Since the institutions under contract are barred from buying from other companies, the contracting company can afford to sell in quantity at much lower prices to large-volume customers than if a large number of smaller institutions were each buying at lower levels. Sometimes an advantage of these contracts may lie in the ability of the manufacturer to deliver supplies and equipment to one central warehouse, where the health care system itself assumes the responsibility and expense of distributing the items to its various offices and facilities. Billing for the large numbers of materials purchased under contract greatly simplifies the process of payment. Because the manufacturer may also have an estimate of the level of certain items that will be needed on an annual basis, the manufacturer is able to produce large quantities quickly and store them for distribution as they are ordered.

Lease-Purchase Agreements

Many sophisticated pieces of laboratory equipment are extremely expensive to purchase and to maintain. Most manufacturers have arrangements by which a health care facility may use the equipment for as long as the laboratory will purchase supplies and reagents for that piece of equipment. Technology is also evolving at such a rate that often what is new today is outmoded tomorrow. Many pieces of laboratory testing equipment are outdated within 2 to 3 years. Creative arrangements are frequently possible as a cost-effective way of gaining access to technology without large capital outlays required to purchase the instruments.

A manufacturer's profits are not usually based on the price of a piece of equipment, and to the extent that they are, the research necessary for designing and producing the machine would require a substantial price tag if the equipment were bought. Competing pieces of equipment also make it a practical practice for manufacturers to provide the equipment in return for an assured level of use of reagents and consumable materials, such as specimen containers. In this type of arrangement, new versions of testing equipment may be procured easily as they arrive on the market, and the lease-purchase contract may be for only 2 years, or may be for longer periods if desired. This makes for excellent business practice for the medical laboratories and entire health systems.

Repeat Testing

It is in the best interest of the laboratory to minimize repeat testing to the fullest extent possible. The need to repeat a test or tests may occur for a variety of reasons. System errors may yield an occasional value that is completely unacceptable, perhaps indicating a level that would not be conducive to the survival of the patient, while the other tests for that patient are normal. Often, results must be evaluated by comparing them with other tests that correlate with the results of a given test. The statistical term "delta checks" is described in Chapter 10, Quality Assurance. This check helps to eliminate errors on patients who have had a certain test done for perhaps several days in a row, and there is no clinical reason in some instances for a change in test values to have occurred. When a mistake is made that may require repeating an entire "run" (or batch of tests), a great deal of time, reagents, and consumables have been wasted, adding to operational costs. Many instruments "flag" results that may be out of the ordinary, which would prompt the technician or technologist to repeat the questionable test. Random errors, or occasional errors that occur even under the best of circumstances, and when instruments seem to be operating perfectly, do occur. This occasional erroneous result will not greatly affect the costs of operation, but it does require that the laboratory worker have the knowledge to perform troubleshooting procedures. Performing preventive maintenance as outlined by the manufacturer on a regular basis will do a great deal to avoid time-consuming repairs causing disruption of services. Recurring problems of a similar nature for a piece of equipment may signal that a breakdown is imminent and may require a service call.

Costs Incurred When Equipment Is "Down"

In all laboratories, the bane of the existence of managers and technical workers is the malfunction of equipment. The large and extremely sophisticated equipment that handles high volumes of procedures each day may unexpectedly cease functioning. In this case, it is helpful when a technologist on site is able to troubleshoot and remedy the problem. Some manufacturers are able to troubleshoot equipment over a telecommunications line. Quite frequently, laboratories will retain old equipment that can duplicate the work of the newer version. It is possible to bring older replacement equipment online quickly to avoid disruptions of services, when the old equipment has been occasionally checked out and otherwise maintained. A disruption of laboratory services will impact the physician and the ability to diagnose a condition, which may be dangerous to the patient's health.

Most larger laboratories have maintenance contracts that provide for on-site repairs and maintenance. Routine preventive maintenance is often a function of laboratory technical personnel and serves to prevent some of the time-consuming and costly malfunctions. Accurate records of daily documentation of repairs and preventive maintenance are required to aid in determining why an instrument might have malfunctioned. Sometimes signs appear in the instrument's operation that may signal an imminent problem with its operation. One of the most important responsibilities of a technologist in a laboratory is to take care of the equipment and to perform all required maintenance procedures to avoid a great deal of inconvenience and perhaps harm to the patients served.

Point-of-Care Testing: A Step Toward the Future?

Because the health care industry is changing rapidly, it is imperative that laboratorians, from management to bench workers, keep their options open as to what is most expedient, cost-effective, and beneficial for the patients. Why is **point-of-care testing (POCT)** included in this chapter? The reason is that the costs per test are higher than the batch tests performed in the laboratory, but personnel costs are low, as those already working in the patient care areas are the ones who perform these tests; thus the tests are at least somewhat cost effective. It is not sufficient to maintain the status quo and those who do not embrace change should not consider laboratory technology as a profession. Changes in methodology for laboratory procedures are emerging rapidly and show no sign of abating. All aspects of the field, including technology, automation, laboratory information systems, robotics, and principles of economics, are evolving daily.

POCT is moving ahead as a major avenue of change. Originally, POCT did not address economic practices, but with the advent of smaller and more portable instruments, more and more procedures may be performed at the bedside of the patient, or in the patient's home. More POCT is not a solution to providing better care to more people, but it may be a possible answer to some of the problems of delivering timely results in laboratory medicine.

Since the advent of modern laboratory testing, particularly in the 20th century, procedures have been performed in a central laboratory by well-trained laboratory workers. Other ways of bringing testing closer to the patient lie in the formation of specialty laboratories situated near the patient treatment area. Even a few decades ago, it was common for some specific testing to be performed in "satellite" laboratories that were at separate locations from the main laboratory. But this differed from POCT, in that procedures were still performed by clinical laboratory technicians and technologists. In contrast, POCT is normally performed close to or at the patient's location and in most instances by nurses and other nonlaboratory personnel. This phenomenon may lead to an increase of testing by nontechnical personnel, as easy to operate and transportable equipment becomes more available. Change is most likely inevitable, and many technicians and technologists, along with some professional societies, oppose the

Table 7-1 Elements of Point-of-Care Testing

Elements Involved in Institutional Point-of-Care Testing
1. Orientation, training, and checkoffs for operators of instruments
2. Documented training in safety procedures for self and patient
3. Observing applicable requirements promulgated by regulatory agencies (government and institutional policies and procedures)
4. Quality assurance program that includes quality control documentation
5. Periodic retraining and assessment of testing personnel
6. Technical support from manufacturers and suppliers
7. Support from institutional technical personnel (biomedical, clinical laboratory)
8. Computer program for input of results from *Quality Control* and reporting of patient results

performance of POCT by nontechnical personnel. However, at this point, most training for performing POCT and maintaining of maintenance records and quality control documentation is still performed by technical laboratory personnel.

Regulation of POCT

POCT at this point is chiefly provided for CLIA-waived procedures, so it is not regulated as stringently as those procedures performed in the clinical laboratory. In explanation, CLIA 88 terms a number of these simpler tests performed on small easy-to-use instruments as "waived" tests, in which the operator needs only basic orientation and training. However, in cases where the instrumentation is used in physician's office laboratories, clinics, and hospitals, certain components related to quality assurance must be observed. Table 7-1 combines all of the elements usually included in the policies and procedures manuals for health care facilities. These activities are points for accreditation agencies to access during their site visits for inspecting operation of the facility.

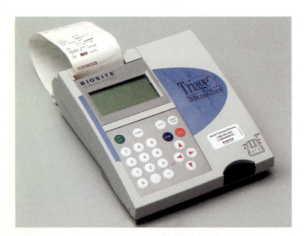

FIGURE 7-1 Triage MeterPlus provides a number of tests related to cardiac health.
Source: Delmar/Cengage Learning.

Where is POCT Performed?

POCT is actually performed in two major sites—that of the home and in critical care units and emergency departments of hospitals. In addition, nursing assistants, EMTs, paramedics, and others often perform glucose testing with small hand-held meters for quick action by the medical team. This type of testing is also used in screening for health risks at health fairs. Basic chemistry tests, such as the determination of cholesterol and glucose levels using small portable instruments such as the one pictured in Figure 7-1, may be simply and conveniently performed in only minutes using whole blood. Patients may even be able to monitor test results themselves in their homes with minimal instruction (Figure 7-2).

Challenges to Health Care Provision

It is to no avail when advanced medical procedures to create a better quality of life and to stay healthier longer are available but few can afford them. As technology creates more sophisticated laboratory testing, surgical procedures, and medications, the costs of these interventions have outstripped the ability of many to pay for them.

During the post–World War II era, those who worked for industrial companies often had employer-provided health care insurance that covered almost all care, and many were thus unaware of the increasing costs for this care; indirect pay made medical care appear to be "free." With the advent in the 1960s of Medicare and Medicaid, federal government programs became available that paid for the care of those who were no longer working or of those who were unemployed, disabled, or extremely poor. These programs led to expectations by some that the federal government should provide health care for all, in a manner similar to that of more socialized countries in Europe and elsewhere. Since 1960, when health care consumed approximately 5% of the nation's budget, the level of the federal budget going for health care has grown to an estimated 17% in 2009.

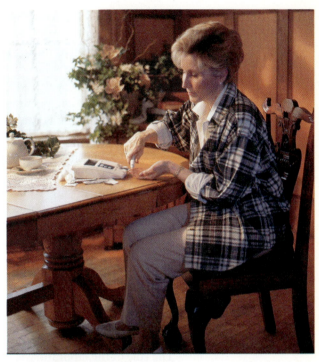

FIGURE 7-2 Patient performing coagulation testing to monitor medication prescribed.
Source: Delmar/Cengage Learning.

To cover their own costs and to remain economically viable, many companies no longer provide health care coverage for their employees. In those that do provide health coverage, the employee often must pay a portion of the premium and an additional co-pay (a preset out-of-pocket payment for a portion of the cost of care).

A segment of the U.S. population believes that a national health care program that insures everyone would be advantageous. However, such a plan may eventually cost more that the current system of private insurance companies that sell health care plans to those who desire them and can afford them. Programs that are provided on a national level almost always exceed the costs estimated when such programs are first legislated into existence. As examples, both Medicare and Medicaid programs are in financial straits and some predict these programs may become bankrupt in a few decades.

Providing health care for everyone is one of the biggest challenges the U.S. and indeed the world will face. Lowering the costs of providing health care by limiting the level of services a patient may receive is a route that may be adopted to rein in the costs of health care. Professional managers of entire health care systems and department heads on lower levels of a business enterprise are often required to assume more responsibility in preparing budgets that include costs of employee benefits. It is imperative that technical professionals such as managers of medical laboratories, pharmacies, and other cost centers become aware of and more educated about control of operational expenses while not sacrific-ing quality and quantity.

Several effective means by which individuals and families can help to con-trol health care costs have been proposed that would not involve sacrificing the advanced level of health care enjoyed in the U.S. today. Most require that indi-viduals assume some personal responsibility for controlling and paying the costs of care. One avenue is the creation of medical savings accounts, encouraged by federal and state governments through tax credits, that would make individuals more likely to prudently seek medical care only when necessary. The other major approach lies in wellness education that begins at an early age. This means of controlling costs might include nutritional diets that are prepared in schools and at home to help individuals avoid obesity and hypertension. A healthful life-style that includes regular exercise and proper rest could go a long way toward controlling health care costs, while retaining the advantages of a country with one of the best health care systems available. Creativity by leaders and personal responsibility for one's health should be the goal of everyone to avoid sacrificing the health of everyone.

The Laboratory Role

The role of the laboratory is included in the demand for more economical medical care. Laboratories have made strides toward providing more economical testing by establishing reference laboratories to do batch tests in large volumes for many lab-oratories at a much lower cost than a single laboratory can accomplish with only a few tests of a given category in a period of time. Mechanization has led to quicker turnaround times, more efficiency, and less costly testing. Health fairs with screen-ing tests have led to the discovery of diseases before symptoms appear, leading to quicker and easier treatment and even cures of diseases that might have become chronic. Contracts are used to control costs for an established period of time, and lease-purchase agreements that require buying of a certain volume of supplies and reagents in return for being allowed to use an expensive piece of equipment for a time are common today. In-house repair technicians, backup equipment for use when a major malfunction has occurred, and POCT have all been advanced to do their respective parts in controlling health care costs.

INTRODUCTION TO LABORATORY FUNCTIONS AND BASIC EQUIPMENT

Testing procedures for each of the major departments within the medical labora-tory may number into the thousands, perhaps tens of thousands, but most hospital-based medical laboratories perform a repertoire of several hundred procedures. Those procedures not performed on a routine basis and in sufficient numbers are commonly sent to commercial reference laboratories or, in the case of a hospital system, laboratories within the system at separate sites that specialize in certain procedures. This can be economical. For instance, a system with five hospitals would send all of a certain procedure to Hospital A and Hospital A would send another set of specialized tests to Hospital C, operating within its own system.

Then tests from this hospital system would be sent to a commercial reference laboratory for those tests that were done at none of the hospitals in the system just described. This could be due to low volume where it would not be cost-efficient to buy equipment for and to retain a person with specialized training to perform only a handful of a certain test per month or even per year. Another reason for sending seldom-ordered tests to an outside laboratory would be a shortage of trained personnel in the region available for performing certain tests. Some specialized tests may require hundreds of thousands of dollars just to set up a section that is ready to perform a certain laboratory test or tests. Some hospitals have data indicating a **breakeven point**—they will assume the testing of specimens previously sent to a reference laboratory when the volume of testing reaches a certain level.

Laboratory Management

In some laboratories, one person serves as both the laboratory manager and the technical supervisor. In the larger laboratories these duties may be split among two or more persons. The laboratory manager falls directly under the laboratory director and may require additional business or management experience along with education and training. The laboratory manager may provide most of the business decisions by receiving requests from the various laboratory departments, and purchases supplies and equipment from a variety of sources, based on contractual requirements, availability, costs, efficiency, ease of use, and operation. In the past, a laboratory manager who might also be called the "chief tech" worked as a bench technologist and handled management issues as part of the job. But in all except the smallest laboratories, these tasks are now handled by a manager who is extremely well-versed in all of the operations of the entire laboratory.

In some extremely large laboratories, the department supervisors may handle their own budgets for supplies and equipment, with oversight by the laboratory manager. As the complexity of clinical laboratories continues to escalate, **financial management** through wise management of resources, including human resources within the laboratory, will undoubtedly receive more attention. Just as procedures are evolving in number, complexity, and sophistication, the required functions of a manager of the medical laboratory are also changing. No longer is it probable that a medical technologist, without further training and even education, will advance to the level of manager, with the required personnel, legal, ethical, and business responsibilities, without education and experience in these areas.

Equipment and Supplies

Equipment and supply lists for the medical laboratory are complex and contain literally thousands of items that are used on a regular basis. While cost is a great part of making decisions, it is not the only factor involved in choosing methodology, which would include both the equipment needed and the supplies required to perform the various procedures. Besides the financial aspects of operating a laboratory, a technical supervisor may work in conjunction with the laboratory manager, setting personnel standards, establishing training and evaluation processes, and monitoring the quality assurance program.

Safety Alert

Centrifuge Safety

Centrifuges may produce several safety hazards when they are used in the laboratory. Standard Precautions must be observed, and the centrifuges become contaminated easily by spills and aerosols produced during centrifugation. Instruction manuals accompanying the instruments will indicate the routine maintenance necessary for adequate performance and the proper manner in which to clean the centrifuges.

General requirements for safe operation include the following:

- The tubes placed in the wells of the rotor must be balanced. Usually, various sizes of tubes will be available to place an equal volume of solution to place directly opposite the specimen. Remember that specimens drawn in similar tubes may vary in volume due to a variety of reasons.

- Tube should remain capped or otherwise covered during the process to prevent aerosolization of the sample.

- Tubes are designed for certain sized wells where the tube is placed, so the correct tube and the correct speed for the particular centrifuge should be observed.

- *Never* open a centrifuge while the rotor is spinning for two reasons. Aerosols may be stirred by the rotation, or tubes may break and throw glass or plastic that might cause an injury.

- Accidental spills should be cleaned immediately according to the protocol established by the laboratory.

Equipment and supplies are ordinarily purchased and stored in quantities that will allow for uninterrupted performance of diagnostic testing. They may include computer costs as well as clerical supplies. Often there are lease-purchase options for large pieces of expensive equipment where the laboratory pays for use of the instrument based on the number of tests performed. Costs for **proficiency testing programs**, quality control programs, and the reporting of patient results to physicians' offices and clinics mandates the establishment of an extremely sophisticated set of procedures to ensure a smoothly running laboratory with as little interruption of results as possible.

Common Equipment Used in Laboratories

Some equipment and supplies are generic (commonly used) in the various departments of the laboratory based on the procedures specifically performed there. Although a few items are commonly used in all the departments, most of the supplies and equipment are used only in one area or department. Storage space is often at a premium, and frequently supplies are handled on an automatic standing order, after a laboratory has determined its usage over a period of time. Some materials have a short shelf life, or must be kept under controlled conditions, such as in a frozen state or in a refrigerator. These items are most often purchased on a regular shipping schedule to eliminate having to destroy outdated materials or to at least limit this sort of wastage of resources. The cost-effectiveness of a well-managed laboratory is often scrutinized by the CEO of the hospital, who may initiate directives to cut costs if the laboratory is not doing an effective job of managing costs.

Many laboratories have procedures in place to continue the workflow even if a major malfunction in equipment or defective supplies occurs. Sometimes a piece of equipment that has been replaced by a later model will be retained for such eventualities. This sometimes requires occasionally "cranking up" the instrument in storage to ensure it will function when it is needed on an emergency basis. In some cases, the laboratory will revert to a manual method that may take longer to perform, until the instrument is repaired or needed supplies are obtained. Medical laboratory workers must be innovative, flexible, creative, and able to "think on their feet" on occasion. This section is devoted to an exploration of some of the most commonly used equipment and supplies on a department basis. The most commonly used items of equipment and supplies will be listed by department, with discussion relative to their use. The purpose of providing the following categories of equipment at this point is to give the student a background in some of the equipment and supplies he or she will be employing when performing the representative laboratory procedures in the next chapters.

A significant number of pieces of equipment are essential to the smooth and effective operation of medical laboratories. In the following description of equipment and their uses, most of these will be found in small to large laboratories. Equipment is needed to procure, prepare, and store samples. Equipment is needed for storage and organization of reagents and other supplies essential for procuring, accepting, and processing patient samples. A great deal of thought and study should be undertaken to make the best decisions related to factors such as manual versus automated procedures, sensitivity and specificity of equipment and test materials, as well as other issues related to the needs of the medical facility.

Centrifuges

A number of types of **centrifuges** are specialized in their uses. They are all used to spin biological samples to separate components within the specimen. Centrifugal forces cause the heavier materials to go to the bottom of the tubes. Samples are centrifuged at speeds that vary by procedure and type of sample. Most commonly, blood is separated for tests where the liquid portion (serum or plasma) is to be used in the procedure. Specimens that require blood cells would not normally require centrifugation. The basic parts of the centrifuge, regardless of type, are similar. The **rotor** is the part that is spun by the motor of the centrifuge, and is controlled by a timer and a speed control.

Centrifuges are differentiated by the jobs for which they were developed. Common centrifuges used for separating blood into solid and liquid components whether as plasma (derived from **anticoagulated specimens**) or serum (obtained from clotted samples) are the most numerous types found in the laboratory, and most laboratories have at least several of each for basic types [Figures 7-3 through 7-7]). A microcentrifuge, or microfuge, is one that is used to spin small tubes at high speeds

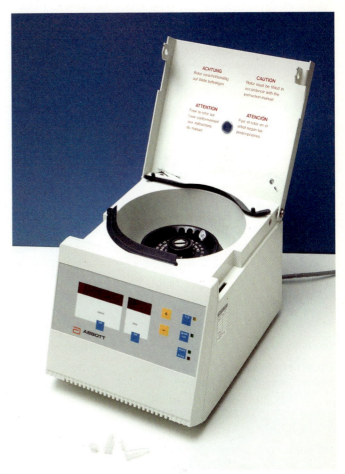

FIGURE 7-3 Microcentrifuge for small types of specimen containers. Source: Delmar/Cengage Learning.

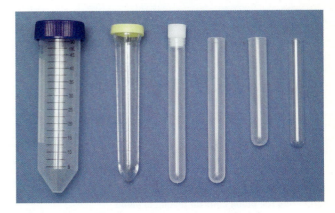

FIGURE 7-4 Test tubes that may be used in centrifugation. Source: Delmar/Cengage Learning.

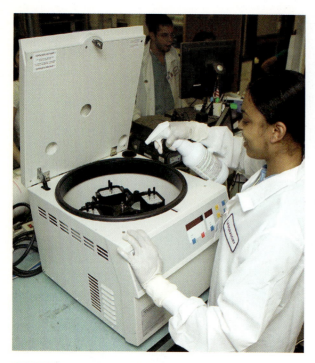

FIGURE 7-5 Disinfecting a clinical centrifuge.
Source: Delmar/Cengage Learning.

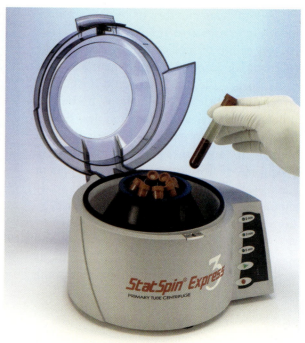

FIGURE 7-6 Balancing specimens in a centrifuge.
Source: Delmar/Cengage Learning.

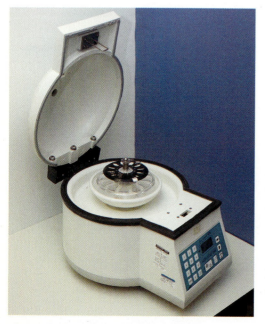

FIGURE 7-7 Serological centrifuge, used for preparing red blood cells for testing in blood banking procedures.
Source: Delmar/Cengage Learning.

that may be as great as 14,000 rpm (revolutions per minute). Other models, called clinical centrifuges, operate in the range of up to roughly 3,000 rpm, and are used to concentrate sediment from urine samples and to separate serum or plasma from whole blood samples. One common specialized centrifuge used in blood banking, or **immunohematology** is the serofuge, for use in washing of red blood cells in small tubes of 2 to 3 mL (see Figure 7-7).

Other centrifuges may be required depending on types of specimens and procedures. Some require high-speed refrigerated centrifuges; some require various types of specimens and differing sizes of collection tubes and containers.

Refrigerators

Basic refrigerators are required for routine use in the laboratory. There are also special refrigerators mainly designed for preserving and storing patient samples and supplies used for various procedures. An example of a specialized refrigerator that requires constant temperature within a certain range and that has alarms built in to prevent the loss of valuable units of blood and plasma is the blood bank refrigerator

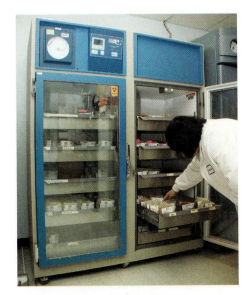

FIGURE 7-8 Blood bank refrigerator designed to store units of blood according to group and type, and special units for patients with unusual blood types or atypical antibodies. Source: Delmar/Cengage Learning.

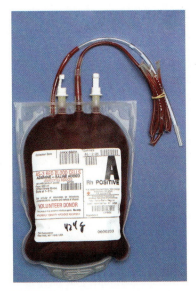

FIGURE 7-9 Blood donor unit to be stored until transfused into patient needing blood. Source: Delmar/Cengage Learning.

(Figure 7-8). This is where units of blood and their components may be stored (Figure 7-9) until they are ready for infusion into the patient. Some freezers are also necessary to provide long-term storage and for supplies that might deteriorate if thawed (Table 7-2).

Microscopes

Microscopes are delicate instruments that are used in many areas of the laboratory, but they must be properly maintained and cared for to gain satisfaction and accuracy from their uses (Figure 7-10). Some are extremely sophisticated, but most are called light or bright-field microscopes, and these contain adapters that enable them to be converted easily for dark-field and phase contrast purposes (Figure 7-11). These modifications are required for performing certain tests.

Table 7-2 Permissible Temperature Ranges for Common Laboratory Equipment

Equipment	Temperature (°C)	Permissible Range (°C)
Refrigerator	6 ± 2	4 to 8
Freezer	−20 ± 5	−15 to −25
Ultracold freezer	−70 ± 5	−65 to −75
Microbiology incubator	36 ± 1	35 to 37
Water bath	36 ± 1	35 to 37

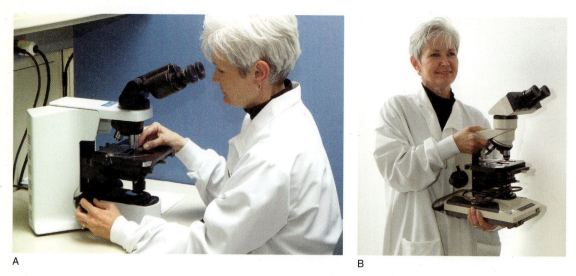

A   B

FIGURE 7-10 (A–B) Caring for the microscope and proper procedure for transporting the instrument are essential. Source: Delmar/Cengage Learning.

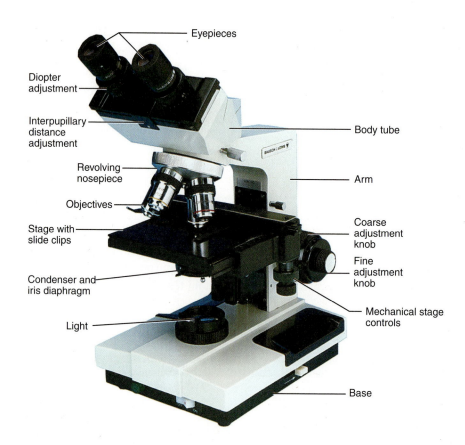

FIGURE 7-11 Binocular brightfield microscope, a basic tool for the medical laboratory worker. Source: Delmar/Cengage Learning.

Autoclave for Sterilizing Certain Pieces of Equipment

Much of the supplies and some equipment components used in the clinical laboratory are sterile if necessary on receipt. To sterilize materials and devices, autoclaves range in size from simple desktop machines to large floor models that will hold large racks of items. Few pieces of equipment require sterilization, but in a few cases pieces of reusable equipment or even reagents that must be sterile require the use of an autoclave (Figure 7-12).

Safety Cabinets and Fume Hoods

These items of equipment are used in the same way, and are similar, except for modifications that better equip them for the purposes for which they are intended. A **fume hood** (Figure 7-13) is used when working with chemicals that may be toxic if inhaled. A **biological safety cabinet** (Figure 7-14) is used for working with microorganisms that have the potential of infecting the laboratory worker.

LABORATORY NEED FOR WATER

Water is the chief solvent in use for a clinical laboratory. Many reagents require dilution of a freeze-dried or dehydrated solute, or reagents may be concentrated and require dilution before use. Several grades are used in the laboratory, and are designated as Type I, II, and III. These three types are recommended by the Clinical Laboratory Standards Institute (CLSI) and the College of American Pathologists (CAP), the latter of which also inspects and accredits laboratories. Type I water is the purest of the three, and all three types are prepared through use of deionizers, distillers, or reverse osmosis. Water from the public water

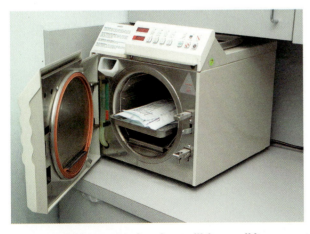

FIGURE 7-12 Table-top autoclave for sterilizing small items.
Source: Delmar/Cengage Learning.

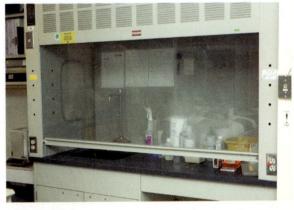

FIGURE 7-13 Fume hood used for working with toxic chemicals that are volatile.
Source: Delmar/Cengage Learning.

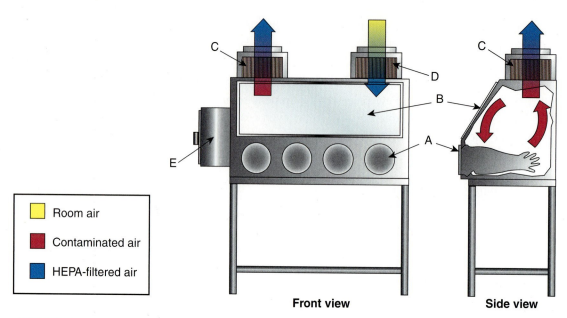

FIGURE 7-14 Diagram of a biological safety cabinet that is designed to filter air passing over the work area under the glass cover of the device. Note opening for arms to be extended into the interior working area.
Source: Delmar/Cengage Learning.

system is never used in making reagents but may be used for the initial washing of laboratory glassware and for cleaning. The three types of water are:

	Method of Preparation
• Distilled water	Water is prepared as a condensate from heated water; most minerals are removed but volatiles such as ammonia, carbon dioxide, and chlorine may remain
• Deionized water	Tap water is passed through resin columns. There are often three or four columns through which the water passes. Charged particles trap impurities, removing them from the water. Not all organic materials such as bacteria are removed in this process.
• Reverse osmosis	This process forces water through a semi-permeable membrane similar to a cell membrane. This procedure removes most bacteria, particulate matter, and organic materials. Small levels of contaminants remain so it does not meet the CAP specifications for Type I or Type II water.

Reagent Grade Water

To make reagent grade water, other steps are required following the above processes. Type I reagent water is the purest grade and is produced by passing distilled water over resin columns and then filters before qualifying as reagent grade water. Type I water is the purest grade and is the only type that is used for preparing standards and controls used in monitoring confidence levels of laboratory test performance. Type I water is used to reconstitute vials of freeze-dried materials so there are no substances that may interfere with the tests being performed.

Type II water may be used where small numbers of bacteria will not interfere with test results. Some procedures in hematology, serology, and qualitative procedures may be performed with the use of Type II water. If Type II water is used in microbiological procedures, it must be sterilized due to the presence of bacteria in this grade of water. Type III water is used as a source for preparing Types I and II water, and for washing and rinsing glassware. However, Type I or II is required as the final rinse following the washing of laboratory glassware. Type I water will absorb gases from the air so it should be used soon after preparation. Types II and III are stored in tightly capped containers to prevent absorption of gases, but unlike Type I may be stored for periods of time.

TYPES OF TESTING

Manual Testing

With the flexible financing available today, most laboratories, even those that are quite small, have a significant amount of automation available for tests that are run in batches on a frequent basis. Manual testing is seldom performed today except when instruments may have malfunctioned and need extensive repair or to confirm a result from an automated system when there is doubt as to the veracity of the result. Many automated instruments take little training to operate. The skills possessed by medical laboratory technicians and technologists are necessary to ensure that all the systems are operating properly and to provide adequate samples that have been properly handled. Some of the instruments will "kick out" results that do not meet certain parameters, and attention is required from the technical personnel. Learning the basics of how tests are performed, even by instruments, is important in the education and training of medical laboratory workers.

Automated Testing

Most automated instruments operate on the same premises as the manual test methodology. Some have evolved into more specific and more sensitive procedures, and instruments have become smaller and simpler to operate. In addition, it is difficult to duplicate the precision pipetting required for both reagents and patient samples by the automated systems, when using manual pipettes for reagents and micropipettes for measuring the patient samples. The most common automated systems used in even the smaller laboratories are the blood cell counter and the chemistry analyzer. The blood cell counter enumerates both red and white cells, and estimates the types of white cells, which is important in both bacterial and viral infections. The shape and size of the blood cells can be determined with these sophisticated cell counters, which evolved from a simple particle counter used by industries to measure the purity of certain chemicals. There is even a simple **spectrophotometer** in the cell counter to measure the hemoglobin level. Larger laboratories may have an automated urinalysis instrument, but to justify this instrument, the volume must be considerable for the system to be economical. Both the blood cell counters and the urinalysis instruments require manual testing of samples if certain parameters are exceeded when evaluated by the instruments.

Automated systems, generally referred to as **autoanalyzers**, have greatly improved the economics of producing test results, as well as the efficiency and accuracy of the laboratory. Autoanalyzers are fast and use small volumes of reagents and other expendable supplies, enabling the laboratory manager to procure and maintain the cost factors to date for each department of the laboratory. Decisions as to whether tests should be sent to a reference laboratory or performed "in-house" are relatively easy to make when figures related to specific test procedures are available at any time. These instruments perform many types of tests in tremendous volumes, economically and accurately, and require little operator action beyond properly setting up the instruments for beginning a "run" of samples and controls.

Student Practice of Procedures

In Chapters 11 through 17 of this book, a select batch of manual test procedures along with an explanation of the clinical significance of the test will be provided. Student technicians and technologists will most likely receive an opportunity to perform some of these basic tests as a valuable component of their education and training. This should occur in the classroom laboratory if there is one in the educational institute. Those who do not have the practice laboratory located at the educational facility will normally have an arrangement with a medical laboratory in a hospital or a large clinic. There a technologist known as a **preceptor** will furnish an orientation to the student, along with supplies, equipment, and instructions for setting up these procedures. The student's performance will be evaluated by the preceptor and sometimes by a clinical coordinator from the educational institute to insure the basic knowledge and practice have been obtained. There will be examples of a number of routine laboratory procedures that are routinely performed in each of the major departments of the laboratory. These procedures are provided for familiarization and are by no means all of the laboratory examinations laboratory technicians and technologists perform.

Representative Procedures

Literally thousands of procedures are performed on a regular basis in the laboratory or referred to a commercial **reference laboratory**. This book is not designed to teach students to perform laboratory analyses, as this set of instructional components will be covered thoroughly by classes in theory before the clinical skills will be taught in depth, and then will be strengthened by clinical applications at medical facilities. The latter chapters of basic procedures are presented mainly for the purpose of introducing the medical laboratory student to a few manual tests performed in each of the major departments of the medical laboratory. Specific department procedures will be presented in more depth normally in specific courses for each laboratory section. Efforts are made to present a variety of techniques for orienting the beginning medical laboratory student. Procedures described are only for a review of the most basic procedures as a means of acquainting the student with examples of what will be expected in the various sections of a typical laboratory. There will be common examples that can be performed manually from each laboratory section. Please keep in mind that most laboratory procedures are performed on automated systems once the student is assigned to a clinical site for training. A classroom laboratory will not have the large automated pieces of equipment, as they are extremely expensive to purchase and to maintain. It is important for the student in clinical laboratory technology training to gain a good grasp of the concepts of laboratory testing by practicing basic manual tests.

SUMMARY

Originally, most consumers of health care services paid for their own care in the form of cash or goods they produced themselves. During chiefly the last half of the 20th century, hospitals and medical clinics became business oriented, and the name of the administrator, who formerly was most often a medical doctor, became the CEO. The facilities were modeled more and more after big business enterprises, and hospitals began to merge and form health care systems with several separate facilities. Then smaller and far-flung clinics associated with the medical centers were established as far-flung enterprises that include ancillary services and quick-access medical clinics to bring in more revenue and to find customers for the larger facilities within their health care systems.

A well-designed and organized student classroom laboratory is preferable for the student to gain familiarity with basic laboratory procedures before being scheduled for clinical practice at medical sites. This will serve to enhance the student's experience in gaining practical job knowledge. For that reason, some of the following chapters will present basic manual laboratory procedures. This practical experience will provide the skills necessary to enable the student to enter the clinical site with confidence and to begin strengthening practical skills when graduating from manual testing to automated testing in the clinical site. In some instances, the malfunctioning of autoanalyzers may force the laboratory workers to resort to manual testing, or manual testing may be required to troubleshoot problems with an automated system or to get the important laboratory tests out in a timely manner.

Students will recognize basic instrumentation and generic supplies that are used in all laboratories. The technical student will understand the reasons for performing manual procedures in some cases versus all tests being performed on automated equipment. This sequential orientation will increase the student's confidence and overall knowledge of the operation of a clinical laboratory at an early stage, allowing for improving the knowledge base and practical application for a successful registry examination experience.

REVIEW QUESTIONS

1. Why would some laboratory procedures be sent to a commercial reference laboratory?
2. What are some basic pieces of equipment that would perhaps be found in ALL clinical laboratories?
3. Why is it important for the laboratory worker to learn the basic manual procedures for a variety of tests?
4. How is automation advantageous to the laboratory?
5. How would using a lease program for an expensive piece of equipment be advantageous?
6. Why do you think medical costs have risen so rapidly in the past 50 years?
7. What is meant by "direct pay" and "indirect pay" for medical services?
8. What are HMOs and PPOs?
9. Where is point-of-care-testing (POCT) testing performed? Is it cost-effective?
10. Describe how repeat testing and down-time for pieces of equipment may affect efficiency and cost effectiveness.

CHAPTER 8

PIPETTING AND USE OF GLASSWARE

LEARNING OBJECTIVES

Upon completion of this chapter, the reader will be able to:

- Identify and describe the importance of accurate measurements of testing reagents and samples.

- Identify the appropriate containers required for measurement of various solutions.

- List key factors that affect the accuracy of measurements using various containers and devices.

- Discuss the reason for and the importance of the maintenance of pipettes and pipetters.

- List the three types of pipettes used in measuring volumes of test reagents for both automated and manual procedures.

- Relate considerations in testing where exact measurements of samples and reagents are required and examples of procedures where a range of accuracy would be acceptable.

KEY TERMS

Acetone
Beakers
Beral pipettes
Bunsen burner
Buret pipettes
Carpal tunnel syndrome
Class A
Colorimetric
Cuvettes
Erlenmeyer flasks
Flasks
Food and Drug Administration
Gilson micropipettes
Glassware
Graduated cylinders

Gravimetric analysis
Griffin beaker
Hexane
Light-guided pipetting systems
Macropipettes
Microliter
Micropipettes
Mohr pipettes
National Institute of Standards and Technology (NIST)
Pasteur pipettes
Pipette calibration
Pipette fillers
Pipette helpers
Pipette tips

Pipettes
Polycarbonate
Polyethylene
Polypropylene
Polystyrene
Polyvinyl chloride
Quantitative pipettes
Semiquantitative pipettes
Serological pipettes
Silica
Teflon
Transfer pipettes
Tygon
Volumetric containers
Volumetric pipettes

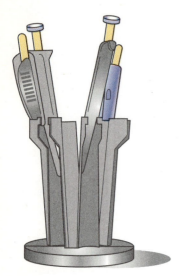

FIGURE 8-1 General measuring equipment.
Source: Delmar/Cengage Learning.

INTRODUCTION

Volumetric containers of varying accuracy and **pipettes** for transferring relatively small amounts of liquids are found in the clinical laboratory. One of the trademarks of laboratories of yesteryear was the presence of a large amount of **glassware** and various measuring devices scattered around. Washrooms were an essential part of the clinical laboratory, and a great deal of time was spent in washing and ensuring that glassware was chemically clean. Laboratory assistants and full-time personnel were involved in washing and drying various pieces of glassware, and even glass pipettes had their own device for washing and rinsing them for reuse. Today, although some glassware is used for a few procedures, pipettes are disposable, and most tubes and containers are made of materials other than glass and are disposed of after one use.

Initially, specialized pieces of glassware were made individually of blown glass, and there were imperfections in the items as well as variations in the volumes and the markings on the pieces of equipment. All of the glassware was made from **silica**, derived from sand. Large quantities of glassware were needed, as most tests were performed individually by manual methods before the advent of automated analyzers. **Cuvettes** for reading specimens in a device called a spectrophotometer were made of high grade glass. These cuvettes required care in handling to prevent scratching and had to be scrupulously cleaned between uses. It was only in the past few decades or so that laboratory pipettes, **flasks, beakers**, and **graduated cylinders** began to be made of plasticized material that gave the appearance of glass but was not truly "glassware." Now, plastic can be manufactured that is clear and has few imperfections that may interfere with the light beamed through the reagent mixture being read on a spectrophotometer. In today's laboratory, almost all devices for measuring and containers for storage are composed of some sort of plastic.

Standardization of Measurement Devices

The **National Institute of Standards and Technology (NIST)** is the federal technology agency responsible for developing and promoting accurate measurements in many disiciplines, including time. The agency provides the standards and technology necessary to ensure significant accuracy in research and testing, such as that of the clinical laboratory. Regardless of the design and purpose of measuring supplies of all sorts, the materials must now meet the specifications set forth by NIST. Those that meet these standards for accuracy are then categorized as **Class A.** Vessels that are used to contain (TC) or to deliver (TD) are designed to transfer or to store a specified amount (volume). Generally, TC devices do not deliver exactly the same volume when the solution is transferred to another container. TD devices, primarily pipettes, indicate that the amount specified for that item will deliver essentially the same amount.

Glassware that does not meet the Class A specifications recommended by NIST may have a tolerance range (range within which it is considered accurate) of more than twice that of an NIST-approved pipette or container. Particularly for pipettes, the tolerance level may be etched or stamped onto the devices. So depending on the intended use, a piece of glassware may be made of varying grades of glass. Where accuracy to a great degree is not required, it is possible to use pipettes and other glassware that are not accurate beyond a minimal standard. Some pieces are more suitable for heating, and others are designed to be disposable due to the materials used in their manufacture. Laboratory plastics might still be called glassware and are often used to replace the actual glassware used in the clinical laboratory. Plastics are highly flexible, somewhat inexpensive, and easily disposed of following use. The drawbacks of plastics are due to the use of large amounts of scarce petroleum products for their manufacture and the need for special handling for the safe disposal of some types. Toxic fumes emitted when plastics are burned may be hazardous to the health of humans as well as wildlife. Some work is being done on biodegradable plastics that will not create environmental contamination.

For safety, it should be noted that glass and plastics that are in direct contact with biohazardous materials are most often disposable. In addition, plastic containers may not break if dropped on a hard surface, but actual glass will almost always break in a laboratory accident, requiring the cleanup of toxic materials in many cases. A number of plastics are manufactured for laboratory practice, and each is practical for certain procedures. The major types of plastics used in a laboratory are **polystyrene**, **polyethylene**, **polypropylene**, **Tygon**, **Teflon**, **polycarbonate**, and **polyvinyl chloride**.

Use and Cleanliness of Plastic versus Glass

Both plastic and glass supplies may require special handling when they are being cleaned. Rinsing glass or plastic supplies after they are used and then washing with detergent designed for cleaning laboratory supplies, followed by rinsing with distilled water, may be sufficient in many instances. Detergents and temperature levels of water for washing the supplies must be compatible with the material from which the supplies are constructed. Glass is required for some procedures while plastics are sufficient for others, depending upon the potential for absorption of chemicals and damage that may occur to the containers when exposed to various chemicals. Plastics may break down when exposed to harsh detergents, so these are considerations to be heeded when washing laboratory supplies. Both plastic and glass containers, tubes, and pipettes should appear spotless on visual inspection if an acceptable process of cleaning was followed.

Although pipettes, both **serological** and **volumetric**, are usually disposable, some laboratories find it useful to wash certain pipettes. Pipettes are washed in special cylindrical washers, if it is necessary to wash them. The ends of the pipettes with the smaller openings are placed toward the top of the wash cylinder and the ends with the larger openings are positioned toward the bottom to facilitate quick and easy drainage (Figure 8-2). For each final rinse, Type I or Type II water is used in a pipette container used exclusively for rinses only, with no detergents added to contaminate the surface of the washer. Some types of plastics have a nonwettable surface and are therefore more easily cleaned. Some organic solvents, stiff wash brushes, and abrasive cleaners should not be used on plastics. Plastics

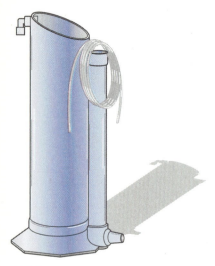

FIGURE 8-2 Pipette washer.
Source: Delmar/Cengage Learning.

also become discolored and brittle over time, and less impervious to chemicals. All plastic or glass supplies should be completely dried after the final rinse and before use.

TYPES OF LABORATORY VESSELS FOR MEASUREMENT AND CONTAINMENT

Laboratory vessels are designed for accuracy only within certain limits. The laboratory containers most commonly in use by a clinical laboratory are categorized essentially by three classifications based on their shapes: flasks, beakers, and graduated cylinders. These containers are generally accurate to within a few milliliters for measuring bulk solutions, so these containers are for measurement of liquids of considerable volume. Volumetric and Erlenmeyer flasks are the types most commonly used in a clinical laboratory, often for measuring solutions for mixing and making working reagents where more than one type of solution is required. For more accurate measurement and extremely small measurements of liquids such as patient samples, pipettes and syringe-type devices are used. Automated analytical instruments that measure reagents, other liquids such as cleaning and rinsing materials, and patient samples will contain both syringe measurements and extremely small but accurate measurement of patient samples.

Volumetric Flask

The volumetric flask, unlike an Erlenmeyer flask or **Griffin beaker**, is used for measurement of a single somewhat-exact volume of liquid and is a TD (to deliver) container. The flask is used to bring a given reagent to a final, accurate volume and should be a Class A (NIST) container. This volumetric flask measures 500 mL ± 0.2 mL, which is extremely accurate for purposes where large volumes of solution are being prepared. To make up a solution, first dissolve the solid material completely in less water than required to fill the flask to the mark. After the solid is completely dissolved, very carefully fill the flask to the 500-mL mark encircling the neck of the flask. Move your eye to the level of the mark on the neck of the flask and line it up so that the circle around the neck looks like a line, not an ellipse (Figure 8-3). Then add distilled water or another prescribed diluent a drop at a time until the bottom of the meniscus lines up exactly with the mark on the neck of the flask. Take care that no drops of liquid are in the neck of the flask above the mark, as they will eventually migrate to the solution below and might bring the total volume to a meniscus that is slightly above the calibration line.

Erlenmeyer Flask

The **Erlenmeyer flask** is a container that is designed to hold different volumes, as opposed to the volumetric flask. These flasks have a narrow neck and mouth that enlarge gradually to a flat bottom (Figure 8-4). They are usually marked on the side (*graduated*) to indicate the approximate volume of contents when filled to

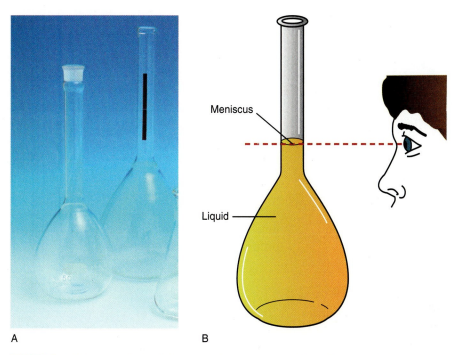

**FIGURE 8-3 (A) Volumetric flasks. (B) Determining measurement in a volumetric flask.
Source: Delmar/Cengage Learning.**

the line. This flask is similar in function to the Griffin beaker but with a narrow neck rather than the vertical walls of the Griffin beaker. This type of top enables the Erlenmeyer flask to be stoppered with a rubber bung or with cotton or steel wool. The contents of an Erlenmeyer flask can be easily swirled or stirred during a procedure without spilling. The flat bottom aids in avoiding tipping over and easily fits onto the ring stand for a **Bunsen burner** or other electronic heating device such as a hot plate.

Griffin Beaker

The Griffin beaker is slightly less accurate for measurements than the Erlenmeyer flask. Usually it also has designations for volumes of a semiquantitative nature on the walls of the beaker (Figure 8-5). These containers are chemically inert and thermally stable, particularly those constructed of glass. A small spout on the lip allows for easy pouring to another container. These containers are most often used for heating materials, melting substances, or mixing liquids that are premeasured and require mixing before their use or where less exactness of the volume of liquid is needed.

Graduated Cylinder

Graduated cylinders are also used for minimally accurate measurements of liquids in larger amounts than the

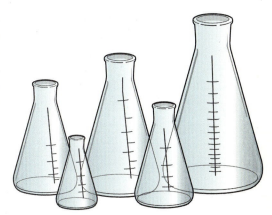

**FIGURE 8-4 Pyrex Erlenmeyer flask starter pack.
Source: Delmar/Cengage Learning.**

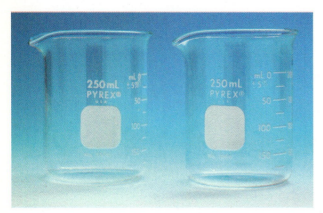

FIGURE 8-5 Griffin beakers of glass with markings.
Source: Delmar/Cengage Learning.

smaller beakers and flasks may accommodate. These devices are long, cylindrical tubes usually held upright by a stable base that is substantially wider than the vertical stem of the cylinder itself (Figure 8-6). The cylinder is marked along its entire length with calibration markers. These containers do not possess the accuracy and precision of volumetric glass and plastic vessels. They may range in volume from 10 mL to 2000 mL (1 L). A reasonably accurate measurement of a 24-hour urine specimen is a common use for this instrument. Another use is for fairly large volumes of materials that must be mixed in certain proportions to each other.

Bottles for Storage

Specialized reagent bottles are available for storage of reagents, but reagents should not be stored for long periods of time. Glass is preferable, and if plastic is used, it should not be used for reagents that may interact with plastic. Normally, only a single day's supply of reagent is prepared for use at one time. Low-quality glass bottles may slowly release ions into the reagents themselves. Bottles are often of amber or brown glass to avoid the deterioration sometimes associated with sunlight and fluorescent lights. Bottles may have various types of closures, such as frosted glass stoppers that fit fairly tightly into the opening, or they may have screw-on caps, preferably of a material that also

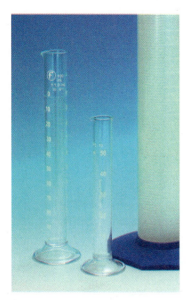

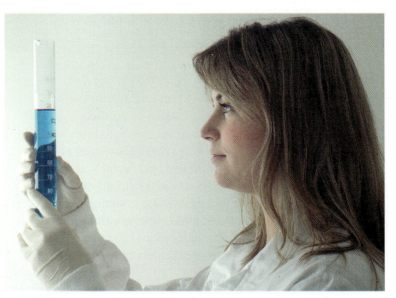

A   B

FIGURE 8-6 (A) Graduated cylinders. (B) Determining measurement in a graduated cylinder.
Source: Delmar/Cengage Learning.

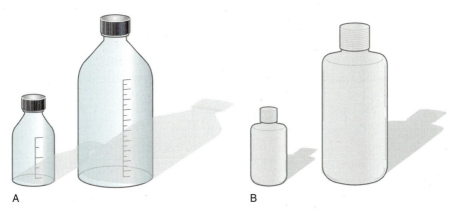

**FIGURE 8-7 (A) Glass and (B) polyethylene storage bottles for laboratory solutions.
Source: Delmar/Cengage Learning.**

will not interact with chemicals. Bottles may be of varying sizes and some have volumetric markings (Figure 8-7), although they are not normally used for measuring solutions but rather for containing, storing, and shipping of reagents, laboratory solutions, and patient specimens.

PIPETTES

Selection of Pipettes

A pipette may also be classified as a pipette, pipetter (usually requires two parts, the pipette tip and a mechanical device), or chemical dropper, and is a laboratory instrument used to transport a measured volume of liquid. Pipetters may be semiautomated or may be operated by electrical means. Pipettes are commonly used in chemistry and molecular biology research as well as for medical tests. They are found in several designs for various purposes requiring differing levels of accuracy and precision, from single-piece plastic pipettes to more complex adjustable or electronic pipettes. All pipettes work by creating a vacuum above the liquid-holding chamber and then selectively releasing this vacuum to draw up and dispense liquids.

Pipettes that dispense between 1 µL and 1000 µL (1 mL) are termed *micropipettes*, while *macropipettes* dispense volumes of liquid greater than 1 mL. **Volumetric pipettes** allow the user to measure one specific volume of solution extremely accurately and then add it to another solution. They are commonly used to make laboratory solutions from a base stock as well as to prepare solutions for titration. Volumetric pipettes are typically marked to indicate one single volume in a particular size pipette (similar to the construction of volumetric flasks). Many different sizes are available. Specialized syringes such as Hamilton syringes are used for small measurements in automated equipment. These syringes measure materials in the microliter category (1 microliter [µL] = 0.001 mL) and are used for the same purposes as pipetters and pipetters. They may have multiple tips for handling several samples simultaneously.

Common Pipettes Used in the Clinical Laboratory

Semiquantitative Measurements

- Pasteur pipettes are used for **semiquantitative** measurements where the amount being transferred is not critical. These pipettes are commonly called droppers or "eye droppers" and are used for transferring small amounts of liquids, often by drops. They are not graduated. Pasteur pipettes may be made of either plastic or glass.
- **Transfer pipettes** are similar to Pasteur pipettes and are used for semi-quantitative measurements. They may be designed for larger quantities than the Pasteur pipette is capable of transferring but can also be used for measuring reagents by the number of drops dispensed. These pipettes are made almost entirely from a soft plastic and their bulbs can serve as a reservoir or liquid-holding chamber.

Quantitative Measurements

- **Serological pipettes** are measuring pipettes that provide a **quantitative** measurement and have graduations extending all the way to the tip. Some are designed as TD (to deliver) and contain a frosted band near the end where a bulb might be placed.
- Mohr pipettes are measuring pipettes that resemble serological pipettes and are used for quantitative measurements. The primary difference between the basic serological pipette and the Mohr pipette is that the graduations on the Mohr pipette do not extend all the way to the tip (usually the last one milliliter). The Mohr pipette is used for "point-to-point" measurements only and not for measuring to the tip of the pipette.
- **Micropipettes** are extremely accurate for quantitative measurements for measuring and transferring very small volumes, such as in patient samples for testing. There are manual versions of the micropipette as well as syringe-type micropipettes, which are found in sophisticated analytical equipment. Manual micropipetters consist of two parts: the device that displaces a certain volume of air and then pulls the same amount of sample into the vacuum of a disposable micropipette tip. The measurements are performed as a small fraction of a milliliter, called a microliter, while reagents are measured in one or more milliliters. The term **microliter** refers to 0.001 mL (µL). Micropipetters provide great accuracy as the primary method for measuring patient samples for testing.

Quantitative Pipettes

Pipettes are designed in a variety of configurations that allow the pipetting of extremely small volumes up to sizable amounts of liquids. These pieces of equipment are usually open-ended glass or plastic tubes used to measure or transfer fairly precise amounts of liquids. They may be either reusable or disposable; increasingly, disposables are being used in clinical laboratories. **Quantitative pipettes** measure volumes to a significantly accurate level. Pipettes that are considered qualitative would most often measure in drops or an approximate value (usually marked on a disposable dropper pipette). Quantitative pipettes range in size from those that measure and dispense extremely small amounts to those that are fairly large that measure and dispense from 1 mL up to 50 mL, based on the particular need for accuracy, sufficient volume, and preservation of samples necessary for the required procedures. The most common are those used to measure 20 mL or less. They may be used in conjunction with automated devices or jar-style measure and delivery methods. As are flasks, pipettes are also classified as Class A or other class, depending on the accuracy of volume needed. The following section describes some of the common types of pipettes and their respective uses.

There are two basic types of **macropipettes**, which are designed to measure amounts greater than 1 mL. One type, the volumetric pipette, has a large bulb and is calibrated for a single volume. Typical volumes are 10, 25, and 50 mL. Alternatively, Mohr pipettes and standard serological pipettes are straight-walled and are graduated for different volumes such as 5 mL in 0.5-mL increments. The single-volume pipette is usually more accurate, with a standard error of ±0.1 or ±0.2 mL.

The pipette is filled by dipping the tip in the solution to be measured and drawing up the liquid with a pipette filler past the inscribed mark. Several pipetting aids will be presented later in this section, which are used for safely aspirating fluid into either of these macropipettes. The volume is then set by releasing the vacuum using the pipette filler or a damp finger until the solution reaches the desired point. While moving the pipette to the receiving vessel, care must be taken not to shake the pipette because the column of fluid may "bounce," causing the loss of a drop of liquid, which would affect the accuracy of the procedure.

Volumetric and Serological Pipettes

Volumetric pipettes are more accurate than serological (also known as graduated) pipettes and contain a bulb that is filled along with a portion of the stem of the pipette, from the meniscus line to the tip (Figure 8-8). The volumetric pipette is intended for delivering only one volume of solution, which may range from 0.5 mL up to 50 mL. The tip is normally touched against the side of the container (not the liquid) to remove a small amount of the residual left in the tip when a solution is being transferred.

Serological pipettes are also categorized with respect to the design and accuracy of the particular type (Figure 8-9). Both serological and Mohr pipettes are used to deliver varying amounts of solution. The serological pipette may be used to measure from point to point and from point to top, as it is graduated to the tip. Mohr pipettes are used for point to point measurements as the last

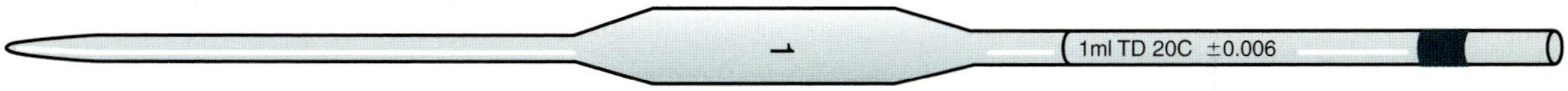

1ml TD 20C ±0.006

FIGURE 8-8 Volumetric pipette with bulb.
Source: Delmar/Cengage Learning.

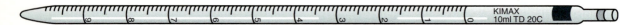

FIGURE 8-9 Serological pipette that is graduated with a frosted ring.
Source: Delmar/Cengage Learning.

milliliter of the pipette is not graduated. When a frosted band is present at the suction end of the stem, this indicates that the contents are to be "blown out" with a pipetting aid for accuracy rather than just draining the solution from the pipette. Suctioning devices or pipetting aids are used with this type of pipette (Figure 8-10).

Mohr Pipettes

Mohr pipettes (Figure 8-11) are graduated pipettes that also use a series of marked lines (as on a graduated cylinder) to indicate different calibrated volumes. However, the graduated lines for a Mohr pipette do not extend completely to the end of the pipette but are designed for measuring from point to point, that is, a 2-mL amount might be measured from the 5.0-mL mark to the 3.0-mL mark. As a rule, measurements performed from one point of the graduation marks to the tip are less accurate than those from "point to point." Mohr pipettes also come in a variety of sizes. These are used much like a buret in that the volume is found by calculating the difference of the liquid level before and after liquid is dispensed. Typically, the precision of a graduated pipette is not as great as that of a volumetric pipette. The vacuum for all of these types of pipettes was originally provided by mouth pipetting of solutions, most often for the measurement of only a few milliliters of material. During the era where most tests were performed manually and as individual tests, it was quite time consuming to pipette all of these reagents and samples accurately. It is inappropriate and unsafe to use the mouth as a source of vacuum to draw the solution into any pipette, as some reagents are quite toxic, and there are many biohazards that could be contracted through mouth pipetting. Several different devices are available for providing a vacuum to aspirate fluids. Most often, a bulb with valves or other device will be used with this type of pipette. Automated instruments will often employ a piston-driven type of aspirating system for measuring both agents and patient samples.

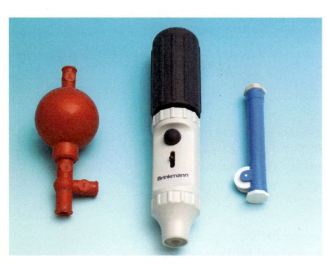

FIGURE 8-10 Pipetting aids for aspirating and dispelling solutions.
Source: Delmar/Cengage Learning.

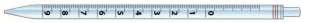

FIGURE 8-11 Mohr pipette without graduation markings near tip.
Source: Delmar/Cengage Learning.

Techniques for Using Quantitative Pipettes

• **To deliver pipette (TD)**

A *to deliver* pipette is indicated with a "TD" inscription near the large open end of the pipette.

Most pipettes are also calibrated at a 20°C temperature for accuracy and standardization. The TD pipette is designed to deliver the volume indicated on the pipette when gravity is used to empty the pipette, leaving a small quantity of solution in the tip. Never should the liquid be aspirated by use of the mouth, nor should it be "blown out" by the mouth from the tip of the pipette. A frosted circle around the large open end of the pipette indicates that it is a "blowout" type, but this is done by use of an instrument such as a bulb or similar device rather than by using the mouth.

- **To contain pipette (TC)**

    A *to contain* pipette is indicated with a "TC" inscription near the large open end of the pipette that indicates that the pipette is designed to contain the volume stated near the end of the pipette. Liquid may adhere to the lumen (open space) within the pipette, and it must be rinsed out to complete an accurate transfer of the solution to be delivered.

Buret Pipettes

Buret pipettes are similar to serological pipettes (Figure 8-12) except for the addition of a valve used to start and stop the flow of the solution. The use of a buret pipette requires slightly more care than other types of pipettes, but when properly used, this type of pipette provides for amazing accuracy to within a small percentage of 1 mL. A buret pipettte delivers a solution in precisely measured volumes with the flexibility to use variable amounts easily. Burets are used primarily for titration, by delivering one reactant to another until the precise end point of the reaction is reached. They are also valuable for delivering accurate amounts of diluents such as reagents to tubes to perform chemical end-point reactions on patient samples. Buret pipettes are not used as often as in the past, when they were commonly used in manual procedures to facilitate the setting up of a number of tests of the same type, allowing a given volume of reagent to be pipetted quickly and easily into test tubes or cuvettes. Samples were then introduced into the measured amounts of reagents by use of a different type of pipette, called a micropipette, to complete a test reaction.

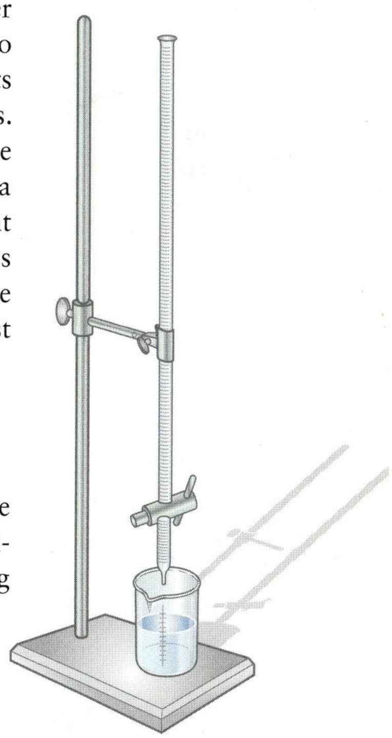

Using a Buret

Be sure the transfer pipette is dry or conditioned with the titrant, so the concentration of solution will not be changed. Before titrating, condition the buret with titrant solution and check that the buret is flowing freely. To condition a piece of glassware, rinse it so that all surfaces are coated with solution, then drain. Conditioning two or three times will ensure that the concentration of the material being titrated is not changed by a stray drop of water. Lubricants that are inert and that will not react with most solvents may be used to lubricate the stopcock, preserving the rubberized sealing washer, as well as allowing for smooth turning of the stopcock.

FIGURE 8-12 Buret pipette with support stand.
Source: Delmar/Cengage Learning.

To fill a buret, close the stopcock at the bottom and use a funnel. You may need to lift up on the funnel slightly, to allow the solution to flow in freely. You can also fill a buret using a disposable transfer pipette. This works better than a funnel for the small, 10-mL burets. Check the tip of the buret for any air bubbles. To remove an air bubble, whack the side of the buret tip while solution is flowing. If an air bubble is present during a titration, volume readings may be in error. Rinse the tip of the buret with water from a wash bottle and dry it carefully. After a minute or so, check for solution on the tip to see if the buret is leaking. The tip should be clean and dry before you take an initial volume reading. When your buret is conditioned and filled and with no air bubbles or leaks, take an initial volume reading. A buret reading card with a black rectangle can help you to take a more accurate reading. Read the bottom of the meniscus. Be sure your eye is at the level of meniscus, not above or below. Reading from an angle, rather than straight on, results in an error of measurement called a *parallax error*. The endpoint should be approached slowly, a drop at a time. Use a wash bottle to rinse the tip of the buret and the sides of the flask. Deliver solution to the titration flask by turning the stopcock. The solution should be delivered quickly until a couple of milliliters from the endpoint, when it is advantageous to slow the flow for better control. The clinical laboratory instructor can show you how to deliver a partial drop of solution when near the endpoint.

Micropipetters and Micropipettes

Micropipetters (to include pipette tips) are designed to deliver extremely small volumes such as a few microliters in most cases and are engineered for precision and accuracy in transferring maximum volumes of up to 1 mL (Figure 8-13). One type of micropipette, the Eppendorf, dispenses varying volumes of liquid from a disposable tip. The pipette body contains a plunger that provides the suction to pull liquid into the tip when a button is pressed. The maximum displacement of the plunger is set by a dial on the pipette body, enabling the delivery volume to be changed. A number of pipettes and pipette tips for single-use that require a reusable pipette are available. The pipettes or pipette tips are normally disposed of following their use.

Mechanics of Micropipetters

Sterile technique prevents liquid from coming into contact with the pipette when disposable tips are used. The liquid is drawn into and dispensed from a disposable pipette tip, which is changed between transfers. Depressing the tip ejector button removes the tip, which is cast off without being handled by the operator and disposed of safely in an appropriate container. The plunger is depressed to both draw up and dispense the liquid. Normal operation consists of depressing the plunger button to the first stop while the pipette is held in the air. The tip is then submerged in the liquid to be transported and the plunger is released in a slow and even manner. This draws the liquid up into the tip. The instrument is then moved to the desired dispensing location. The plunger is again depressed to the first stop, and then to the second stop, or "blowout," position. This action

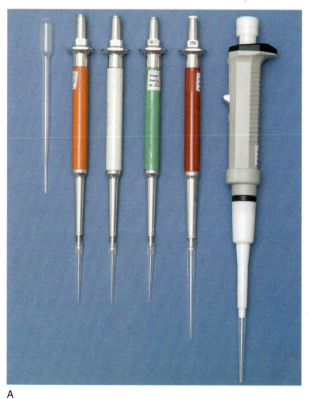

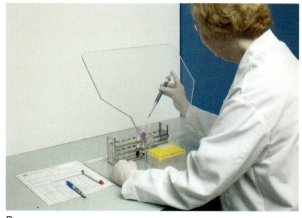

A   B

FIGURE 8-13 (A) Micropipetters with disposable transfer pipette tips. **(B)** Using micropipetter behind clear safety shield.
Source: Delmar/Cengage Learning.

will fully evacuate the tip and dispense the liquid. The volume in an adjustable pipette is variable as the volume in the tip can be changed via a dial or other mechanism depending on the model. Some pipettes indicate the selected volume in a small window for reference.

Semiquantitative Pipettes

For the most part, **semiquantitative pipettes** are not used for accurate measurement but rather for the general transfer of variable amounts from one tube or container to another. Some of these pipettes are etched with markings indicating 0.5- to 1.0-mL volumes, but these are not considered as accurate measurements. They are used only for transfer of approximate volumes of solutions. These basic disposable pipettes designed for estimated amounts are designed for use with a rubber bulb that fits tightly on the large end of the pipette or, in some cases, is built into the pipette. Both types of pipettes are disposable, but the rubber bulb that is required to be fitted onto the pipette is not disposable.

Pasteur and Beral Pipettes

There are two basic types of semiquantitative pipettes that require the use of a bulb for aspirating solutions. The differences between these two types of transfer

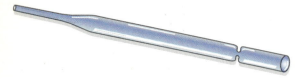

FIGURE 8-14 Pasteur pipette, disposable.
Source: Delmar/Cengage Learning.

pipettes lies in the fact that one uses a separate rubber bulb for aspiration, while the other uses a single piece pipette with the aspirator bulb built into the pipette. The Pasteur pipette (Figure 8-14) uses a separate rubber bulb for aspirating solutions for transfer from one container to the next. Pasteur pipettes are not calibrated for any particular volume and are essentially large droppers that can be used to remove liquid from one container and add it to another. It is not necessary to use a different Pasteur pipette for each test when placing drops of a specific reagent into a number of tubes or other containers. The Pasteur pipette can potentially be reused unless it becomes chipped or contaminated during the procedure.

The second type, the **Beral pipette,** is a one-piece pipette, usually made from flexible soft plastic (polyethylene) that has a built-in bulb on the end (Figure 8-15). Where accurate measurement is not required, the soft plastic bulb can also be filled with fluid to obtain larger volumes than the stem itself would accommodate.

Characteristics of Semiquantitative Pipettes

Originally, pipettes were made of glass and were not disposable. The disposable pipettes in use currently are more common in chemistry procedures when using aqueous solutions. Glass and plastic graduated serological pipettes that may be disposable, as well as disposable Pasteur pipettes, require the use of some kind of additional suction device (Beral pipettes have a built-in suction bulb). This is typically a pipette bulb, which is a rubber bulb that sucks the liquid into the pipette by negative pressure and also allows one to drain the pipette in a controlled fashion. Pasteur pipettes may also be known as droppers or eye droppers

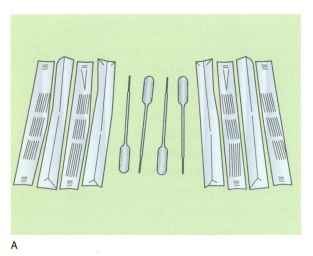

A

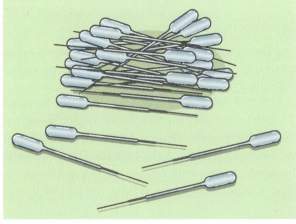

B

FIGURE 8-15 (A) Beral disposable one-piece pipettes may come individually wrapped when clean or sterile pipettes are required. **(B)** For general use that does not require sterility, Beral pipettes come in bulk packages.
Source: Delmar/Cengage Learning.

and are used to transfer or dispense small quantities of liquids. They are usually glass tubes tapered to a narrow point and fitted with a rubber bulb at the top. Pasteur pipettes come in various lengths. They are sold in boxes of hundreds and are generally considered cheap enough to be disposable. However, so long as the glass point is not chipped, the Pasteur pipette can potentially be washed and reused indefinitely. The term *eye dropper* also may refer to early models of fountain pens, which had to be refilled with some kind of Pasteur pipette before the invention of rubber sacks, piston devices, or the modern ink cartridge.

Plastic Beral pipettes are used in a similar manner to Pasteur pipettes and are also referred to as transfer pipettes. They have their stems and bulbs in the form of a single piece made of plastic and are of different sizes depending on the purpose for which they are being used. The volumes are usually marked on the stem, although the markings are usually simple etched lines and are not particularly accurate.

Plastic Pasteur pipettes are often used in biology where most media are aqueous, and solvent resistance is not important. Most organic solvents, such as hexane and acetone, cannot be used in plastic Pasteur pipettes. They dissolve the plastic in these instruments, rendering them inadequate for many types of applications. The pipettes are also hard to wash and are usually discarded with other biohazard or toxic waste after each use. Plastic bulb pipettes are considered not precise enough to be used for even reasonably accurate measurements, whereas their glass counterparts can be extremely precise in some instances. The longer and thinner the tip of a glass pipette, the more accurate is the measurement. Usually these pipettes will be used in conjunction with a scale to accurately measure a volume of fluid.

Piston-Driven Air Displacement Pipettes

Gilson micropipettes are the most accurate and precise pipettes. They are more commonly used in biology, although they are frequently used by chemists as well. These pipettes are designed and manufactured for accurate and precise liquid sample measurements, and are accurate for volumes from 0.2 μL to 10 μL. The plastic pipette tips are designed for aqueous solutions and are not recommended for use with organic solvents which may dissolve the plastic. These pipettes operate by piston-driven air displacement. A vacuum is generated by the vertical movement of a metal or ceramic piston within an airtight sleeve. As the piston moves upward, driven by the depression of the plunger, a vacuum is created in the space left vacant by the piston. Air from the tip rises to fill the space left vacant, and the air is then replaced by the liquid, which is drawn up into the tip and thus available for transport and dispensing elsewhere.

PIPETTE ACCESSORIES

Pipette accessories come in a variety of designs (see Figure 8-10). They are used to facilitate the safe and efficient filling of pipettes.

- **Pipette fillers** are used to fill the pipette easily, avoiding the need for mouth pipetting.

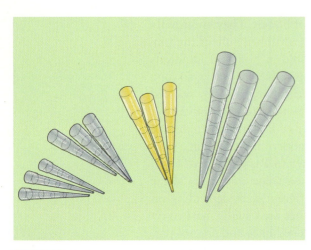

FIGURE 8-16 Pipette tips used with pipetters for extremely small amounts.
Source: Delmar/Cengage Learning.

- **Pipette helpers** are battery operated and are designed to be used with disposable pipette tubes. These disposable pipettes cannot be calibrated and their accuracy is determined by that of the printed graduations on them and the accuracy of the pipette helper itself.
- **Light-guided pipetting systems** are pipetting accessories that are computer based and use flat-screen LCD monitors or LED arrays to light up source and destination wells in microplates or vials for accurate well-to-well pipetting. Some of these systems use text-to-speech to alert the operator during plate or volume changes when pipetting specimens or reagents according to laboratory protocols.
- **Pipette tips**. The pipetters and injection-molded plastic disposable tips (Figure 8-16) together form a reliable pipetting system. It is recommended to use the original manufacturer's tips to guarantee the precision and accuracy of the pipettes. The precision-made pipetter tips provide excellent reproducibility and accuracy. Pipetter tips are available in autoclavable boxes, refills, and bulk packaging. Nonsterile, presterilized, and filtered tips are usually available in single trays and certified for all practical purposes as contaminant and endotoxin free.

ACCURACY IN PIPETTING

Proper care and maintenance of pipettes and pipetters are mandatory to ensure accurate functions of and measurement of solutions. Pipettes and pipetters are generally useful for a period of about 3 years. Wear, fatigue of components, and buildup of materials affecting performance of the pipettes eventually cause them to fail. Calibration and maintenance on a regular schedule will lengthen the useful life of these devices.

Steps to Ensure Accuracy in Pipetting Procedures

Besides the proper calibration of pipetters, a number of other considerations and processes should be observed to achieve optimum accuracy and reproducibility. Consistency of procedures leads to accuracy. The following steps will also eliminate or at least minimize differences that might be present when more than one operator performs the same types of procedures.

- Operator consistency of steps is mandatory to achieve repeatable results. The necessity of operator practice and development of good pipetting practices and habits is absolute. Light-guided pipetting aides may be used to help reduce errors and will speed up liquid handling practices.

- When aspirating a liquid, the tip of the pipette must be submerged 3 to 4 mm below the surface of the liquid, at approximately a 90-degree angle.
- When dispensing a sample, a pipette should be held at a 45-degree angle with the tip placed against the side of the receiving vessel. Glass vessels are preferable as the surface tension of the glass enhances the complete emptying of the tip, avoiding some errors of measurement and resulting in greater accuracy of testing.
- The tip must never be wiped off or blotted in any way, even from the exterior, while liquid is in the tip. These actions tend to attract and thus bleed off some of the liquid, resulting in decreased accuracy and reproducibility.
- A dry tip should be moistened for each aspiration by drawing up and dispensing the chosen volume a minimum of three times. This action reduces the surface tension on the inside walls of the tip and also provides the proper level of intertip humidity, which reduces evaporation of the sample liquid.
- Most pipettes are calibrated "to deliver" (TD) and not "to contain" (TC). If the pipettes are TD pipettes, they should not be rinsed following the delivery of their contents. If the pipette is labeled TC, it should be rinsed to obtain the correct amount of material. If the fluid to be measured is quite viscous or sticky (such as glycerol solutions), the pipette must be calibrated, and in this case the outside of the tip must be carefully wiped with lint-free tissue to remove the liquid adhering to the tip. Care must be exercised not to touch the opening of the pipette tip, a process that may require some practice. Accuracy in delivering liquids with high or low viscosity may require a "positive displacement" or piston-driver type pipetter, which is quite distinct from an air displacement pipetter.
- To achieve maximum accuracy, and especially when calibrating the pipette, relative humidity in the room environment should be maintained between 50% and 75%, and in no case should the humidity be allowed to drop below 50%. Maintaining the correct humidity limits the rate of sample evaporation, which can cause significant errors, especially at lower volumes. Sample evaporation is a problem in dry climate areas and in winter months when humidity is lower than at other seasons. Humidifiers may be necessary to provide for an environment conducive to an acceptable accuracy level for calibrating sensitive pipetters.

Factors Leading to Errors in Pipetting Procedures

The importance of fastidious operator skill cannot be overstated. A high-quality, well-calibrated pipette in the hand of an uninterested or untrained operator is an unreliable instrument. Four basic factors can negatively affect the accuracy and reproducibility of even highly trained laboratory workers, and these factors must be allowed for or minimized to achieve optimal accuracy.

1. Heat can be transferred to the instrument and its metallic components inside the instrument. This can occur through such innocuous sources as heat from the operator's hand in contact with the handle of an instrument and transferred to the metallic components in the instrument. Continuous operation of a pipette for long periods of time may also result in significant heat buildup inside the instrument, causing expansion of sensitive parts involved in calibration. Increases in heat may reduce the accuracy, consistency, and reproduction of data by the instrument. Since the volume that is delivered depends in part on the piston sizes and the tension of the springs that provide the movement for the piston, an action that provides negative pressure results in aspiration of a fluid. Changes in the size of each of the components will change the volume dispensed, and even minimal changes result in inaccuracies for such a sensitive procedure. This effect is more pronounced in low-volume instruments. Additionally, the expansion of a metallic component that interacts with a nonmetallic one that does not expand as readily in the presence of heat may cause the instrument to seem to stick, hang up, or react more slowly. Pipettes with thin handles are particularly susceptible to this phenomenon. Plumper handles are both more ergonomic and less likely to suffer from heat transfer problems. The best technique for maximum accuracy is to use multiple pipettes and rotate them often, storing them between uses in a stand that holds them vertically.

2. Operator fatigue is an often-overlooked but crucial component when seeking maximal accuracy and repeatability. Human beings are not robots, and repetitive motions cause stress in human joints and muscles. Even a well-trained and experienced operator will see a decrease in accuracy and replicability as length of time on a workshift increases. It is for this reason that pipette calibration service providers that are dedicated to excellence limit the number of pipettes that can be calibrated by an individual technician to a daily maximum. Each pipette, and each customer, deserves a high level of care in the treatment of the instrument. Additionally, some dedicated professionals train themselves to pipette ambidextrously, allowing them to reduce arm and finger strain by alternating hands. Another solution is choosing an electronic pipetter, which significantly reduces hand fatigue. Once the operating button is touched, the pipetter always operates the same way, producing user-independent accuracy and precision.

3. Long-term pipette operation can lead to repetitive strain injuries (RSI), such as carpal tunnel syndrome. These injuries may cause significant reductions in accuracy and repeatability by altering the proper pipetting techniques that are crucial to achieving optimal accuracy. Preventive measures include learning to pipette with both hands and alternating hand usage, taking frequent breaks while pipetting, and choosing the most ergonomic (ease and safety of handling) pipette available. Instruments with plumper handles are generally superior in this regard. On the other hand, electronic pipetters, which operate with a light touch, reduce RSI significantly.

4. Let the pipette "rest" for at least one minute after a volume change is made. This does not apply to single-volume instruments, also called *set volume* or *fixed volume pipettes*. A change in the dispensed volume of an adjustable

pipette involves modifying the internal tensioning of a spring that governs the piston's travel distance. Springs subjected to changing tensioning behave more smoothly and consistently when they are allowed to enjoy an interval of rest as they settle into their new configuration. A pipette that is left idle for at least 1 minute after a volume adjustment will perform more accurately than one that is used too quickly. This is especially important when calibrating a pipette.

Pipette Calibration

Pipette calibration, along with other maintenance, is periodically required for pipettes used in diagnostic testing, such as that performed in a clinical laboratory, to provide continued accurate, consistent, and repeatable operation and measurements. The intervals between calibration vary depending on several factors, which include but are not limited to:

- *The skill and training of the operators.* Skilled operators tend to operate the instrument more correctly and make fewer accuracy-robbing mistakes.
- *The liquid dispensed by the pipette.* Corrosive and volatile liquids tend to emit vapors, which ascend into the pipette shaft even under proper operating conditions and may corrode the metal piston and springs, or the seals and o-rings that provide an airtight seal between the piston and the surrounding sleeve.
- *Proper and careful handling.* Pipettes that are frequently dropped, are subjected to careless handling or horseplay, or are not properly stored in a vertical position will tend to degrade in accuracy over time.
- *The accuracy required by the instrument.* Applications requiring maximum accuracy also demand more frequent calibration. Instruments used for purely research applications or in educational settings generally require less frequent calibration.

Under average conditions, most pipettes can be calibrated semiannually (every 6 months) to provide satisfactory performance. Institutions that are regulated by the U.S. Food and Drug Administration generally benefit from quarterly calibration, which is every 3 months. Critical applications may require monthly service, while research and educational institutions may need only annual service. These are general guidelines, and any decision on the appropriate calibration intervals should be made based on knowledge and skill. Also, considerations of the brand and type of pipette in question (some are more reliable than others) should be included in the decision to calibrate pipettes. The conditions under which the pipette is used and the operators themselves are also important factors to consider.

There are two basic methods of calibration for pipettes. One type of calibration is accomplished through means of gravimetric analysis. This requires dispensing samples of distilled water into a receiving vessel placed on a precision analytical balance. The density of water is a well-known constant, and therefore the mass of the dispensed sample provides an accurate indication of the volume that is delivered. Relative humidity, room temperature, and barometric pressure based on altitude above sea level and weather conditions are factors in the accuracy of the measurement. These factors are usually combined and computed by a complex formula where the raw mass data output of a balance provide an adjusted and more accurate measurement. Properly calibrated microbalances, capable of reading in the range of micrograms (10^{-6} g), can also be used effectively for gravimetric analysis of low-volume micropipettes.

The second method, a **colorimetric** method, is the most common method for calibration and uses precise concentrations of colored water to affect the measurement and determine the volume dispensed. A spectrophotometer is used to measure the color difference before and after aspiration of the sample, providing a very accurate reading. This method is more expensive than the more common gravimetric method, due to the cost of the colored reagents which are extremely precise in their concentrations, and is recommended when optimal accuracy is required. This method is also recommended for extremely low-volume pipette calibration, in the 2-μL range, because the inherent and uncertain factors involved with the computation of the gravimetric method, performed with standard laboratory balances, become significant.

SUMMARY

Practically all laboratory procedures, even those of a qualitative nature, require at least minimal accuracy of measurement. Some laboratory tests require almost absolute accuracy to obtain results that are accurate and consistent from operator to operator and from test kit to test kit. A number of factors including cleanliness are involved in ensuring accuracy. Glassware such as the various types of containers found in a clinical laboratory normally are used to measure volumes that will cause little variance when there is as much as a small percentage of deviation from the desired volume. Glass and plastic flasks, beakers, and graduated cylinders only require cleaning to remove residues of materials and to prevent contamination of reagents and test procedures when solutions are measured.

Pipettes that are used manually to contain and to deliver, such as serological (Mohr) pipettes, must be scrupulously cleaned and rinsed after each use if they are not disposable. These are usually constructed of plastic and, under ordinary laboratory conditions without extreme variables in temperature and humidity, allow for an acceptable level of accuracy. They are both used for measuring relatively large volumes but the Mohr might be considered slightly more accurate, as it measures from point to point and the serological pipette measures to the tip of the pipette, which is less accurate than point to point. TD (to deliver) and TC (to contain) pipettes, when used in the prescribed manner, will provide remarkable accuracy in measuring volumes of reagents and other solutions. Most procedures in current use are performed on instruments with built-in pipettes that require little care beyond routine cleaning. Out-of-range controls that are performed with each batch of tests might signal changes in the pipettes requiring recalibration, additional cleaning, or replacement of the pipettes due to wear on the components of the syringe-type measuring devices.

Micropipettes are used for extremely small volumes of materials, usually standards and controls, as well as patient samples. Those found in autoanalyzers may measure amounts of sample as small as 2 to 10 µL. This type requires a pipetter that may be adjustable to several volumes or may be fixed in the volume aspirated. Accuracy levels for these sensitive pieces of equipment are remarkably good. Piston-driven pipettes are found in technically advanced automated equipment and require calibration and cleaning on a regular basis.

REVIEW QUESTIONS

1. A 24-hour urine specimen is received in the laboratory. It is to be measured to within a few milliliters of an exact volume. What type of laboratory container would be best for measuring the volume of urine?

2. A volume of 200 mL of a 50:50 ratio of reagents A and B are to be mixed to prepare a working solution for a certain laboratory procedure. Which container would be most appropriate for preparing this reagent?

3. Describe the difference between a serological pipette and a Mohr pipette.

4. Why is it necessary to dispose of damaged glassware?

5. A patient's sample requires the most accurate method of measuring due to the extremely small volume used. Which pipette would be most useful for this measurement?

CHAPTER 9

LABORATORY MATHEMATICS

LEARNING OBJECTIVES

Upon completion of this chapter, the reader will be able to:

- Compare and contrast pH as to alkalinity or acidity.

- Compare molality with molarity.

- Describe the preparation of a serial dilution of serum.

- Discuss significant figures and their purpose.

- Discuss the grades of water used for preparing medications and laboratory solutions.

- Identify the purpose for using logarithms.

- List the three basic units of the metric system.

KEY TERMS

Acidity	International System of Units (SI)	Normality
Alkalinity	Inulin	Normal solution
Anemia	Kilogram	Percent solution
Beer's law	Kilometers	Significant figures
Celsius	Liters	Solute
Centimeter	Meters	Solvent
Deciliter	Molality	Specific gravity
Fahrenheit	Molal solution	Spectrophotometer
Grams	Molarity	Urinometer
Hemoglobin	Molar solution	

INTRODUCTION

All accredited medical laboratory programs are required to ensure that a background in mathematics is included in the curriculum for the program. Most colleges require at least one course in college-level algebra, which of course requires general knowledge of mathematics. While most calculations for medical laboratory procedures are performed automatically, it is frequently necessary to perform manual calculations. For tests that are not performed on automated systems and for those where an estimate of the values of certain procedures is part of a review of the results, some knowledge of mathematical functions is required.

In some instances, equipment may malfunction and become completely inoperable so it is mandatory that the technician or technologist be able to calculate results when a procedure is performed manually.

Several common calculations are used in the medical laboratory on a frequent basis. Some of these formulae will have been taught in basic chemistry classes as well as in mathematics classes. But it will do well to refresh the student's memory since a number of calculations will be performed manually for various test procedures. The chemistry and serology departments are the laboratory areas most likely to require an analysis by use of mathematics, although hematology will also require some basic mathematics functions. Just a few of the many mathematical functions which exist are presented in the following pages. A number of these calculations will require a knowledge of the metric system. This is necessary to calculate values that are consistent with the factors of measurement used by laboratory equipment and that can be compared with values from another laboratory, possibly even from another country.

Significant Figures

Significant figures refer to the minimum number of digits that are required to accurately provide a meaningful laboratory value. It is important to realize that constituents tested for in all clinical departments of a medical laboratory are often measured in minute quantities. For some procedures, decimal places at least to the tenth will be significant in these determinations. The term *significant figures* refers mostly to a value expressed in scientific notation, for example, 222.4×10^4, which would give an amount of 2,224,000. The whole number would be unwieldy to manipulate in performing calculations so it would be expressed in scientific notation. Almost no clinical laboratory values are expressed in such high denominations, so you will seldom see laboratory values expressed in scientific notation, although research laboratories are likely to use them. Therefore, except in only a few instances, significant numbers for clinical laboratory results are not as important as they for the precise equations for research in physics and chemistry.

In the medical laboratory, significant figures are often thought of as the number or numbers following the decimal. In some laboratory procedures, figures following the decimal point require rounding up or down. For instance, a glucose expressed in milligrams/deciliter (mg/dL) of 109.4 would simply be reported as 109, but a glucose of 109.7 would be documented as a glucose of 110 mg/dL. Some procedures are measured in much smaller denominations than the example of a blood glucose. An example of a value that would be important if expressed in tenths of the units reported would be that of hemoglobin, a laboratory test for the oxygen-carrying iron pigment on the surface of red blood cells. This test is most commonly used to determine if some type of anemia (an insufficient level of hemoglobin) is present. A normal hemoglobin of 12.6 grams/deciliter (g/dL) would not be rounded and would be reported as 12.6 g/dL. In the case of the first example using the blood glucose determination, a value would be interpreted as normal if it were either 109 or 111, so a figure following a decimal point is not significant. In some tests, a gain or loss of one or two digits is inconsequential, but in others, a tenth of a milligram or gram may be of clinical importance.

Logarithms (Negative or Inverse)

Logarithms are not used often in today's laboratory, but certain elements of these mathematical functions are common in laboratory practice, although they are not fully understood by many laboratory workers. An example of a common laboratory calculation using logs of a number is the determination of the pH of a solution (acidity or alkalinity). The pH of a solution is based on the numbers of hydrogen ions (H^+) in the solution. Keep in mind that a neutral solution would have a pH of 7.0, while an acid solution would have a pH less than 7.0 and an alkaline solution would have a pH greater than 7.0. The *character* of a log (number to the left of the decimal) may be positive or negative, and the *mantissa* is the part of the logarithm to the right of the decimal point. Log tables are in the appendix of this book, or may be derived from a calculator with that function. A sample calculation of the pH of a solution is as follows:

Where "X" = log of 2.61 and
"N" = 5 (derived from the superscript of -5),
the equation for determining the pH of a given solution is:

$$pH = x - \log N$$

The hydrogen ion concentration of a solution is 2.61×10^{-5}
From a logarithm table, N is equal to (0.4166) and $x = 5$.
Therefore, the pH for the solution given is:

$$pH = 5 - 0.4166 = 4.5834 \text{ (round to 4.58)}$$

LABORATORY AND SCIENTIFIC SYSTEMS OF MEASUREMENT

Basically, two systems of measurement are used in the world today. One is the English system, which the United States has used since the country was established. The second is the metric system, which is much more accurate for scientific work than the English system for specific measurements of all types. The English system was based on the average anatomical features of the human body. For instance, a yard was the distance from the nose to the end of an outstretched hand, a foot was the length of a bare foot, and an inch was the length of one bone in the finger. Because there are size differences between individuals, the amount of material measured would vary with the size of the individual. Although this system has been standardized, it remains difficult to use.

The International System of Units (SI) was developed in 1960 and is used in science and for many procedures performed by the clinical laboratory. SI is an advanced, more extensive measurement system based on the metric system. Built on the convenience of the number 10, SI is derived from the meter-kilogram-second system rather than the centimeter-gram-second system, where some variations in units were present.

SI measurements are precise and reproducible measurements that provide consistency in the diagnosing of diseases in patients as well as in the preparation of quality control functions. Units of measurement are created as scientific advances

Critical Reminder

Three Basic Types of Measurements

1. *Length or distance*

   Measured in *meters*, which may be divided into units smaller than 1 meter by the addition of a prefix (Table 9-1). See Figure 9-1 for a comparison of the common English system of inches and a contrasting scale of millimeters. Figure 9-1 shows a comparison of a nonmetric or English-style ruler and the metric scale on the opposite side of the ruler, which shows that 1 inch is equal to 2.54 centimeters (cm) (25.4 millimeters [mm]). Both of these units of measurement are commonly used in the clinical laboratory.

2. *Weight or mass*

   Measured in *grams* (g), which may be divided into units smaller than 1 gram by the addition of a prefix (Table 9-1). Most electronic scales can be adjusted to provide measurements in both ounces (English system) and grams (metric system). See Figure 9-2 for two types of analytical laboratory balances used for accurate measurements in both English and metric methods.

3. *Volume*

   Measured in *liters* (L) as the base unit. Again, a prefix may precede the base unit to measure units either smaller or greater than 1 liter, that is, 1 mL is 1/1,000th of 1 liter.

occur and definitions are modified through nearly international agreement. Three countries (Myanmar, Liberia, and the US) have not entirely embraced the new system except for certain areas such as clinical laboratory science. In the United States, the National Bureau of Standards sets the official units of measurement by law, under very strict standards and environmental conditions.

Basic measurements used in the medical laboratory relate to length, weight (mass), and volume. Measurements used by the MLT/CLT student will include such measurements as the concentration of solutions, which includes both weight and volume measurements. Temperature and units of time in seconds are also standard measurements used in the laboratory.

The two devices commonly used for measuring length and weight (mass is similar) are shown in Figures 9-1 and 9-2. The analytical balances are more commonly used in the clinical laboratory and the metric ruler would be most often used in the anatomic laboratory.

Elements Used in the Metric System

Length (distance), volume (displacement), and weight (includes mass, slightly different from weight) are all types of measurements you will use, as well as time and temperature. The units of the metric system used for the three basic types of measurement are **meters** for length (distance), **grams** for weight (mass), and **liters** for volume (displacement).

Temperature and time are also measurements you will use. For the most part in the clinical laboratory, temperature is measured in degrees **Celsius** (formerly referred to as centigrade), but sometimes in degrees Kelvin (absolute temperature) for the most advanced scientific studies.

Various facilities make decisions as to whether a 12-hour or 24-hour time system is to be used. The 24-hour system is most

Table 9-1 Useful Prefixes

The most often used prefixes in the clinical laboratory when weighing or measuring volumes:

Prefix	Meaning	Prefix	Meaning
Deca	Refers to 10	Deci	Refers to one-tenth (0.1)
Hecto	Refers to 100	Centi	Refers to one-hundredth (0.01)
Kilo	Refers to 1,000	Milli	Refers to one-thousandth (0.001)

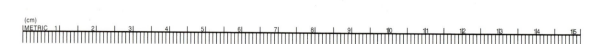

FIGURE 9-1 Comparison of nonmetric (*top scale*) and metric (*bottom scale*) rulers.
Source: Delmar/Cengage Learning.

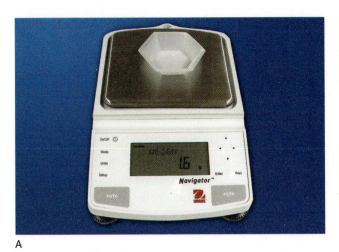
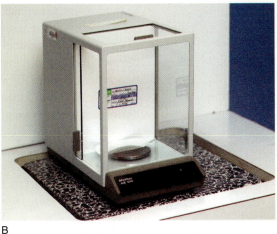

A   B

FIGURE 9-2 (A) Compact portable electronic scale. (B) Cabinet balance.
Source: Delmar/Cengage Learning.

common in medical facilities as it prevents confusions with times that are A.M. and
P.M. Midnight is 0000 hours, noon is 1200 hours, and afternoon and evening hours
are added to 12 (noon). Thus, 1:00 A.M. is 0100 hours, and 1:00 P.M. is 1300 hours
under the 24-hour system.

Useful Metric Terms

The metric system uses decimal notations in increments of 10. Units that are
smaller than the three basic units may be obtained by dividing by increments
of 10, or multiplying by a *power* of 10. As an example, the prefix *kilo* refers
to "1,000," so a kiloliter would be 1,000 L. Other useful prefixes are shown
in Table 9-1. Table 9-2 shows conversions in size by use of scientific notation,
which helps to avoid using numbers with many zeros.

CONVERTING UNITS OF MEASUREMENT

Converting One Metric Unit to Another

When performing laboratory determinations, it is often necessary to convert from one
metric unit to another. If one knows the equivalents, it is quite simple, much more

Table 9-2 Scientific Notations (Units Increased or Decreased by Powers)

This table shows the consistent gains and decreases in size or number, as the prefixes change in
relation to the scientific notations.

10^n	Prefix	Decimal	10^n	Prefix	Decimal
10^{-12}	pico	.000000000001	10^{12}	tera	1,000,000,000,000
10^{-9}	nano	.000000001	10^{9}	giga	1,000,000,000
10^{-6}	micro	.000001	10^{6}	mega	1,000,000
10^{-3}	milli	.001	10^{3}	kilo	1,000
10^{-2}	centi	.01	10^{2}	hecto	100
10^{-1}	deci	.1	10^{1}	deca	10

so than with the English system. For example, the technician or technologist might need to know how many milligrams are in grams, or a fraction of a gram, since the measurement may involve a value of less than a gram. The prefix *milli-* literally means "one-thousandth." For example, 700 milligrams (mg) would indicate 700 thousandths of a gram, which is 70% of a gram, since 700/1,000 equals 70%.

To *convert measurements from a smaller unit to a larger unit*, such as milligrams to grams (weight), the decimal in the original unit would be moved to the left. For example, because there are 1,000 milligrams in a gram (1 mg = .001), the decimal would be moved three places to the left to indicate 1 gram. A value of 1,200 mg, then, could be converted to grams by moving the decimal three places to the left from the end of 1,200 to make the value 1.2 grams.

To *convert measurements from a larger unit to a smaller unit*, such as liters to milliliters (volume), the decimal would be moved to the right. An example would be that of the conversion of 3.5 liters to milliliters (mL) by moving the decimal to the right three places: 3.5 L to 3500 mL. One should begin to remember some of the basic names and abbreviations used for the various units, such as the designation mL for milliliter, which is also synonymous with a cubic centimeter (cc). Pipettes are devices designed in most cases for measuring liquids in milliliters. Reagents or chemicals used to test for certain components of blood are measured in milliliters or fractions of milliliters. Patients' samples are much smaller in newer procedures and are measured in thousandths of milliliters called microliters (μL).

Converting mg/dL to mmol/L or from mmol/L to mg/dL is often necessary when the clinician to whom the result is reported requires it. Certain countries use mmol/L instead of mg/dL. To get the equivalent mmol, you can multiply, for instance, a glucose value in mg/dL by the conversion factor of 0.05551 (example: 110 mg/dL × 0.05551 = 6.1 mmol/L) (Table 9-3). Or, you can use an easier but less precise way by dividing the mg/dL value by 18 to get the equivalent number in mmol/L (example: a glucose of 110 mg/dL will be divided by 18 = 6.1 mmol/L). Factors for converting from mg/dL to mmol/L or vice versa require a different factor for each analyte tested for.

Table 9-3 Conversion Factors from mg/dL to mmol/L (for Glucose Only)

mmol/L	mg/dL	mmol/L	mg/dL	mmol/L	mg/dL
0.06	1	6.7	120	16.0	288
0.28	5	7.0	126	16.6	300
0.55	10	7.2	130	17.0	306
1.0	18	7.5	135	18.0	325
1.5	27	7.8	140	19.0	342

NOTE: These factors are for glucose only. Other analytes will be entirely different.

Converting English Units to Metric Units

In the medical laboratory it is often necessary to convert English units to metric units to complete an equation. Table 9-4 is an easy-to-understand reference for these conversions. There are often conveniently located charts in medical

Table 9-4 Common English Units and Their Equivalent Metric Units of Measurement

	English Unit	English Abbreviation	Multiplication Factor	To Obtain Metric Unit	Abbreviation for Metric Unit
Length/ Distance	1 mile	mi	1.8	1 kilometer	km
	1 yard	yd	0.9	1 meter	m
	1 inch	in	2.54	1 centimeter	cm
Weight/ Mass	1 pound	lb	0.454	1 kilogram	kg
	1 pound	lb	454	1 gram	g
	1 ounce	oz	28	1 gram	g
Volume	1 quart	qt	0.95	1 liter	L
	1 fluid ounce*	fl oz	30	1 milliliter	mL
	1 teaspoon*	tsp	5	1 milliliter	mL

*Also may be called apothecary (pharmacy) units.

laboratories and on scientific calculators to accomplish this task. Scientific research has always used a metric system mainly because of the global aspect of this type of work, but it is imperative that the clinical laboratory worker feels equally comfortable with both metric and English units of measure. Because the English system does not allow for merely moving a decimal place to the right or left, it is necessary to memorize some English units and their equivalent metric units. We are most likely to round off English system factors as it is simply too cumbersome to carry out the functions for several decimal places. The most common equivalents of English and metric system units used are given below.

Common English Units and Metric Equivalents

Length

1 inch   = 2.54 centimeters (*centi*- means "100th" and is 1/100th of 1 meter)

1 foot (12 inches) = 12 × 2.54 or 30.5 centimeters (cm)

Distance

1 mile   = 1.6 kilometers

There are 5,280 feet in 1 mile, so it is more convenient to convert this measurement to kilometers (rounded-off), since 1,000 meters equals 1 kilometer.

Weight/Mass

1 pound   = 454 grams (rounded off)

1 kilogram   = 0.454 pound

1 pound   = 16 ounces (oz), so dividing 454 grams by 16 oz gives 28 grams per oz

Volume

1 quart (qt)   = 0.95 liters (L)

1 fluid ounce   = 30 milliliters (mL)

1 teaspoon (tsp) = 5 mL

Common Metric Equivalents

Mass

1×10^{-3} kg	= 1 gram (g)	.001 kg
1×10^{-3} g	= 1 milligram (mg)	.000001 g
1×10^{-3} mg	= 1 microgram (mcg)	.000000001 mg
1×10^{-3} mcg	= 1 nanogram (ng)	.000000000001 mcg

Volume

10^3 mL	= 1 L
10^3 µL	= 1 mL
10^2 mL	= 1 dL (10 squared = 100 mL, or 1 dL [deciliter])

Converting Temperature from Degrees Fahrenheit to Degrees Celsius

Temperature conversions are also required in many chemistry calculations. Degrees Celsius (°C) is the standard method of temperature measurement for scientific operations. Most households in the United States still use the **Fahrenheit** (°F) scale for body temperature measurement, and household appliances most often use the Fahrenheit scale (Figure 9-3).

Formula for Converting Fahrenheit to Celsius

Values for conversions where C = 32° and F = 56° are as follows:

C = 5/9 (F − 32)	Example 5/9 × (56 − 32) = 0.556 × 24 = 13.3°C
F = 9/5 (C) + 32	Example 9/5 × 32 + 32 = 1.8 × 32 + 32 = 89.6°F

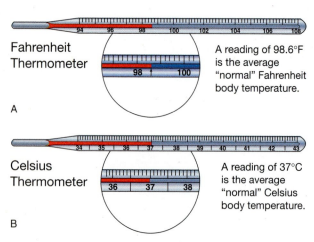

A

B

FIGURE 9-3 (A) Fahrenheit and **(B)** Celsius Thermometers used in measuring body temperature.
Source: Delmar/Cengage Learning.

A chart is in many cases the most convenient for conversions from Fahrenheit to Celsius and vice versa. Some common numbers that may be converted are shown in Table 9-5.

INTERNATIONAL SYSTEM OF UNITS (SI)

Although an attempt to standardize the reporting of laboratory results by using SI units has been underway for at least 40 years in this country, a great deal of resistance has been encountered. Tests were performed and reported as milligrams or grams per deciliter before the SI system came to the forefront in many countries. The SI system uses actual cell counts and millimoles of the measured material (analyte) per liter. Sometimes a facility will report the values in both denominations, but conversion from the previously-used method to the SI units is possible. With global relationships in business and in medicine, as well as differences in the reporting of values even in the United States, it is necessary to become familiar with the two basic methods of reporting values, particularly in chemistry tests. The clinical laboratory worker may be considered as a valuable reference resource for explaining the units used for reporting the various values. Sometimes report forms will document the results of laboratory procedures in both denominations. Values frequently encountered in the SI system are shown in Tables 9-6 and 9-7.

Table 9-5 Temperature Conversion Chart, Fahrenheit to Celsius

°F	°C	°F	°C	°F	°C	°F	°C	°F	°C	°F	°C
32	0	90	32.2	100	37.8	105	40.6	110	43.3	115	46.1
70	21.1	95	35	101	38.3	106	41.1	111	43.9	116	46.7
75	23.9	97	36.1	102	38.9	107	41.7	112	44.4	117	47.2
80	26.7	**98.6**	**37.0**	103	39.4	108	42.2	113	45	118	47.8
85	29.4	99	37.2	104	40	109	42.8	114	45.6	119	48.3

NOTE: 98.6°F and 37°C = normal (average) body temperature of a human.

Table 9-6 Values in the SI System

Blood cell counts are sometimes reported by both units of measurement.

Previously Used Nomenclature	SI System Nomenclature
Micron (µm)	Micrometer (µm), or 10^{-6} m (meter)
Cubic micron (formerly used for blood cell size)	Femtoliter (fL) or 10^{-15} L
Angstrom	Nanometer (nm) or $\times 10^{-9}$ m
Lambda	Microliter (µL) or 10^{-6} L

Table 9-7 Examples of SI Units in Blood Cell Counts

Example of reporting a complete blood count with red blood cell (RBC) indices (size and concentration of hemoglobin).

Constituent	Conventional Unit	SI Unit
Red and white cell counts	#/cu. mm (mm³)	Cells/microliter or liter
Hematocrit (% of red cells/whole blood)	Percentage, i.e., 36%	Decimal, i.e., .36
Hemoglobin	g/dL	g/L
MCV (mean corpuscular volume)	μ^3	fL
MCH (mean corpuscular hemoglobin)	Uµg	pg
MCHC (mean corpuscular hemoglobin concentration)	%	g/dL or g/L

PREPARING SOLVENTS FOR USE IN THE MEDICAL LABORATORY

Concentration refers to the amount of **solute** (material being dissolved) in a **solvent** (substance, usually a liquid, in which another substance is dissolved). Many reagents come with the mixtures already prepared under strict conditions and accurate measuring. However, it is sometimes necessary for the laboratory worker to prepare solutions of a given concentration. Of extreme importance along with the accurate measurement of both solute and solvent is the purity of the chemicals. Water is often the solvent for chemicals used in the medical laboratory, and a method of manufacture is used to prepare extremely pure materials when required. Chemicals with a purity designation of USP and NF grade (see Table 9-8) may be used to manufacture medications as they are pure enough not to cause injury to the patient who will receive the medication. Laboratory grade chemicals, including water, must be AR or ACS, or have the term "for laboratory use" printed on the label of the container. These chemically pure reagents help to avoid erroneous results based on reactions occurring other than with those analytes (chemical constituents) being tested for.

Reagent Grade Water

The quality of water needed in the laboratory varies by the purpose for which it is used. Preparation of reagents and solutions, reconstituting of lyophilized specimens, and sample dilutions must meet certain specific requirements for purity level. Water used in a laboratory should be free of interfering substances, and those preparing these various dilutions and reconstitutions must be aware of the purity of water needed. Errors that are clinically significant may be obtained from test results if water impurities are not removed prior to use.

There are three basic levels of water purity established by the National Committee for Clinical Laboratory Standards and the College of American Pathologists (CAP). Type I water is used quickly as it may absorb carbon dioxide. Types II and III may be stored in glass and polyethylene containers but are used as quickly as feasible due to possible contamination with airborne microorganisms. Reagent water is normally used as soon as prepared, as purity cannot be maintained for a considerable length of time.

Table 9-8 Grades of Chemicals

AR	Reagent grade or analytic reagent	High degree of purity, used in preparing reagents in clinical laboratory
CP	Chemically pure	Sufficiently pure for some purposes, but impurities not provided; not used for research
USP	May be less pure than CP reagents	Specifications established by the United States Pharmacopeia
NF	Similar to standards for USP	Specifications set by National Formulary

Type I

Type I is the purest type of reagent water for certain procedures where maximum quality is required and where measurements of analytes are in nanograms (ng) or subnanograms.

Type II

This type of water may contain microorganisms but is suitable for most procedures in the clinical laboratory and other clinical test areas.

Type III

Type III water may be used in urinalysis procedures, and in washing and rinsing laboratory glassware. However, a final rinsing with Type I or Type II water may be necessary based on methods for which this glassware will be used.

Methodology for Preparing Pure Water

Water obtained from areas with industrial contamination of water and soil, such as inorganic and organic materials from farming, may contain materials that no single purification system can remove. Sometimes more than one method is used to prepare water for laboratory use, such as deionization and distillation. For instance, distilled water may be treated by a deionization process to obtain a higher degree of purity. The presence of ionizable materials in water can be measured by the conductance or electrical resistance of the water being tested. Most deionizers and distillers have purity meters which warn the user if there is an unacceptable level of contaminants.

Deionized Water

Substances that can ionize (form charged particles) are passed through resin columns that contain both positively and negatively charged particles. The ions in the water will combine with the particles in the resin columns but some organic and other substances that do not ionize will not be removed, and will require other removal methods. Type I water is produced by this method.

Distilled Water

Distilled water is made by a simple process of boiling the water and allowing the steam to condense on a surface. Distilling water removes minerals found in natural water sources. This process produces Type II and Type III water. The method eliminates microorganisms but the water may contain carbon dioxide, chlorine, and ammonia.

Other Methods of Purifying Water

Water of higher purification may be produced by using both deionization and distillation, while other methodologies are also available. *Reverse osmosis* is a process where water is passed through a semipermeable membrane under pressure, which removes roughly 90% of the impurities from dissolved solids such as minerals, and perhaps 98% of organic impurities, including microorganisms and other undissolved materials. Reverse osmosis does not remove carbon dioxide and other dissolved gases, and removes only a tenth of ionized particles. *Filtration* removes insoluble materials, and activated charcoal, clays, and other materials can be used to remove organic materials. These methods result in the production of Type I water.

MEASURING SOLUTION STRENGTH

A concentration of an analyte (material being tested for) is expressed in several ways. The most common methods for measuring concentrations or strength of the reagent's active component would be expressed as a percent solution, either molar, molal, or normal. These terms for measurement mainly relate to preparing basic chemical solutions but are no less important when performing chemical reactions on body fluids. The amount of specimen and the amount of analytes in the specimen is based on concentration, and calculating the results often requires a factor for the dilution of the ratio of sample and reagent.

Percent Solutions

Percent solutions refer to the amount of solute expressed as parts per 100 parts of solution. As an example, a 10% solution would have 10 parts of solute and 90 parts of solvent, making a total of 100 parts. Rarely, one will have the situation where there would be 10 parts in 100 parts of solvent. This situation would be expressed as 10 in 100, as the total volume would then be 110 parts. Therefore, this would be different from a 10% solution. For general laboratory use, percent solutions are most often used in performing tests that require they be made fresh by the laboratory worker. Figure 9-4 shows two methods of preparing percent solutions. *A* is a weight-to-volume (w/v) problem, and *B* is a volume-to-volume (v/v) problem.

Molar Solutions

A molar solution refers to a type of reagent sometimes prepared for use in the clinical laboratory. Molarity refers to the number of moles (mol) of solute per liter (L) that are dissolved in a solution. Commercially prepared chemistry reagents for performing clinical chemistry tests are often made as a molar solution. Test results may be based on the amount of solute called a substrate that is found in specific amounts in the reagent. One mole of a substance, which is its gram molecular weight (gmw), when dissolved in 1 liter (L) of solvent is a molar solution of 1 mol/L, or 1 M. The SI unit of measurement for many chemistry procedures is based on millimoles/L (10^{-3} or thousandths). Sometimes, for analytes found in very small amounts in the human body, the reagents will be in micromoles/L (10^{-6} or millionths), and nanomoles/L (10^{-9} or billionths). Figure 9-5 shows the information needed and the calculations for preparing a molar solution of sodium hydroxide (NaOH).

A

Problem:	Prepare 500 mL of 0.85% saline.
Solution:	1. A 0.85% solution contains 0.85 g of the solute in every 100 mL of solution. 2. Therefore, to prepare 500 mL, 5 × 0.85 g, or 4.25 g, of sodium chloride (NaCl) must be used. 3. To prepare the solution: a. Weigh out 4.25 g of NaCl. b. Fill a 500 mL volumetric flask approximately half full with water. c. Add 4.25 g of NaCl and swirl gently to dissolve. d. Add water to the flask's fill line.

B

Problem:	Prepare 500 mL of 10% bleach solution.
Solution:	1. A 10% solution of bleach contains 10 mL bleach (hypochlorite) per 100 mL of solution. 2. Therefore, 500 mL of solution would contain 50 mL of bleach (5 × 10 mL). 3. To prepare the solution: a. Place 450 mL of water into a flask or bottle. b. Add 50 mL of bleach. c. Carefully mix; label the container.

FIGURE 9-4 (A) Percent solution as a weight-to-volume measurement; **(B)** percent solution as a volume-to-volume measurement.
Source: Delmar/Cengage Learning.

Problem:	Prepare one liter of a 2 M solution of NaOH.
Solution:	The gram molecular weight of NaOH is 40. A 2 M solution of NaOH contains 40 X 2 g/L. One liter of a 2 M solution contains 80 grams NaOH in one liter of solution
Explanation:	As described previously, 1 gmw is 1 mole of a substance. For sodium hydrox-ide, 1 mole equals 40 grams as derived by adding the molecular weights for the three atoms: 1 mole of sodium (Na) is 23, 1 mole of oxygen (O) is 16 grams, and 1 mole of hydrogen (H) is 1. **Solution:** 80 g NaOH/40 (gmw) = 2.0 mol/L or 2 molar solution or 2 M

FIGURE 9-5 Preparation of a 2 M solution of NaOH (sodium hydroxide).
Source: Delmar/Cengage Learning.

Molal Solutions

Molality is sometimes confused with molarity. Molality is always used as weight per weight, where a relationship is established between the weight of the solute and the weight of the solvent. Therefore, molality is unlike molarity as it is always expressed as moles per kilogram of solvent, or mol/kg.

Normal Solutions

Normality differs from molarity and molality by using the term *equivalent weight,* which is the gram molecular weight divided by its valence, or the number of units or ions that can combine with or replace 1 mole of hydrogen ions (H⁺). The SI does not recommend normality as a measurement unit in reporting test results. In previous years, when normality was used routinely, electrolytes such as sodium, potassium, and chloride were reported as milliequivalents per liter (mEq/L). The proper SI methodology for reporting these electrolytes is now millimoles per liter (mmol/L).

pH-Adjusted Solutions

Although it is rare that a laboratory worker finds it necessary to prepare a solution of a specific pH, sometimes an acid or alkaline solution may be required. Some requirements for preserving a sample or preparing a volume of solution with a certain pH may be necessary, and it is well that a laboratory worker be familiar with this procedure.

The pH of a solution is based on the hydrogen ion (H⁺) concentration, which indicates the acidity or alkalinity. For basic estimates, pH (sometimes called litmus) paper may be used. A color chart is usually provided with litmus paper for this purpose. This is sufficient for measuring the pH of a urine specimen, as is found on the pad on a urine chemistry dipstick, but is not sensitive enough to provide accuracy for laboratory reagents in many cases.

Principle of Adjusting pH

A neutral pH is 7.0, which is the pH of pure water. The hydrogen ion concentration and the hydroxyl (OH⁻) ion content are equal. Values above a 7.0 pH are alkaline. Human blood is slightly alkaline (7.35–7.45), which is a critical value needed for the body's metabolic processes to continue. Values below 7.0 are termed acidic. A number of substances are used to adjust the pH of a solution. Fruit juices, vinegar, and hydrochloric acid (also called hydrogen chloride and HCl) will serve to acidify solutions. Baking soda, sodium hydroxide (NaOH), and potassium hydroxide (KOH) will make solutions more alkaline. HCl is rich in hydrogen ions, and sodium or potassium are rich in hydroxyl ions, so they are most commonly used to adjust the pH of solutions.

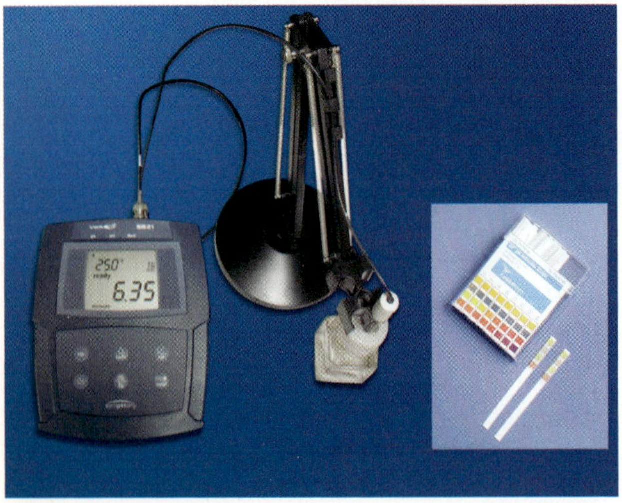

FIGURE 9-6 pH meter along with pH indicator strips used for basic screening tests for pH.
Source: Delmar/Cengage Learning.

pH Meter

The pH meter (Figure 9-6) reflects the hydrogen ion content by comparing it to a reference electrode, in which the electrical potential across a membrane in the electrode is measured. These instruments are extremely sensitive and accurate, providing the value for the pH on a dial or screen, measured to the hundredths (i.e., 7.82) and on some instruments even to the thousandths. pH meter probes that are placed into the solution being analyzed must be cleaned with distilled or deionized water between uses but are not stored in water. Electrodes are calibrated by the use of known values of pH solutions or standards, with both acid and alkaline solutions used in the adjustments of the instrument.

Specific Gravity

Specific gravity refers to the concentration of a solution. This calculation may also be thought of as the density of a solution and is based on the comparison of pure water to a solution with dissolved substances in it. *Density* is described as the ratio of the concentration (the amount of solutes dissolved in the solvent) of a material at a certain temperature. Occasionally, it is necessary to determine the specific gravity and to adjust a reagent to a specific level when performing certain procedures, such as a flotation test for parasitic ova. Urine specimens in the laboratory are commonly tested for specific gravity. This is estimated by the use of a test that is not specifically a test of the density but compares well with an actual specific gravity. This test measures the presence of ionic concentration of the urine specimen by color changes on a chemically-treated dipstick. This method is acceptable for determining that the pH range is normal. A **urinometer**, a modified cylinder with a flotation device, gives an accurate specific gravity when the conditions of temperature and cleanliness of the device are acceptable (Figure 9-7); it compares urine with pure water. Most urinometers are designed for optimum performance at ambient or room temperature (RT) of 26–27°C, but some are gauged for 20°C. An example of the calculation of the specific gravity (density) of a given solution would be as follows:

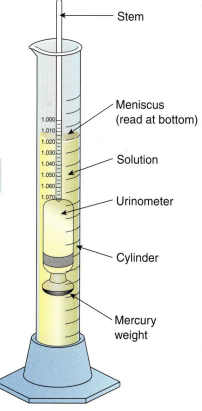

Weight of solution for analysis/Weight of pure water (1.000) = Specific gravity

Another method for determining specific gravity is the use of a refractometer, where dissolved solids bend light waves; it compares a solution with air (Figures 9-8 and 9-9).

Differences between Values by Three Types of Specific Gravity Determinations

Except in rare circumstances, a specific gravity measured by any of the three methods above is acceptable because, in most cases, differences between the three methods are negligible, although each relies on a different measurement principle.

- Urinalysis dipstick—Measures dissolved ions
- Urinometer—Compares solution with pure water
- Refractometer—Measures specimen against air

FIGURE 9-7 A urinometer is sometimes used to determine the specific gravity of a urine specimen.
Source: Delmar/Cengage Learning.

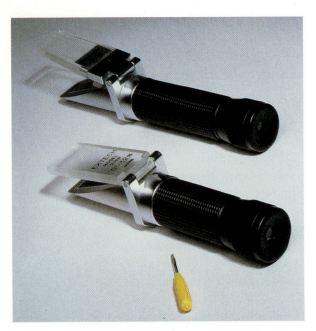

FIGURE 9-8 Refractometer that compares solutions with air.
Source: Delmar/Cengage Learning.

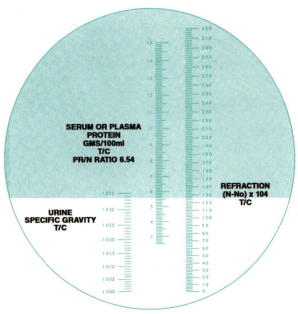

FIGURE 9-9 Refractometer scale showing a specific gravity of 1.034; note the scale for serum or plasma protein.
Source: Delmar/Cengage Learning.

PREPARING SOLUTIONS FROM A MORE CONCENTRATED STRENGTH TO A MORE DILUTE STRENGTH

Some reagents are labeled as dilute, concentrated, saturated, or supersaturated. This does not indicate a definitive measure as to the concentration of a reagent. Temperature, presence of other ions (charged particles), and other factors greatly affect the amount of solute that can be dissolved in a solution. These terms are more qualitative than quantitative in nature. A dilute specimen contains little solute, while a concentrated solution contains much more. A supersaturated solution contains a great deal of undissolved solute particles. Physical tests (also called colligative properties) may also be used in diagnosing the disease state of a patient. For example, the osmolality or high level of ions that are present in urine or plasma is determined by the effect they have on the temperature at which the solution freezes.

Calculations for Obtaining the Desired Solution Strength

Most solutions can be bought from commercial suppliers. However, some solutions come as concentrates, and it is necessary to prepare them according to the strength needed. In addition, some solutions must be prepared as "working reagents" by adding two or more solutions together. These reagents may be required to be fresh, as the reactivity may be lost on standing for a period of time. In Figures 9-10 and 9-11, two methods of preparing solutions are provided.

Problem:	A buffer is made by adding 2 parts of solution A to 5 parts of solution B. How much of solution A and solution B would be required to make 70 mL of the buffer?
Formula:	$\dfrac{\text{Total volume required (C)}}{\text{parts of A + parts of B}}$ = volume of one part (V)
Solution:	$\dfrac{70 \text{ mL required}}{2 \text{ parts of A} + 5 \text{ parts of B}} = V$
	$\dfrac{70}{7} = 10 \text{ mL} = V$
	2 parts of solution A = $2 \times 10 = 20$ mL 5 parts of solution B = $5 \times 10 = 50$ mL
Answer:	The buffer would be made by mixing 20 mL of solution A with 50 mL of solution B to give a total volume of 70 mL.

FIGURE 9-10 Preparing a solution using proportion.
Source: Delmar/Cengage Learning.

Problem:	Prepare 100 mL of 0.1 M HCl using 1.0 M HCl.
Formula:	$C_1 \times V_1 = C_2 \times V_2$
Solution:	$(1.0 \text{ M}) (V_1) = (100 \text{ mL}) (0.1 \text{ M})$
	$V_1 = \dfrac{100 \text{ mL} \times 0.1}{1.0}$
	$V_1 = 10 \text{ mL}$
Answer:	10 mL of 1.0 M HCl is added to 90 mL of H_2O to make 100 mL of 0.1 M HCl solution.

FIGURE 9-11 Preparing a solution using the formula $C_1 \times V_1 = C_2 \times V_2$, where C = concentration and V = volume.
Source: Delmar/Cengage Learning.

Dilutions

The term *dilution* refers to a concentrated material that may need to be diluted to meet the requirements for a certain procedure. This would also be relevant if a patient sample were of such a concentration for a constituent such as glucose, that the method used for determining the level would be higher than the procedure could accurately handle (called *linearity*). The stock solution provided would need to be diluted with a solvent such as water where the total volume of the concentrated solution along with the volume of the diluent (solvent) would be compared with the concentration of the stock solution. This is called the *dilution factor*. As the dilution factor increases, the concentration of the solute (concentrated stock solution) decreases. An example for diluting a stock solution would be as follows:

1. What dilution factor would be needed to prepare a 50 mEq/L solution of NaOH (sodium hydroxide) from a 2,000 mEq/L stock solution by diluting with distilled water?
   Solution: 50 mEq/2,000 mEq = 5/200 or 1-to-25 dilution factor or 1:25
2. If 100 mL of the 50 mEq solution is needed, the dilution ratio of stock concentrate to total volume must be observed. The ratio of the dilution needed is 1 mL of stock to 25 mL of the diluent.

   Solution: $\dfrac{1}{25} = \dfrac{x}{100}$

Therefore, $25x = 100$, so $x = 4$. In order to maintain a total volume of the desired 100 mL, 96 mL of diluent would be added to 4 mL of the stock concentrate.

Serial Dilutions of Sample

It is sometimes necessary to quantitate the level of a component of the blood serum or plasma by diluting the sample and then reacting the diluted samples. For example, to quantitate the level of antibodies against a certain antigen, a serum sample would require serial dilutions growing less and less concentrated, and then reacting the diluted samples with the antigen. The last tube showing a reaction would be the end-point and the results would be a semi-quantitative result. The increasing dilution levels must be consistent, e.g., they must increase from 1:2, 1:4, 1:8, etc., or 1:10, 1:20, 1:40, etc. See Table 9-9 for an example of the dilutions for a two-fold dilution series.

Procedure for Serial Dilution

From Table 9-9, the procedure is as follows:

1. 1.0 mL from tube 1 mixture will be added to tube 2.
2. After mixing, 1.0 mL from tube 3 will be added to tube 4, and so on, until all tubes have been treated. Note that each tube will contain 1 mL when the mixture from the preceding tube is added.

Table 9-9 Serial Dilution Starting with a 1:2 Dilution

Table shows dilution factors when diluted specimens from previous tube are added to the next tube.

	Tube 1	Tube 2	Tube 3	Tube 4	Tube 5	Tube 6	Tube 7	Tube 8	Tube 9*
Resulting ratio	1:2	1:4	1:8	1:16	1:32	1:64	1:128	1:256	1:512
Serum	1.0 mL	…	…	…	…	…	…	…	…
Diluent	1.0 mL	1.0 mL	1.0 mL	1.0 mL	1.0 mL	1.0 mL	1.0 mL	1.0 mL	1.0 mL
Diluted sample—from previous tube	…	1.0 mL	1.0 mL	1.0 mL	1.0 mL	1.0 mL	1.0 mL	1.0 mL	1.0 mL

*The last tube will contain 2 mL, so 1.0 mL must be discarded.

1. Set up 9 tubes, each containing 1.0 mL of diluent.
2. Transfer 1.0 mL of patient serum to tube 1.
3. Mix the serum and diluent, and transfer 1.0 mL of the mixture to tube 2.
4. Repeat the procedure, transferring 1.0 mL each time after mixing with diluent.
5. Discard 1.0 mL from the last tube.
6. When dilution series is complete, each of the nine tubes should contain 1.0 mL.

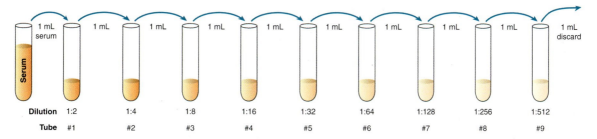

FIGURE 9-12 **Setting up and performing a two-fold serial dilution.**
Source: Delmar/Cengage Learning.

3. The last tube will contain 2.0 mL, so 1.0 mL must be discarded from this tube, since the addition of any indicator cells, etc., would change the dilution of the last tube (Figure 9-12).

Interpretation

Each sample after the first tube will have 1.0 mL added to an equal amount of diluent. This will effectively cut by one-half the strength of the preceding tube from tubes 2 through 9. If a reaction occurred in tubes 1 through 5, the result would be reported as positive at a 1:32 dilution.

BEER'S LAW

Beer's law is used when a **spectrophotometer** measures the amount of light absorbed when the beam is directed through a solution that may be colored or where a reaction may occur at a wavelength not visible to the naked human eye. These values are measured with an ultraviolet wavelength and are often used for enzymatic reactions where an enzyme reacts with a substrate contained in the reagent. Many reactions follow **Beer's law** (that the absorption coefficient is directly proportional to the concentration of a solution) when a given wavelength is established under conditions of temperature, pH, length of the light wave, and the depth of the chamber in which the reacting substances are placed (this is often standardized at 1 cm).

Automated instruments and manual spectrophotometers use this law for many common analyses of constituents in the human blood and other body fluids. When a manual assay is being performed, the amount of concentration in a patient's sample is compared with a known standard. A simple Beer's law graph (Figure 9-13) indicates absorbance in nanometers (nm). A spectrophotometer is used to measure the absorbance of the standard and the absorbance

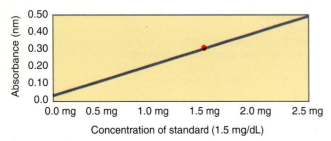

FIGURE 9-13 Beer's law graph.
Source: Delmar/Cengage Learning.

of the blood sample. The operation of a spectrophotometer is indicated in Figure 9-14. As shown by the line in Figure 9-13, a standard with a concentration of 1.5 mg/dL gives a spectrophotometric reading of 0.30. If an unknown sample is read under the same conditions, and the unknown sample yields a 0.42 absorbance, calculations for the value of the unknown would be as follows:

Absorbance of unknown/Absorbance of standard × Measured concentration of standard = Value of unknown

$$0.42/0.30 \times 1.5 \text{ mg/dL} = 2.1 \text{ mg/dL}$$

KINETIC ENZYME CALCULATIONS

For enzyme calculations, conditions are extremely important in determining a factor for obtaining the value for an enzymatic reaction. A common enzyme is alkaline phosphatase; bone tissue is rich with this enzyme. The reaction is a rate reaction that should be linear as the enzyme reacts on the specific substrate. This examination is also performed on a spectrophotometer, but instead of measuring the color development as is done for some end-point determinations, this procedure measures the rate of change for a specific period of time, which may vary by instrumentation and by manufacturer of the reagent. The purpose of showing this representative calculation for determining enzyme concentration in serum or

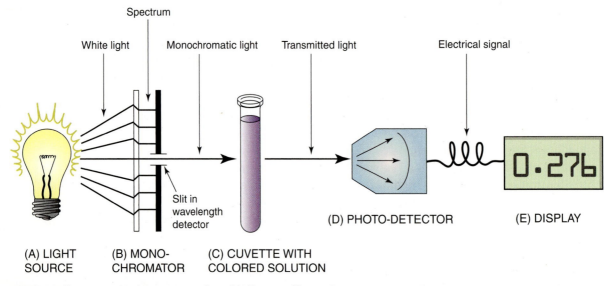

FIGURE 9-14 How a spectrophotometer works, with diagram of internal parts.
Source: Delmar/Cengage Learning.

plasma is to indicate the importance of standard conditions for the process to take place as well as the extremely accurate measurement of the enzyme substrate of 18.75 millimoles. Many chemistry determinations utilize this method for accuracy, speed, and specificity. The conditions and the determination of the factor are presented below.

Assay Conditions

Chemistry reactions often must have specific conditions to work properly in a reasonable amount of time or at all. When laboratory determinations are performed, the conditions are engineered for accuracy, speed, and specificity. The following set of conditions are required for most chemistry procedures and are often programmed into the chemistry analyzers. Each reaction will have some differing parameters, such as wavelength, test volumes, reaction time, and temperature (Table 9-10).

> **Explanation of a Rate (Kinetic) Reaction**
> U/L = Delta (common term for changing absorbance) change per minute × Factor

Delta absorbance (Δ) is the change in absorbance as measured for a period of time with use of the spectrophotometer. This is a rate (also called kinetic) reaction for a specific substrate reacted on by a specific enzyme. Some medical tests are reported in units per liter (U/L).

CLEARANCE TESTS

Some tests are developed to show how well certain body organs are removing certain toxins and waste products that affect a patient's health. The kidneys and liver are the two organs that are most responsible for this task. The kidneys reabsorb most of the components as they remove certain elements or excess water. Some organic components are not reabsorbed to a great extent. One of these is *creatinine*, a byproduct of energy conversion in the muscles. A creatinine clearance test is extremely important in diagnosing certain kidney diseases, and requires the analysis of both urine and blood creatinine. One other clinical

Table 9-10 Example of Assay Conditions for Basic Kinetic Chemistry Reaction

The requirements for a test reaction called a *rate* or *kinetic reaction* are specific. Most procedures will provide an assay sheet with the information necessary to manually calculate a value or to be programmed into an autoanalyzer.

Wavelength	405 nm	Temperature (constant)	37 °C
Reagent volume	1 mL	Sample volume	25 µL
Total test time	4 minutes (approx.)	Millimolar absorptivity of substrate	8.5
Cuvette dimensions	1 cm (square)	Units	U/L

component that may be tested to determine the clearance rate for the kidneys is that of inulin, a polysaccharide derived from plants. Inulin clearance is used less frequently than creatinine clearance.

Calculations for Determining the Factor from Data in Table 9-10

$$U/L = \frac{\text{Delta absorbance } (\Delta) \times 1.025 \times 1000}{8.5 \times 0.025 \times 1.0} = \text{Factor of } 4824$$

The factor of 4824 is multiplied by the Delta absorbance (Δ) for each unknown value for the clinical laboratory value for each patient.

For the creatinine clearance test, a 24-hour urine specimen is collected and stored in a cool environment to retard bacterial growth and alteration of the urine specimen. Creatinine determinations may be performed on either plasma or serum samples as well as urine specimens. The calculation of a creatinine clearance reveals the glomerular flow rate of the kidneys as they remove materials from the blood. Normal values for creatinine clearance are approximately 110 to 120 mL/min. A factor may be used for surface body area, since the amount of creatinine removed is proportional to muscle mass. A sample calculation with arbitrary values is shown here:

Clearance Test for Assessing Kidney Function

Total 24-hour urine volume = 1,650 mL
Minutes (60 minutes × 24 hr)/day = 1,440
Serum creatinine = 2.2 mg/dL
Urinary creatinine = 165 mg/dL

$$\text{Creatinine clearance} = \frac{\text{Urine creatinine} \times \text{Urine volume (mL)}}{\text{Serum creatinine} \times \text{Minutes}}$$

$$\text{Clearance with above data} = \frac{165 \times 1,650 \text{ mL}}{2.2 \times 1,440 \text{ min}} = 85.9 \text{ mL/min}$$

SUMMARY

It is important for the clinical laboratory student to have a strong grasp of mathematics, including knowledge of and calculations using both the English and the metric systems. Many of the calculations during analysis by instrument will be performed automatically by computers within the analyzer. However, there are basic calculations and methods of measurement that will help in troubleshooting malfunctions of instruments and in analyzing reagents for problems. In some instances, instrument failure may require that the laboratory worker perform calculations manually.

When taking licensure and registry boards, mathematic calculations must be performed to ensure competency in manipulating figures, which indicates an understanding of the scientific and chemical aspects of the reaction taking place in the procedure. But the most important factor in support of having a firm understanding of math lies in the conversions from one system of measurement to another. A good background in math makes this translation relatively simple, and most laboratory workers eventually become as familiar with metric measurements as with English measurements.

REVIEW QUESTIONS

1. Name at least two cases when common math skills are needed in a clinical laboratory.
2. Why are international standard units, or SIs, used in the laboratory?
3. Describe a rate reaction that is performed for the determination of a particular enzyme.
4. Describe how Beer's law operates.
5. Define molar, normal, and percent solutions.

QUALITY ASSURANCE

LEARNING OBJECTIVES

Upon completion of this chapter, the reader will be able to:

- Compare the meanings of accuracy and precision and know how each is measured.

- Discuss the term "clinical significance" and relate it to the reporting of laboratory results.

- Identify four components of quality assurance.

- Describe how a Levey-Jennings chart would indicate deterioration or changes in reagents and equipment.

- Compare the use of *F*-tests and *t*-tests.

- Provide the three major values used in computing an average value for a set of control values.

- Discuss the meanings of standard deviation and coefficient of variation.

- List the three categories of errors that may routinely occur in the performance of laboratory tests.

- Compare and contrast sensititivity and specificity.

KEY TERMS

Accuracy
Analyte
Analytical error
Clinically normal persons
Clinical significance
Coefficient of variation (CV)
Continuous quality
  improvement (CQI)
Cumulative sum (CUSUM)
  control chart
Efficiency
F-test

Levey-Jennings charts
Mean
Median
Mode
Normal distribution frequency
Percentage
Population norms
Postanalytical error
Preanalytical error
Precision
Predictive value
Proficiency testing (PT) programs

Quality assurance
Quality control programs
Random error
Reproducibility
Screening tests
Sensitivity
Shift
Specificity
Square root
Standard deviation
t-test
Trend

INTRODUCTION

Many components and departments of a modern health care facility are required to have programs to provide continuous monitoring of all facility processes and systems. The laboratory in particular is involved with providing documentation of effective and accurate functioning in the provision of diagnostic testing. The common term *quality control* (QC) and the activities involved in quality control programs were thought for many years to be sufficient for providing for accuracy in the laboratory. Eventually it was realized that QC provides for precision, or reproducibility, whereas proficiency testing (PT) is now used for monitoring accuracy, although the two go hand in hand. Quality assurance (QA) became the new buzzword, and the Clinical Laboratory Improvement Amendments (CLIA) required programs to ensure quality results through systematic procedures to improve the quality of laboratory services. Operational changes were called for. Although larger organizations already had a version of QA as mandated by their accreditation agencies, smaller laboratories and physicians' office laboratories (POLs) began to scramble to initiate a QA program or to improve on what they had and to document their activities for accreditation site visitors to review.

Quality Assurance in the Medical Laboratory

Quality assurance is a general term that includes many components. While QC is of the utmost importance in the medical laboratory, it is by no means the only aspect of quality assurance. Quality assurance may be thought of as the global aspect of an institution, and QC for the laboratory is a vital piece of the institution's quality assurance program. Quality assurance is a focus of The Joint Commission (TJC; formerly, Joint Commission on Accreditation of Healthcare Organizations [JCAHO]) and federal requirements under the CLIA 88 regulations. Quality assurance, also sometimes known as quality assessment, among other terms, includes QC and PT programs.

Personnel Qualifications and Proficiency Testing

Some personnel, depending on the state in which they work or the facility in which they are employed, are required to meet certain standards, although there is a great disparity between requirements for education and training in various institutions. Continuing and inservice education are a must, with facilities often required to provide for both types of education and training. To further ensure accuracy other than by having only qualified, trained personnel, PT may also be required to ensure accuracy. Certain agencies provide programs where *blind samples* of assayed specimens that have been tested multiple times by more than one method to establish ranges for acceptable performance are prepared for periodic testing. The blind samples are then sent to subscribing laboratories. Results submitted from participating clinical laboratories must fall within the established ranges to document accuracy in test performance. Failure to achieve acceptable results may lead to pro-hibiting the laboratory from performing certain tests or, in extreme cases and with repeated failure, could result in closing of the laboratory. *Quality systems* in some cases replaced quality assessment and are used to evaluate policies, methods of performance, and processes necessary to provide for quality results in tests performed.

All of these programs, by whatever moniker they are known, have a common goal. The desired result is that all laboratories adopt sufficient policies and systems to ensure accurate and timely laboratory results, to provide for and protect the health of the patient.

QUALITY IMPROVEMENT

Quality improvement is a term that some facilities use to describe their ongoing efforts to improve the quality and level of services provided to patients and clients. With the increasing importance of this concept not only in the health care environment but also in industrial and business applications, the term **continuous quality improvement (CQI)** now is often used to describe ongoing measurable changes that are deemed improvements. The medical laboratory with quality control programs makes it easy to statistically document improvement. In the case where there is a decline in expected results, there are problems that need addressing. Some aspects of quality assurance include components that are not statistically measurable but that show a qualitatively positive condition. The use of competent personnel, usually determined by hiring only certified, registered or licensed workers, should be a main concern of a medical facility. Risk management and utilization reviews are other areas where hospitals may effect positive results in quality assurance programs. A *quality management system* is another approach for the laboratory to focus on providing consistently accurate cost-effective results that positively benefit the patient. The box on the next page lists key components in any quality assurance program for the clinical laboratory.

EFFECTIVE QUALITY ASSURANCE PROGRAMS

Certain common factors are involved in an effective quality assurance program. Although all aspects of the functions of the clinical laboratory and the health care facility as a whole should be considered, QC is the basic component of a quality assurance program that gains the most attention in the laboratory. This is true because no patient results can be released unless certain parameters of QC have been achieved for each "run" of samples.

Spectrophotometry for QC

Both patient specimens and QC samples are treated in the same manner. Colorimetric end-point determinations use a principle that measures the intensity of light transmitted through the sample and reagent combination following a reaction between the two. In this method, the resulting reaction produces a characteristic color, which differs by the specific test type being performed. Some enzymatic reactions are used in the end-point methods, but most enzymatic reactions are measured as a rate reaction at a wavelength not visible to the naked eye (ultraviolet range). This reaction is measured in the same way as the end-point methods except that the reaction is ongoing while the sample is being read, giving a rate change for a given amount of time, while the end-point reaction is allowed to complete the reaction, usually 5 to 10 minutes.

Reading of QC samples uses the spectrophotometer in chemistry and in some other areas of the laboratory as well. Maintenance and care of the spectrophotometer are necessary on a routine basis to maintain good QC. Deteriorating and dirty spectrophotometers will adversely affect QC results, leading to the conclusion that the QC sample itself is inaccurate through contamination or faulty reconstitution. When light of an appropriate wavelength strikes a cuvet that contains a colored sample, some of the light is absorbed by the solution; the rest is transmitted through the sample to the detector. The proportion of light that reaches the detector is known as percent transmittance (%T) and is represented by the following equation:

$$\text{Intensity of light transmitted through sample} / \text{Intensity of light striking sample} \times 100 = \% \ T \ (\text{transmittance})$$

The general rule in regard to Beer's law is that as the concentration of colored solution in a cuvet is increased, the %T is decreased. Control samples may contain both end-point reactions and kinetic rate reactions. Other methodologies, such as those using ion-selective electrodes, are not discussed here.

QC Terminology

QC programs are an integral and vital component of quality assurance programs and are required as a condition of both accreditation and licensure for the medical laboratory. A number of terms have evolved relative to QC programs over the years and it is necessary to understand the meaning and the intent of the functions that these terms denote (Table 10-1).

The following is a list of three of the most common charts used in a QC program. Any or all of these may be used in the laboratory.

- **Levey-Jennings charts** show daily values in a graph form. The mean will be shown across the middle of the chart. Both negative and

Table 10-1 Quality Control Terminology and Definitions

Terms generic to all quality control programs in a clinical laboratory setting are as follows:

Term	Definition
Accuracy	Accuracy is how close a measurement is to a value verified by other analytical methods.
Analytical error	An analytical error occurs during testing. For example, in an autoanalyzer, a hundred samples may be relatively accurate, and one sample may be extremely abnormal; often the cause is never determined.
Average for a laboratory test	Also known as a mean; chiefly associated with control specimens; determined by the sum of all the determined values divided by the total number of values.
Coefficient of variation (CV)	The coefficient of variation (CV) is a calculation that shows variability between measurements for the same laboratory test performed more than once. It is normal to have some variability due to variables such as changes in electrical voltage, age of the spectrophotometer bulb, and standard errors in pipetting. ESSENTIAL TO REMEMBER: CV is always measured as a percentage!
Control specimen	Contains known concentration of constituents being measured; may be assayed or unassayed; used to measure precision (reproducibility). Originally these results were displayed on Levey-Jennings charts but are now stored in computerized documents that are filed for review as necessary.
Normal frequency curves	Established for each constituent measured, including calculated ones.
	Gaussian curve—graph (sometimes called a bell curve) that plots the distribution of determined values around the mean value of the control specimen (also called normal frequency curve).
	Levey-Jennings chart most common: provides the days of the month, along with 1 and 2 SDs delineated on the chart.
Population norms	Laboratory test values for an entire ethnic or geographic group.
	Moving averages over a period of time (months to years) should equal zero. Each day a quality control value is either positive or negative, and should "balance out" over a significant period of time. Shifts and trends would adversely affect the moving averages due to multiple and sequential positive or negative values.
	The normal range is determined by repeat testing and the history of the values determined. The normal or reference range aids in identifying the abnormal or diseased patient. A large number (100 to 300) of healthy individuals is tested, and the mean, median, and mode of each type of procedure is calculated, along with the SD (1 and 2 SD).
Postanalytical error	A postanalytical error occurs following the completion of testing. It most often involves handling and transmittal of the report.
Preanalytical error	A preanalytical error occurs before testing is completed, and may include patient misidentification, improper sample collection, or improper standardization of instrumentation.
Proficiency programs	External programs are sent to laboratories that, as a part of being licensed or accredited, are required to participate in a proficiency testing program. While controls evaluate precision, meaning reproducibility, proficiency testing (PT) programs assess accuracy. Test results from groups of laboratories throughout the country that employ similar procedures with similar equipment and supplies are compared. These results are usually also furnished to state laboratory licensure offices for action if results are not within an established range.
Quality control charts	Contain constituents in both normal levels and abnormal levels—sometimes three-level controls; may be assayed and unassayed; sufficient stock on hand to handle the annual historical workload; inconvenience; run at intervals; time or specimen numbers.
Quality control programs	Internal and external programs both may be used to efficiently cover the 24-hour schedule. As an example, a commercial (externally purchased) set of controls may be used in the morning, and an internal specimen from a patient may be used a number of hours later to determine if any malfunction with an instrument has occurred.
Random error	A random error whose cause cannot be definitively identified is usually environmental or operator generated.

(Continues)

Table 10-1 Quality Control Terminology and Definitions (*Continued*)

Term	Definition
Sample	Subgroup of a population; such as women, Native Americans, etc.
Shift	An abrupt change from the established mean is a shift; may be positive to negative values, or vice versa, but will all be on one side of the mean (e.g., all values for a glucose with a mean of 100 will provide measurements of 98, 95, 96, 91, etc.).
Shifts and trends	Large number of assays more meaningful.
	Ensures that results obtained are probably accurate, and that instruments and reagents are working adequately.
Standards	Primary standard—a substance that can be accurately weighed or measured to produce a solution of an exactly known concentration that is free of impurities; NIST provides standard practices and quality control for calibrating measuring devices and purity of solvent in which a substance is dissolved.
Systematic error	Related to instrument, reagent, and technological causes.
Trend	When a control value moves in the same direction (increases or decreases) for 6 consecutive days, it is designated a trend.

positive values (above and below the mean) should be seen over a period of time, such as for the month.

- *Twin-plot graph of Youden, modified by Tonks,* uses two control values by the same method or one control value using two methods. The variances should be virtually the same for the two controls and for the one control analyzed by two different methods.
- *CUSUM graph* is a cumulative method in which the mean result is subtracted from each control result as it is obtained, producing either a positive or a negative value each day. The resulting value is added to the total of the previous days to give a cumulative difference from the mean. Another similar method used in some laboratories is *Bull's moving averages.* These data are often managed cumulatively by automated equipment, and deviations outside the norm would be brought to the attention of the operator of the equipment.

Quality Control Concepts

The previous introduction to terms related to QC, a vital component of quality assurance, laid the groundwork for the calculations to determine precision. **Precision** relates to **reproducibility** of results when the conditions under which the procedures are performed are the same in all cycles of testing (from day to day, for example). An integral calculation used in calculating standard deviations (SDs) for groups of specimens relies on using the **square root** of the differences of results from the mean value. Even the most basic calculators usually have a key for easily calculating square roots.

Certain essential calculations are used in providing QC data to evaluate the precision of test procedures on a daily basis. This might be done automatically by the large autoanalytical instruments in use in most laboratories, but it is essential that the laboratory worker be familiar with the statistical terms shown in the Critical Reminder box on the following page.

Critical Reminder

Primary Measures of Quality Assurance

Precision   Refers to *reproducibility* and is determined by a set of control samples

Accuracy   Refers to any deviation from the *true result*, and is measured by proficiency testing that is obtained from an external commercial companies

STANDARD DEVIATION AND NORMAL FREQUENCY DISTRIBUTION

When the methods and tools presented in this section are used, it is easier to determine factors contributing to poor QC. When QC is out of range, results necessary for following a patient's diagnosis or care are delayed.

Random Error

Random error is just what the term implies: an error that occurs for no known reason and may be based on any number of factors. Quite often a random error is not even detected unless it occurs with controls and not with a patient sample. The reason for the error is often not determined. Statistically, random errors occur as a fraction of a percent for all tests performed. Random errors are often discovered when a particular result does not match the clinical picture or does not correlate well with tests for other **analytes** (constituents of body fluids tested for) for a specific patient.

Random errors are difficult to detect and analyze. They may result from various environmental factors, differences between operator functions, fatigue of certain components that affect high or low levels, transient interference, and almost any other factor that could be included in operation of high technology equipment.

Degree of precision is best expressed in terms of standard deviation, which is also the distribution of random error. This denotes the dispersion or variability in a distribution of results. **Normal distribution frequency** refers to a curve or bell-shaped curve, which may also be called the Gaussian random variable distribution.

Standard Deviation (SD)

Basically, the **standard deviation** is used as a measure of the variation in a distribution of values around the mean value for a group of the same tests. From the mean value, the standard deviations are calculated by taking the sum of the squared differences for each individual test from the mean value and dividing it by $n - 1$, where n is the number of tests performed. The square root of the figure derived from this process is equal to 1 SD and is doubled to determine 2 SD ranges. The mean, median, and mode are all common statistical terms that will be further discussed along with the detailed procedure for determining standard deviations.

To determine standard deviation, start by determining the mean of a group of tests (such as those for glucose) by adding all of the test values together and dividing by the number of tests performed. For each determination you do after this, subtract your test results from the mean. This number may be positive or negative. Square the differences and then use a calculator

Critical Reminder

Statistical Terms Used in Quality Control Calculations

Mean—average of all values (total of all values divided by the number of analyses) frequently used in calculations

Median—middle value within the range

Mode—most frequently occurring value

NOTE: In a good QC program, the mean, median, and mode should be virtually the same.

to obtain the square root of this *total* after dividing by *n* (the number of determinations) minus 1. This gives 1 SD, so you would multiply the calculated value by 2 to get 2 SDs, and by 3 to get 3 SDs. Look at the normal frequency distribution curve, also called the Gaussian or bell-shaped curve, in Figure 10-1 for a graphic picture of the distribution of results when performing a specific procedure on a number of different "runs" or sets of values that are run simultaneously.

A Gaussian distribution curve enables one to readily see the distribution of values for 1, 2, or 3 SDs. Slightly more than 95% of the values obtained will fall within 2 SDs of an established mean average for controls used to measure precision (see Figure 10-1), and approximately 99.7% will fall within 3 SDs. Each procedure is evaluated on this basis. Most automated analyzers in the modern medical laboratory perform these statistics through computations by each instrument's internal computer system. As samples are run over a period of time and larger numbers of determinations are made, the SD values should become narrower and narrower. This is particularly true for a laboratory that conscientiously performs routine maintenance and cleaning of equipment. Improvement in the value of SDs should be the goal of every medical laboratory. As a general rule, a laboratory that performs a procedure by the same method for a significant length of time will realize that the SDs have grown progressively smaller.

Critical Reminder

Statistically, in the normal frequency distribution (Gaussian) curve (Figure 10-1) approximately 95% of values should fall within 2 standard deviations of the mean and 99.7% will fall within 3 standard deviations of the mean. That means that 0.3% of results will be attributed to random error. This statement is true for any procedure performed.

Critical Reminder

Usually charts are drawn where acceptable results for QC programs will be within ±2 SDs. The values for 3 SDs are often included because 99.7% of results will fall within 3 SDs. Observe the Westgard rules for accepting or rejecting patient results based on QC results.

Spread of Data on the Scale

The term "spread of data" most often refers to the range incorporated within 2 SDs and in most cases will include the 3 SD range, because control values may occasionally extend into the 3 SD range for a single determination, while the other controls are within 2 SDs. This term is graphically seen on a Gaussian distribution curve.

Variance from Mean (SDs)

The acceptable **variance** from the mean value is 1 SD and this figure doubled is the value for 2 SDs. This is the basic figure used to determine precision based on QC samples for any test.

The **variance** (SD^2) of the samples in Example 10-1 is:

$SD^2 = 35.625/18$ (total values) $- 1$ or $(n - 1) = 35.625/17 = 2.0956$

The square root of 2.0956 = 1.4476, which is rounded to 1.45, or 1 SD

2 SDs $= 2 \times 1.45$, or 2.9

Example 10-1 Variances from the Mean Squared

Follow these calculations where variances from the mean are squared. The variances from the mean were designed to show a consistent variation from the mean, using both positive and negative values. An equation after this example shows how both SDs and CVs are determined.

Variance from Mean	Squared Values	Variance from Mean	Squared Values	Variance from Mean	Squared Values
Day One 0.25	0.0625	Day Seven 1.75	3.0625	Day Thirteen −1.00	1.0000
Day Two 0.50	0.2500	Day Eight 2.00	4.0000	Day Fourteen −1.25	1.5625
Day Three 0.75	0.5625	Day Nine 2.25	5.0625	Day Fifteen −1.50	2.250
Day Four 1.00	1.0000	Day Ten −0.25	0.0625	Day Sixteen −1.75	3.0625
Day Five 1.25	1.5625	Day Eleven −0.50	0.2500	Day Seventeen −2.00	4.0000
Day Six 1.50	2.250	Day Twelve −0.75	0.5625	Day Eighteen −2.25	5.0625

NOTE: The variances from the mean value are treated the same, whether *values are negative or positive. A negative value, when squared, becomes a positive value.*
The sum of the squared differences for this set of samples is 35.625.

How to Calculate the Standard Deviation

Table 10-2 is a simplified set of procedures to obtain a 1 SD value. Working through steps 1 through 7 of Example 10-2 is good practice for finding the standard deviation values needed for QC records.

Sample Calculation of a Standard Deviation

Using the steps in Table 10-2, calculate the standard deviation for the values given in Example 10-2.

Step 1 *Calculate* the mean value.
Determine the mean from values obtained on days 1 through 20.

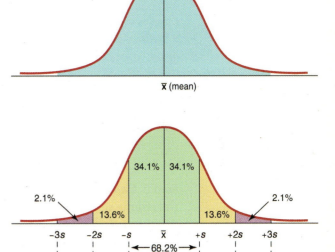

FIGURE 10-1 Normal frequency distribution curves.
Source: Delmar/Cengage Learning.

$$\frac{92 + 93 + 92 + 90 + 89 + 87 + 88 + 89 + 88 + 92 + 88 + 91 + 90 + 88 + 87 + 93 + 90 + 92 + 92 + 89}{\text{Mean } \textbf{20} \text{ of } 90.05 \text{ (Round to 90)}}$$

Mean Value = 90

Table 10-2 Calculating Standard Deviations

Step	Activity	Example of How to Obtain Values
1.	Determine the mean of the control values.	When 10 laboratory values are obtained, add them all together. Then divide the sum of the ten values by 10. This is the mean.
2.	Calculate deviations (±) from the mean.	Calculate the amount **each** laboratory value deviates from the mean, plus or minus.
3.	Square the deviations from the mean.	Multiply each variance by itself.
4.	Add all the squared deviations.	Calculate the sum of all the squared deviations.
5.	Divide sum of squared differences by $n - 1$.	The sum of the squared differences is divided by the total number of values (procedures) minus 1.
6.	Take the square root of the quotient from step 5.	Calculate the square root of the figure obtained

Example 10-2 Graph for Normal Control in Daily Glucose Tests

A **normal level** control (80–105 mg/dL) was tested at the beginning of the morning shift at a local hospital. The reagent used was of the same lot number, the instrument operator was the same, and all conditions were controlled to ensure the results would not be affected by environment or by any condition that could be controlled. These simulated daily results are taken from the Levey-Jennings chart in Example 10-3.

Day 1 92	Day 6 87	Day 11 88	Day 16 93
Day 2 93	Day 7 88	Day 12 91	Day 17 90
Day 3 92	Day 8 89	Day 13 90	Day 18 92
Day 4 90	Day 9 88	Day 14 88	Day 19 92
Day 5 89	Day 10 92	Day 15 87	Day 20 89

Step 2 *Calculate* deviations from the mean (negative and positive numbers are treated the same) by subtracting each of the 20 values from the mean.

$$+2, +3, +2, 0, -1, -3, -2, -1, -2, +2, -2, +1, 0, -2, -3, +3, 0, +2, +2, -1$$

Step 3 *Square* the deviations from the mean.

$$4.0, 9.0, 4.0, 0, 1.0, 9.0, 4.0, 1.0, 4.0, 4.0, 4.0, 1.0, 0, 4.0, 9.0, 9.0, 0, 4.0, 4.0, 1.0$$

Step 4 *Add* all the squared deviations.

$$76$$

Step 5 *Divide* the sum of squared differences by $n - 1$.

$$76 \text{ divided by } (20 - 1) = 4.00$$

Step 6 *Take the square root* of the quotient determined by dividing the sum of squared differences by $n-1$.

> Square root of 4.00 = 2.00 (1 SD)

Step 7 *Calculate* 2 SDs and 3 SDs from 1 SD.

> 1 SD = 2.00   2 SDs = 4.00   3 SDs = 6.00

Equation for Calculating a Standard Deviation and a Coefficient of Variation

The following formula is a simplified explanation of the calculations just explained at length, using the values provided in Example 10-2. Both the standard deviation and the coefficient of variation are indicated. Consult the lengthy explanation and then recalculate the values by using the simple equation presented here.

Calculating the Standard Deviation (SD)

> The **variance** (SD^2) of the samples in Example 10-2 is:
>
> $SD^2 = 76.0/20$ (total values) $- 1$ or $(n-1) = 76/19 = 4.00$
>
> The square root of 4.00 = 2.00, or 1 SD
>
> 2 SDs = 2 × 2.00, or 4.00

How to Calculate the Coefficient of Variation

The coefficient of variation (CV) is always expressed in a **percentage** form. It is based on the percent value that **each** individual control value differs from the mean. It is another way to express the degree of deviation from the mean.

Coefficient of Variation

> **Coefficient of variation** (CV) = SDs/sample mean × 100%
>
> For the set of sample values from Example 10-2,
>
> CV = SD (2.00) divided by the mean (90) × 100 = 2.22%

CUSUM: ANOTHER QUALITY CONTROL TOOL

A term that is not often heard in the forefront of quality control is that of a **cumulative sum (CUSUM) control chart** in which the cumulative sums of deviations from the mean value are recorded manually or by computer programs within analytical instruments used in laboratory testing of control samples. This tool is used not only in clinical laboratories but also in industrial plants as a component of quality control programs. The control charts developed by Dr. Walter Shewhart for detecting statistical control of a process are simpler to operate but not as efficient in detecting small shifts in the mean of a process.

Measuring the small, sustained shifts in a process that would be important in determining shifts and trends is simplified when using the CUSUM system. Essentially, the system measures the totals of the positive movements above the mean of a control sample and the totals of the negative movements. Over a period of time, these totals should be virtually equal when equipment and supplies are performing adequately. This process might be compared with the game of golf, with par being the mean and each shot over is a +1 and each shot below par is a -1, with a cumulative score being determined at the end.

Using the values provided in Example 10-2, a CUSUM determination would be performed by calculating the cumulative sum of the variances from the mean of 90, yielding the following data:

Value	Variance	Cumulative Sum	Value	Variance	Cumulative Sum
92	+2	+2	88	-2	-2
93	+3	+5	91	+1	-1
92	+2	+7	90	0	-1
90	0	+7	88	-2	-3
89	-1	+6	87	-3	-6
87	-3	+3	93	+3	-3
88	-2	+1	90	0	-3
89	-1	0	92	+2	-1
88	-2	-2	92	+2	+1
92	+2	0	89	-1	0

LEVEY-JENNINGS CHART

The Levey-Jennings chart is the most common chart used in the laboratory. A quick glance at the control results shows any shifts or trends developing, signaling an impending systematic failure. These charts are seldom found on display but can be visualized on computer screens of the various analyzers, especially for chemistry procedures.

WHEN PATIENT RESULTS MAY BE REPORTED

Generally, patient results may be safely reported when the controls show no signs of shifts or trends (Figure 10-2) or when none of the control values fall outside the acceptable range. A student will find that a multitude of factors may

Example 10-3 Levey-Jennings Chart—Plotting of Daily Normal Control Values

Three levels of control samples were performed for a 20 day period. The following values are those from the normal control vial.

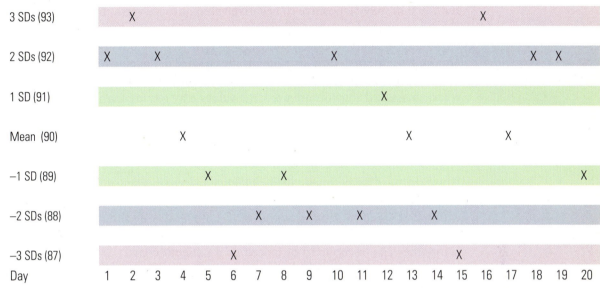

3 SDs (93)	X														X					
2 SDs (92)	X		X						X								X	X		
1 SD (91)											X									
Mean (90)			X							X			X							
−1 SD (89)					X		X													X
−2 SDs (88)						X		X		X			X							
−3 SDs (87)					X									X						
Day	1	2	3	4	5	6	7	8	9	10	11	12	13	14	15	16	17	18	19	20

For simplicity in depicting a typical Levey-Jennings chart, the standard deviations (SDs) shown were not calculated from any data presented, but for ease of understanding, they were chosen arbitrarily as whole digits with some deviating from the norm by more than 2 SDs. The CUSUM determination is performed by subtracting each result from the mean; the above figures resulted in a +2 SD, which is an acceptable value. In the CUSUM process, the lower the value of the sum of the differences of all the determinations, the better. Optimally, there should be equal differences of both + and − values, indicating no shifts or trends.

affect the results of laboratory tests. Although there are random errors at the rate of approximately 0.3% of tests performed, it is generally safe to assume that patient results are relatively accurate when all the controls are within an established range. Again, random errors are those for which no definite cause can be established. Correlation of results and knowledge of the patient's medical condition is often sufficient to resolve many of these errors. Simply rerunning a patient sample where all other test values are normal often will provide a clinically consistent result.

Acceptability of Patient Testing

There are general and simple rules to follow when determining if patient values are valid.

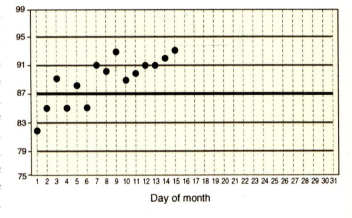

FIGURE 10-2 Levey-Jennings QC chart showing normal distribution for days 1 through 6, a shift for days 7 through 9, and a trend for days 10 through 15.
Source: Delmar/Cengage Learning.

When all control values are within ±2 SDs, all data are accepted. If one or more controls are within 2 and 3 SDs, repeat the errant sample using new control(s). Frequently in laboratory medicine, both a normal and an abnormal control will be analyzed. If both of these controls are out of range, the appropriate action would require a rejection of all results followed by troubleshooting protocol. When a control value moves in the same direction (increases or decreases) for 6 consecutive days, it is termed a *trend*. An abrupt change from the established mean is a *shift*. A shift may be positive to negative values, or vice versa, but it will all be on one side of the mean.

QC records are evaluated under Westgard rules or possibly another similar program. Many analytical instruments are capable of flagging results that fall outside of the parameters established by the manufacturer of the controls. In the case where unassayed controls are used, the values may require manually placing data into the instrument after a period where sufficient values have been performed.

Westgard Rules (Multirules)

Westgard rules (sometimes called *challenge rules*) are a set of rules to determine if a method is out of control. This occurs when at least two controls are not within 2 SDs and the third is within 3 SDs. Preferably all three levels of controls will be within 2 SDs. Results of laboratory tests must meet the following criteria before they can be reported or placed on a patient's chart.

Westgard Rules

1. The *warning rule* is broken when one control measurement exceeds the ±2 SD guideline. The other rules must now be tested by examining other control values in the run (within run) and in previous runs (across runs) before making a decision on the acceptability of the patient results. If any of the remaining rules are violated, the laboratory professional must thoroughly examine the test's analytical procedure, troubleshoot steps in the procedure, and or perform instrument maintenance, etc. before making any decision about releasing the results or re-running the test.

2. The *within-run only rule* detects random error for a control but may also point to systematic error. The run is considered out of control when one control value exceeds the ±3 SD limits. But random errors may occur with no warning and for unknown reasons. Repeating a control when it is out of range often remedies the situation. Note that random errors for patient specimens are not detected as this refers only to controls.

3. The *two-consecutive control rule* is designed to detect systematic error and can be applied within and across runs. It is violated when two consecutive control values exceed the same ±2 SD limit.

4. The *range rule* is applied within the same run only to detect random error. It is violated when the SD difference between two consecutive control values exceeds 4 SDs. The 4 SD spread may occur across the mean value and include both a positive and a negative value from the mean.

5. This rule detects **systematic errors** and may be used both within and across runs performed the same day or succeeding days. It is violated within the control material when the last four control values of the same level exceed the same ± SD limit. It is violated across control materials when the last four consecutive controls for different levels exceed the same ±1 SD.

6. This rule also detects **systematic error** and is applied both within and across separate runs. It is violated within the control material when the last 10 values for the same control level are all on the same side of the mean. It is called a shift if violated across control materials when the last 10 consecutive values, regardless of control level, are on the same side of the mean. The number of values considered can be decreased if three or more levels of control are run.

7. The term *Delta checks* refers to the difference between a patient's present laboratory result and a previous result that exceeds a predefined limit. Delta checks are done on samples from patients who have repeat analyses of tests that have relatively stable parameters from day-to-day operations. These parameters may be in chemistry or hematology predominantly, and are for patients who have at least a several-day hospitalization period. Delta checks are investigated by the laboratory internally to rule out mislabeling, clerical error, or possible analytical error. Therefore, failures discovered by Delta checks may be preanalytical or systematic. Actions to verify reasons for a failure may be the repeat of the sample, repeat of the previous sample from the same patient, or a manual method of determining the veracity of the results. In addition, a call to the physician or nurse may confirm that a preanalytical error occurred due to the specimen being drawn from an IV line, mislabeling of the sample, or a drastic change in the patient's condition. Documentation on the patient's report should indicate what actions were taken and that the specimen was rerun for verification.

Quality Control for All Types of Tests

Clinical laboratories perform qualitative, semiquantitative, and quantitative tests on a variety of biological specimens. A qualitative test is defined as one in which a particular characteristic of the specimen is determined to be either present or absent and is most often reported as positive or negative. Quantitative tests determine the amount of a particular substance or property by an instrument, with the result expressed numerically. Some tests are defined as providing semiquantitative results. For instance, if a very small amount of protein is found in a urine specimen, it might be reported positive as a trace amount. CLIA 88 requires that a laboratory must establish and follow an appropriate QC program for all testing performed by the laboratory.

Establishment of Control Limits for Quantitative Tests

For quantitative methods, laboratories may use either "assayed" or "unassayed" control materials. *Assayed* controls are defined as such when the manufacturer of the materials has established the acceptable limits for the control test results. Generally, the limits represent a 2 to 3 SD range. If the laboratory is using assayed controls, the results obtained from testing the control material **must** be within the assayed limits or range. If control results fall outside the limits, the laboratory **must** take corrective action. Some laboratories will establish over time a narrower range established by the manufacturer of 2 SDs using the assayed control materials. However, the new limits must be within the range given by the manufacturer, which would always be the case as the range would grow smaller as the number of data points from testing of controls increases.

Unassayed controls are controls tested by the laboratory at a specified frequency and time period to establish the acceptable limits or range. To establish the acceptable limits or range, new lots of control material should be analyzed for each analyte in parallel with the assayed control material in current use. Once the SDs are established for the unassayed control when both the assayed and unassayed controls are performed together, the laboratory may convert to using only unassayed controls and therefore using its own established values. At least 20 sets of data and preferably more than 20 separate runs should be obtained. The common practice is to set the limits or range at 2 SDs. As a general rule, the SDs as stated before should become smaller as the laboratory produces more sets of test results for the various procedures being performed.

For quality assurance and as part of the laboratory's QC program, the laboratory must have a plan or procedure for accepting the results obtained from QC materials, as well as the course of action to be taken when results fall outside acceptable limits. QC rules should be incorporated into the laboratory's procedure or plan, to determine if the QC results are within an acceptable range. These rules can be designed to detect inappropriate bias or imprecision that may affect the quality of patient test results. A variety of control rules have been used to monitor the quality of laboratory testing. These rules generally use Gaussian statistics and assume a Gaussian-type distribution of data. Control limits are usually the mean ($\bar{x}$) of individual control values obtained over various periods of time, and the limits are customarily based on multiples of the SD.

Due to such large number of control rules and their various ramifications, Westgard developed a shorthand notation for the representation of these rules. Most of these rules are incorporated into the computerized equipment, where the instrument operator enters data for analysis and the compilation and storage of QC data. Many of these instruments will "flag" results outside the acceptable range, and will give a cautionary message if results from a patient's values would be a critical value or if some malfunction was noted by the instrument during the procedure. In general, only approximately 4.5% of control results should be found outside the ±2 SD limits as seen on the distribution curve shown earlier. The lower control limits are calculated from the formula $\bar{x} - 2$ SDs and the upper limit from $\bar{x} \pm 2$ SDs. For QC purposes, a value that is too high is no worse than one that is too low. Whenever a new control observation is obtained, it is compared to the mean ±2 SD control limits. If an observation is outside these limits, it may indicate an accuracy or precision problem. As you can see from the "targets" in Figure 10-3, accuracy and precision are two different things; accuracy indicates whether the true measurement of a component has been achieved, whereas precision indicates reproducibility.

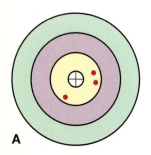
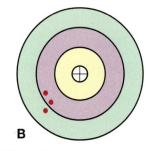

A   B

FIGURE 10-3 (A) Accuracy versus (B) precision.
Source: Delmar/Cengage Learning.

ANALYZING QUALITY CONTROL RESULTS

The list of rules described previously indicate *how* to determine if patient results can be safely reported or if a problem exists. This section is a more in-depth discussion of the rules and the corrective action to take when Westgard rules are violated.

Most QC rules will detect both random and systematic error, *but a preanalytical error might not be uncovered unless a repeat specimen is drawn*. Remember, there are preanalytical factors, analytic, and postanalytical issues that may adversely affect the results that are reported. It would be well to remember factors involved with all three aspects of testing to be more effective as a professional.

Only a few control rules have adequate sensitivity for the detection of both random and systematic errors. Effective QC procedures require sensitivity to both types of error and should have an acceptable false rejection rate, which should be a low value. Improved sensitivity to both random and systematic error may be accomplished by combining QC rules. QC procedures using a combination of rules are called "multirule control procedures" or are multirule procedures such as the ones developed by Westgard. Multirule procedures combine both the rules and the order in which the rules are applied to the control data. According to CLIA 88 requirements, if control results fall outside an established range of acceptable values, the technician or technologist must take action to rectify the problem. It is also mandatory that any action taken to correct the problem be documented. It is easier to correct a systematic problem or a random error immediately following the discovery of the problem.

Remember that control results must fall within acceptable limits before any patient results may be reported. Sometimes physicians will demand results even before remedial action has been taken and the results repeated and verified, but officially no results may be disseminated until QC results are acceptable. It is important to repeat the original patient test results if it is determined by the remedial action that the patient test results could be affected. Guidelines that are readily available for the laboratory's technical workers should be in place defining the corrective action that should be taken as found in the following list.

Steps to Follow When Control Results Are Out of Range

It is essential to arrive at a point as quickly as possible where patient results can be released. The following steps start with the simplest remedy first and progress to more time-consuming procedures that tend to further delay the dissemination of laboratory results that may affect a patient's treatment. The steps should be done in the order provided.

Remember, if the first step corrects the problem, no further action is required. Fortunately, the first two steps will eliminate the errors in most cases. Controls and sometimes standards must be reconstituted and allowed to stand for up to 30 minutes before they are ready for use. This delays the test results for quite a period of time, so if step 1 corrects the problem, much time can be saved, thus the reason for following the correct order for action.

Sequential Steps for Out-of-Range Controls

1. Repeat the test procedures using the same control or calibrator material (standard).
2. Repeat the procedure(s) with a new vial of control or calibrator material.
3. Insure all reagent lot numbers match the assay sheets in place and that expiration dates have not been reached.
4. Look for variations in results such as shifts or trends, or obvious instrument malfunctions.
5. If a new batch of control or calibrator material (standard) is available, repeat the testing using the new lot.
6. Routinely perform the basic preventive maintenance for each instrument on a regular basis, but repeating this process when an error is discovered often uncovers a problem that just occurred.
7. Recalibrate the instrument if required before performing repeat testing of the control material.
8. Open new test reagents and calibrate the instrument before performing repeat testing if required.
9. Call for service from the manufacturer's technical service department.
10. Notify the immediate section supervisor, who may contact the laboratory manager.
11. Thoroughly document corrective action taken as laboratory inspectors will investigate this area.

In summary, a "quality" QC program ensures that steps and documentation have been taken when results do not meet the guidelines for the QC program. This ultimately proves that the laboratory is reporting accurate and reliable patient test results. Remember, control results may be above or below the target value. In either case, the results are equally in error and must be evaluated in the same manner.

Reject the Test Run and Do Not Report Patient Results

The accompanying Critical Reminder states five shortened versions of Westgard rules for rejecting the run (batch of specimens) for a laboratory procedure.

COMPARISON OF PRECISION

It is sometimes necessary to perform certain statistical processes when two versions of a laboratory procedure are being compared. Obviously, it would be important to determine which method would be most accurate. The *t-test* is a procedure in which two versions of a *single* test such as a glucose determinations, are being compared. If the results are the same (null hypothesis), factors other than accuracy would be used to determine the method to choose. Another test, the *F-test*, is used

---

Critical Reminder

When a Run Should Be Rejected

1. When one control exceeds the established mean by ±3 SDs
2. When one control exceeds the mean by 2 SDs in the same direction (±) for two consecutive times or on two controls in the same run
3. When two controls in the same run have a difference between the established values by 4 SDs (i.e., one control is +2 SDs and the other is −2 SDs)
4. When four consecutive controls exceed the mean by 1 SD or more in the same direction (on the same side of the mean value; this is called a shift)
5. When 10 consecutive values fall on the same side of the mean

for comparing two *different* tests, rather than two different methodologies. The precision for the two tests might be different, and the test with the greatest degree of precision would most likely be chosen. The *t*-test and the *F*-test are the two most common methods for comparing precision (reproducibility) for two methods and two different procedures (Table 10-3).

Predictive Value

Predictive analysis is important in that it attempts to match laboratory test values with the actual incidence of disease in a given population. False positive results in a population with a low level of a certain disease state would incorrectly increase the percentage of persons deemed to have the disease.

Sensitivity and specificity are important in this area. These concepts are discussed later in this chapter in the section on clinical and statistical significance. Briefly, a test that is too sensitive would yield an increased number of false positives where extremely low levels of a certain metabolite may be present, and a test that is not specific may measure entities unrelated to a disease process. If a condition has a low prevalence (number of cases of a specific disease present in a given population) and the test methodology is not 100% specific, false-positive results will be higher than the **predictive value**. The predictive value refers to a test result that might be substantially elevated or found at a lower level than would be expected for certain disease states. Procedures should be highly specific to avoid large numbers of false positives, because some tests will yield a positive result in the presence of chemicals found in certain foods and medications. False positives may cause undue mental stress and treatment for a disease that is not present.

On the other hand, if a test is not specific enough, false positive results may arise due to other conditions. An example of this is the common test for syphilis. It is a serological test that may provide false positives for a number of illnesses not related to syphilis. But **screening tests** for large populations must be sensitive enough to identify those who *may* have the disease, and further definitive testing and physical examinations could then be performed only on those who might have the ailment. Most laboratory procedures will include information regarding

Table 10-3 Types of Comparisons for Laboratory Procedures by Analysis of Results

t-Test	The t-test measures reproducibility and is also called the paired t-test. This process compares the accuracy of **two methods** because it tests the difference between the mean value for each testing method. Remember that there are numerous methods for performing any laboratory test. The reference or current method is considered to reflect true value. A null hypothesis results when there is no difference in the two methods.
F-test	The *F*-test measures method accuracy (accuracy of test results is determined by performing proficiency testing). The *F*-test compares the precision or reproducibility for **two procedures**. The SD of the method showing the larger variance divided by the SD of method showing smaller variance = % difference.

NOTE: *Method* refers to how a test is performed. *Procedure* refers to a different test, e.g., a total protein and a calcium.

medications and other concurrent conditions that may cross-react with the procedure and give a falsely positive result.

Predictive value is not the only criterion of laboratory test usefulness and may at times be misleading if used too rigidly. For example, a test may have excellent characteristics as a screening procedure in terms of sensitivity, low cost, and ease of technical performance but may also have a low positive predictive value. Whether the test is useful would depend on other factors such as the type and cost of follow-up tests necessary in case of an abnormal result and the implications of missing a certain number of persons with the disease if some less sensitive test were used.

Sometimes, reasons for circumstances where predictive value are misleading or difficult to establish. If the medical laboratory worker is calculating the predictive value of a test, he or she must first know the sensitivity and specificity of that test. This information requires that some accurate reference method for diagnosis must be available other than the test being evaluated. A standard against which the test in question can be compared is sometimes called a "gold standard." An example of a gold standard is the use of a complex procedure called an electrophoresis for total protein. This test would not be used for normal testing procedures but could be used to evaluate a simple and quick method such as dye-binding. In some cases, this is not possible. There may not be a more sensitive or specific test or test combination available or the test being evaluated may itself be the major criterion by which the diagnosis is made. In other words, if it is not possible to detect all or nearly all patients with a certain disease, it will not be possible to provide a truly accurate calculation of sensitivity, specificity, or predictive value for tests used in the diagnosis of that disease. The best one can obtain are estimates, and these vary in their reliability.

Calculation of Predictability Values

This is most often achieved by computer analysis, either by automated entry of data or by manual entry of data by the technician or technologist. The student should become familiar with the computer terms commonly used in the process. Almost all laboratory equipment now has computer processes for operating the mechanical aspects of the procedure, as well as interpreting the results from raw data. Patient values can then be read as meaningful figures before transmitting them to the appropriate clinical areas for use in diagnosing and treating the patient. QC records typically are recorded for long-term management in the Laboratory Information System (LIS) for reference when errors such as shifts and trends occur. Repeat occurrences of the same or similar problem might herald a pending problem of a certain type.

WHAT IS MEANT BY REPRODUCIBILITY AND ACCURACY?

Reliability of laboratory tests may be greatly affected by the level of technical performance within the laboratory. The effect of these technical factors is reflected in test reproducibility and accuracy. Reproducibility (precision, or inherent or built-in error) is a measure of how closely the laboratory can produce the same answer when the test is performed repeatedly on the same specimen. In theory, exactly the same answer should be obtained each time. But in actual practice this does not happen due to equipment and human imperfections and differences between operators. If all tests were 100% reproducible from day to day, there would be no need for running control samples except at the initial use of a piece of equipment. Variations are anticipated and accepted, hence, a "range" for acceptable quality control results. A theoretical frequency distribution for a set of data that are normally variable is often represented by a bell-shaped curve, with data equally arranged on either side of the mean. This is sometimes called a Gaussian distribution.

As was seen in the definitions of QC terminology, control specimens are used for measuring precision, or reproducibility, of the QC system. Precision does not mean the same thing as accuracy. Accuracy is provided through a PT program where a commercial company provides specimens with known values. Each laboratory reports its values, and all of the individual values from the various procedures are measured against all other laboratories around the country that use similar equipment and supplies. Both accuracy and precision are important. One without the other is not a satisfactory condition (Figure 10-4).

Variation from the average (mean) value is expressed in terms of standard deviation (SD). The laboratory frequently converts the SD figure to a percentage of the mean value and calls this the coefficient of variation (CV). The majority of tests in a good laboratory can be shown to have reproducibility expressed as CV in the neighborhood of 4%. This means that two thirds of the values

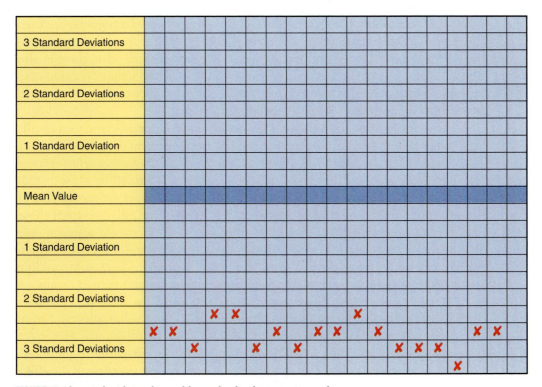

FIGURE 10-4 Levey-Jennings chart with precise but inaccurate results.
Source: Delmar/Cengage Learning.

obtained are actually somewhere between 4% above and 4% below the true value. Because ±2 SDs (which includes approximately 95% of the values) is most frequently used to determine acceptable limits or normal ranges, plus or minus twice the CV similarly forms the boundaries of permissible technical error. In the example above, a resulting deviation of up to ±8% would therefore be considered technically acceptable. For some assays, particularly those that are very complex and where automated equipment is not used, variations greater than ±8% may be permitted, particularly for low-volume testing.

The experience and diligence of a conscientious technical worker, the reagents involved, and the equipment used will all affect final procedure results and will ultimately affect the reproducibility that is reported as the CV. As a general statement, it is assumed that the worse the reproducibility is (expressed as higher CVs), the less chance there is for producing an accurate result. But good reproducibility in itself will not ensure accurate results. Reproducibility, is good, but all of the results may still be inaccurate while showing excellent reproducibility.

These considerations mean that a small change in a test value may be difficult to evaluate because results could be due to a laboratory artifact rather than to disease or therapy. Larger alterations or a continued trend of change are much more helpful. *Accuracy* is defined as the correct value, where a result or value that is obtained for the assay is the one that should have been produced by testing.

So, reproducibility of accurate results would be the desirable situation in day-to-day operations, and would detect changes in reagents and systems being used. Reproducibility is measured by QC samples, while PT programs are used to determine accuracy. Shifts and trends are determined from QC samples, and may help to avoid costly equipment failure. Besides inherent error, there is also the possibility of unexpected error of various kinds, such as preanalytical human mistakes when obtaining the specimen, during performance of the test, or when reporting the result, even when automation is used.

Those responsible for reviewing QC values have reported erroneous results in a range of 0.2% to 3.5% of reported values from different departments of the laboratory. The laboratory will analyze appropriate control specimens (assayed or unassayed) with each group of patient specimens. It should be obvious that any technical factor that might affect a procedure and produce erroneous patient results could also yield control specimen results that are different from those expected. Random errors cannot be avoided but in the best-case scenario they can be minimized. Random error affects only a fraction of a percent of patient values and might or might not affect the control sample values, but random error with controls is much more easily discernible than with patient results.

The observant medical laboratory worker will watch for and repeat any tests where patient results do not fit the clinical picture. Other values obtained from the patient's sample may be flagged by the Delta checks mentioned earlier for patients with repeat testing when significantly different test patterns are noted. Preanalytical errors such as testing a specimen from the wrong patient, the effect of specimen hemolysis (breaking down of red blood cells), or lipemia (presence of large amounts of fats in blood) are commonly found. Inaccurate pipetting and improper mixing when the procedure requires the use of a whole blood specimen will produce poor results. In addition, postanalytical clerical errors are the most common type of errors that occur, even when the equipment and supplies are in good order. In the experience of most medical laboratory personnel, the majority of clerical difficulties are associated with patients who have the same last name, unless bar code identification bands are correctly used. But there have been some reports of bar codes being erroneously read by the computer scanner.

Before the widespread use of computerized reports and bar codes affixed to samples at the time of collection, there were many more errors than are seen today. Examples of errors from pre-computer days were:

- Displaced decimal point mistakes
- Patients who moved from one room to another
- Transfer of results to the wrong person's laboratory report form
- Direction of a patient's report to another patient's medical records

Many of these errors have been greatly minimized through the use of identifying bar codes affixed to both specimen and laboratory request or drawing list, eliminating misreading errors that may occur when the name of the patient is written manually. The physician who receives unexpected laboratory results (or sometimes even the degree of abnormality of results) should interpret the result in the context of the clinical picture. He or she should ask for a repeat test if a single result in a battery of tests is abnormal, and neither the clinical picture, medical condition, or the other values support the unexpected result. This should not be interpreted as meaning that unexpected test values should be ignored. But when there is doubt as to the validity of the results, the values for laboratory tests should be verified, and if no errors affecting the laboratory test results are uncovered, a more extensive workup or therapeutic action may be warranted.

When an astute technician or technologist conscientiously reviews a report and has doubts about questionable results, the procedure should always be repeated before results reach the physician. If possible, the repeat test should be performed on the original specimen or, if that is no longer available, a new specimen should be obtained and tested without delay. The greater the time lapse between the original and the new specimen, the more difficulties will be encountered in differentiating an error in the original specimen from a true change that may have occurred since collecting the initial specimen. One of the most frustrating issues a laboratory director is forced to face is when a question or complaint about a laboratory test result is presented several days or even weeks after the test was performed. Specimens may have been discarded and the patient may no longer be available for a routine re-collection. Then it is usually too late for a complete investigation of the problem. Sometimes it requires voluminous research and additional work, because an entire group of other patients may have also shown erroneous results that were accepted by the physician and therapy initiated on the basis of erroneous results.

NORMAL REFERENCE RANGES

The most important single aspect of laboratory test interpretation is the concept of a normal range, where test values that fall inside the range are considered normal and those occurring outside the range are considered abnormal. The established range and those patients falling even slightly outside the range are of great importance to the physician and the patient. The first step usually used to establish normal ranges is to assume that all persons who do not demonstrate clinical symptoms or signs of any disease are normal, even if one or more test results fall outside the "normal" range. For some tests, *normal* is defined as the absence of clinical evidence associated with one particular disease or chronic condition. A second assumption commonly made is that test results from those persons considered normal will have a random distribution. Factors that would place a significant group of these values toward either the low or the high side of the normal range may be present. Then a Gaussian (random) distribution that resulted from a slight distortion of the mean from the previous level would yield a new mean value located in the center (median) of the value distribution where it is possible that no abnormality would be observed from results with slight elevations or decreases in value.

In a truly random or Gaussian value distribution, 68% of the values will fall within ±1 SD above and below the mean, 95% within ±2 SDs, and 99.7% within ±3 SDs (see Figure 10-1). The standard procedure is to select ±2 SDs from the mean value as the limits of the normal range. Accepting ±2 SDs from the mean value as normal will place 95% of **clinically normal persons** within the normal range limits. Conversely, it also means that 2.5% of clinically normal persons will have values above and below this range. Normal ranges created in this way are a deliberately thought-out process.

A wider normal range of ±3 SDs would place almost all normal persons within the normal range limits and this would require a wider swing from the mean value for determining if results are abnormal. However, this would place some diseased persons with only a small test abnormality into the expanded normal range of ±3 SDs and thereby decrease test sensitivity for detection of disease. On a practical basis, most patients who are suffering from a particular disease will not have borderline results but will have results that may be several times the normal mean rather than minimal changes in most analytical tests.

A patient may exhibit results that are outside the normal range and actually be free of disease, at least relative to the test performed. There are several reasons for this. For instance, genetic variations within a specific ethnic group may be found, with no clinical reason or outward manifestation for the abnormal analyte for a specific patient. Ranges have been established for indigenous population groups from specific areas of the country or the world. Because the population of the United States is quite homogeneous, normal values were developed from a cross-section of the entire population. Racial differences may be averaged into the mean. However, the mean value for that particular group may be low or high within the normal range, or the numbers for each cultural or ethnic population might have been insignificant and too small to affect the mean value to any great extent, if at all.

Other factors that influence differences in the mean value for normal ranges for most analytes relate to diet, culture, lifestyle, and gender. Long-term diets rich in certain foods may cause a significant difference in values (e.g., the Northwest with a diet rich in salmon or the Southeast with a diet rich in fried foods). The normal ranges include both males and females where some constituents of the blood may be significantly different based on gender. So a female at the low or high end of the normal range for females may fall slightly outside the normal range. Normally the physician will discount any findings that are minimally outside the normal range if the results are insignificant in value or if clinical findings, physical findings, signs, and symptoms are absent.

Problems That Occur from the Use of Normal Ranges

Difficulties occur when the normal ranges are adhered to so closely that perfectly normal patients may be required to undergo the expense and discomfort of further testing because one test was outside the "normal range" by a small amount. All living organisms have differences, and some individuals in a population will be slightly different in their metabolic processes, which may be of a genetic or environmental nature, rather than due to a disease. Possible misuses of normal ranges include the following:

1. A supposedly normal group used to establish normal values would most often contain a small but definite group of clinically normal persons with subclinical manifestations of disease. Some who report themselves as "normal" may have an undetected disease while nevertheless being included in the data used to establish the values. This would have the effect of having abnormal persons erroneously considered normal. This will affect the normal range through the inclusion of test results from persons not suspected of having any disease. But if large numbers of subjects are used to determine a mean for normal values, a few diseased subjects may have only a minimal impact on the population mean. In the same manner as including both males and females and various population groups to determine the mean, the normal limits would be widened with resultant overlap between normal and abnormal persons. For example, tests for plasma glucose specimens from a small group of clinically normal blood donors might be used to obtain the normal range for a new instrument with reagents that differed from those previously used. The range might be 75 to 101 mg/dL, and possibly very close to the values listed in the package insert for the new reagents and instrument. Subsequent test results from a larger group of donors that included those with low normal values and high normal values may be influenced inordinately if the expanded group had a larger number of subjects with a low plasma glucose. Typically when developing a new population norm for any analyte, each test is performed individually. Discarding abnormally low and abnormally high results would yield a normal range very different from that of a small group with a wide variation in values, which might be "normal" for those individuals. Optimally, if the group had an equal number of high values compared with low values, the results would provide a more realistic mean.

2. Normal ranges should never be derived from a small number of individuals. If normal ranges are calculated from a number of values too small to be statistically reliable, a large percentage of individual patients may fall into the abnormal range. This often occurs when a laboratory procedure is rarely

ordered in a particular laboratory and the range is calculated from a small number of procedures spread over a significant time span. Most laboratories now refer these seldom-performed procedures to commercial reference laboratories that accept specimens from across the entire country, giving a more accurate snapshot of what a normal range would be.

3. A number of different factors may affect results in nondiseased persons. The population from which specimens are received for normal range determination may not accurately represent the segment of the population that is being tested. There may be differences due to age, sex, locality, race, diet, sampling from an upright versus reclining position, the length of time the tourniquet is left on the arm, specimen storage time, and many other factors, such as condition of the sample. An example is the erythrocyte sedimentation rate (ESR) in which the normal values by the Westergren method for persons under age 60 years, after correction for anemia, are 0 to 15 mm/hr for men and 0 to 20 mm/hr for women; for patients over age 60, normal values are 0 to 25 mm/hr for men and 0 to 30 mm/hr for women. There may even be significant variation for certain times of the day and for some analytes from day to day in the same person. One example of the effect of timing is that of cortisol. Cortisol peaks around 8:00 AM and falls to its lowest levels during the late evening. This would be a preanalytical issue to consider when patient results inexplicably are out of the normal range and differ from previous results.

4. Normal values obtained by one analytical method may be inappropriate when used with another method. For example, there are several well-accepted techniques for assay of serum albumin. The assay values differ somewhat because the techniques do not measure the same thing. Dye-binding methods measure dye-binding capacity of the albumin molecule, biuret procedures react with nitrogen atoms, immunological methods depend on antibodies against antigenic components, and electrophoresis is influenced primarily by the electric charge of certain chemical groups in the molecule. In fact, different versions of the same method may not yield identical results, and even the same version and method, performed on different equipment, may display variance.

5. Normal values supplied by the manufacturers of test kits frequently do not correspond to the decrease in test values after change from upright to supine position, or when a tourniquet has been left in place, constricting the blood flow, for more than 30 seconds or so.

ERRONEOUS SAMPLES

A multitude of factors may affect the patient's sample and alter the results. Some may be easily identifiable and others may be virtually impossible to pinpoint. While many of these problems are preanalytical in nature, they are not by any means exclusively preanalytical. The quality of the sample with respect to timing of the test, preparation of the patient for the test, use of the correct vacuum tube, and drawing of the sample in the right order, as well as proper identification of the sample, are all examples of erroneous samples.

Effects of Position on Laboratory Values

As pointed out previously, variations may be observed in common procedures due to differences in anatomical positioning while the specimen is being collected. Differences occur due to fluid shifts in the body that occur with various positions. It takes as much as 20 minutes or more to equalize fluid shifts due to changes in position. Keeping the tourniquet on for more than a minute will also cause hemoconcentration and will increase certain values. This would be a pre-analytical issue to consider when results are out of range.

The position of the body for even a short period before blood is collected and the position of the body during collection can be significant. Patients who are having certain tests performed should be told to avoid prolonged standing before the venipuncture. Standing for more than a few minutes will cause capillaries in the tissues to allow only protein-free fluid or more watery substances to pass through the small venules. A person who is lying supine and then returns to a sitting or standing position will cause blood plasma to filter into surrounding tissues, resulting in a decreased level of blood plasma of up to 10%. This would result in an increase in values for those components normally tested for that are bound to protein such as aldosterone (regulates sodium), bilirubin, calcium, cholesterol, iron, and renin. Renin and aldosterone may affect blood pressure directly, so there might be a change in blood pressure as well as laboratory results. Potassium is also greatly increased if the patient had been standing during the past 30 minutes, due to a release of intracellular potassium from muscle cells. High-density lipoprotein (HDL) values may vary by up to 15% by going from a supine position to that of standing.

Other Factors Affecting Laboratory Values

Pregnancy affects laboratory values because numerous physiological changes are taking place in many of the body's systems. Body fluid levels increase during pregnancy, diluting red blood cells and other components and contributing to lower than normal values. Smoking dehydrates the smoker, and the resulting hemoconcentration may raise many values, particularly cholesterol, glucose, triglycerides, and white blood cell counts. Smoking also lowers the levels of most of the immunoglobulins (proteins that contribute to immunity). Youngsters who smoke may also alter their thyroid-stimulating hormone (TSH) and growth hormone (GH).

Stress can cause increases in white blood cell counts and cortisol, and decreases in serum iron. As one would predict, changes in temperature and humidity affect body fluids. Acute heat will cause tissue fluids to move into the vascular system, increasing volume and diluting components of the blood. Excessive sweating will also cause hemoconcentration if fluid replacement is not provided. These environmental factors account for differences in values for population groups in diverse geographic locations with extremes in weather conditions.

Types and Characteristics of Samples

Samples vary by methodology and the test being performed and erroneous results may be obtained if the wrong specimen or improper collection is performed.

Timely collection and proper transport are extremely important if accurate results are to be produced. When analyzing specimens, results must be precise, sensitive, accurate, and specific. Ingestion of certain foods and certain medications may alter dramatically the values obtained from blood testing. A number of laboratory determinations require an overnight fast, and those who are being tested after a fast must be informed of the possible effect of eating or of chewing gum or tobacco. Certain values are higher at certain times of the day or night, and it is vitally important to collect the specimens at the proper time or the results will be useless for determining if abnormalities are present. Specific and consistent levels must be maintained for certain medications as the therapeutic range is very narrow for some types of drugs. Some medicines are also toxic at certain levels and may cause permanent damage or even death if the values rise above those levels. Therefore, timed specimens are drawn for a number of medications. An example is a group of drugs called generally "hospital antibiotics" because they are only administered to an inpatient, normally by IV injection. For many of these, peaks and troughs are established where the concentration is within a therapeutic range but is not allowed to rise to a toxic level.

CATEGORIES OF ERRORS

Errors fall into three categories and they may affect patient care if they result in the reporting of erroneous results. Errors may occur before testing begins (preanalytical), during the test procedure (analytical), and following completion of the test (postanalytical) with handling of the data. Remember that analytical errors may occur during performance of the tests, and in an autoanalyzer, a hundred samples may be relatively accurate, and one sample may be extremely abnormal, and often the cause is never determined.

Preanalytical

Errors caused by the failure to adhere to all of the procedures required to ensure that the sample was adequate and was properly identified fall into this category. Preanalytical errors occur outside the laboratory during the collection of specimens, such as mislabeling the tubes, using the wrong preservative required for a particular procedure, collecting blood in the wrong tube(s), having inadequate volume of a specimen, or collecting a specimen from the wrong patient. Other preanalytical errors include mistakes by the physician by requesting the procedure on the wrong patient or hospital medical personnel failing to submit a timely request to the laboratory. Another common error in this category is that of the patient who should be fasting but eats a meal or is given a meal by the hospital personnel or a visitor. Errors of this nature are among the most difficult to determine and to remedy. The delay in obtaining meaningful results often results in an increased hospital stay or failure to initiate needed treatment and may even cause permanent damage to the patient.

Analytical

These errors occur inside the laboratory after the specimen is collected and properly transported to the laboratory and even to the correct department. These usually involve human or instrument failure, and sometimes are caused by the quality or condition of the standards and reagents used to calculate the results for the procedures. Disturbances to the electrical supply for the equipment, weakening of instrument components due to age, and failure of the laboratory worker to detect malfunctions are common areas that result in poor or negative results. Even during the best instrument operation and when everything seems to be running smoothly, and even if all instructions have been followed, a random error may occur. Although the result from a random error is the type of error most difficult to determine, in most cases a laboratory procedure that shows an abnormality will be accompanied by other abnormal results. An astute technologist should be able in most instances to review all the results and look for supporting tests to support the value or to determine if a result is a random error. An unresolved random error may cause unwarranted delay in treatment or treatment for a condition that does not exist.

Postanalytical

An example of a postanalytical error is when the correct result was obtained but was incorrectly recorded or was applied to the wrong patient. This may cause the wrong treatment or failure to treat a patient who needed therapy. Many of these problems have been eliminated by more specific identification of the patient and linking of the results by numerical means rather than by names. This does not eliminate the human error in which a report is placed on the wrong chart and the physician or other clinician reads the results but does not verify the name.

INTERPRETATION OF RESULTS

A postanalytical error with correct results may affect the patient's well-being but is beyond the purview of the laboratory. The clinician (usually a physician) makes a determination as to whether the results are normal or expected based on the patient's clinical condition. Changes in test values that are significantly different from previous results indicate that a patient's condition is changing. If results are inconsistent with clinical findings, physical assessments, and signs and symptoms, it is possible that either the diagnosis was in error or the results are in error. This requires follow up by the clinician responsible for the patient's care, but may require that a medical laboratory worker do some research to determine if a problem occurred in the performance of the test(s).

Determining if Results Are Normal

A Gaussian distribution curve is a bell-shaped curve divided into equal halves on the upper and lower sides of the mean. Each side is then divided into 1 SD, 2 SD, and 3 SD values. Results within 2 SDs should include 95% of tested subjects (1 of 20 patients would be outside normal range) even if clinically normal. The normal range may have limitations, e.g., a patient with cholesterol within the normal range may suffer from coronary heart disease or a patient with an elevated serum cholesterol may have no level of coronary disease. So it can be assumed that a normal range does not mean an "ideal" range.

Clinical versus Statistical Significance

There are two major types of variations: analytical and biological. *Analytical variation* would occur due to functions of the machines, reagents, and other conditions difficult to determine. *Biological variations* occur due to differences between groups of peoples based on genetics and on lifestyle factors such as diet and cultural practices. For example, a physician would have to weigh any biological differences with the test results before forming informed conclusions regarding the health of an individual. Clinical significance has little to do with statistics and is subject to a medical professional's interpretation and judgment. Therefore, results can be statistically significant yet clinically insignificant.

To determine if figures are clinically significant, the SDs for repeated measurements on a single QC specimen are compared with the SDs for repeated measurements made at weekly intervals within a group of healthy subjects over a period of 10 weeks, which allows for seasonal variations. While clinical significance derives from a calculation for statistical significance, it is usually a matter of clinical judgment. In clinical trials for certain medications or procedures, results are treated as significant when the chance that the difference between two groups occurred is less than 1 time in 20.

Clinically Consistent

If the value derived does not match the clinical diagnosis, research to find an explanation must be pursued. Was the sample identified correctly? What was the method of collection? Did a repeat sample give similar results? If not, the diagnosis may be in error. This is the reason that laboratory workers must have an adequate knowledge of anatomy and physiology, and of disease states that may affect other values. It requires experience and observation before the critical thought processes reach the point that the technologist or technician is able correlate sets of values, often from different departments of the laboratory.

SPECIFICITY AND SENSITIVITY

Specificity is the measure of the incidence of true negatives in persons known to be free of a disease. If a certain procedure is specific in measuring for a disease, persons with clinical manifestations of the disease should test qualitatively positive, and in quantitative tests, results should be considerably elevated or decreased.

Sensitivity is incorporated into test procedures where changes in certain metabolic processes in the body can be measured at levels that are clinically significant. Sensitivity should not be so great that an analyte normally found in low levels in the body will give a false positive result. But a procedure must be sensitive enough to detect levels that indicate the presence of a certain disease when low levels are clinically significant. When the sensitivity of a procedure is optimal, only levels that are in a certain range indicating a specific disease will yield a result that will be helpful in diagnosing the presence of a disease or medical condition requiring medical attention.

EFFICIENCY

Efficiency of methodology should be chosen by selecting the test method with the greatest number of correct results when divided by the total number of tests. An efficient method for most purposes in the medical laboratory would consider economical measures such as cost of reagents, time for each test (dwell time), and even ease of operation of equipment and storage of supplies.

REPORTING OF RESULTS

Results are most often reported directly via computer to patient areas and even to physicians' offices. Simultaneous storage of patient results and dissemination to a patient's chart, whether in a hospital, clinic, or private physician's office, are done quickly and effortlessly. Point-of-care testing, also called near-patient testing, requires that all personnel who perform procedures with bedside equipment perform function checks and QC, which is stored in the instrument and in some cases is transmitted to the laboratory's LIS. Remember that point-of-care testing is most often performed by those other than medical laboratory personnel.

COMPUTER PROCESSES WITHIN THE CLINICAL LABORATORY

There are defined processes by which data are entered into a computer system. The data are often stored as information in a form that are not readily readable by the laboratory worker. Computers process and correlate data to provide reports that may be distributed to the clinicians for their review. Some of the terms used in computer procedures are hardware, CPU (central processing unit), memory, storage media, along with input and output devices. In the laboratory, a large amount of data are produced and disseminated on a constant basis. An LIS is normally installed in any laboratory of even modest size. Information is coordinated by the system to achieve delivery of patient reports in a timely manner and in an organized format. This would not be possible without highly sophisticated computer systems capable of receiving data input from a large variety of instruments as well as from manual entry of data produced when manual methods of testing are performed. The following components are required to operate these large systems.

Central Computer Memory

Many of the calculations and storage of QC data and patient results are accomplished within the central memory of the instruments. Some facilities use storage for permanent records on tape drives or other forms of memory for long-term record keeping. When storing large amounts of data, tape can be substantially less expensive than disk or other data storage options. Permanent storage has been greatly facilitated by improved computer hardware and software over the past few years and more innovative methods will undoubtedly follow.

Software for Mechanical Functions and Calculation of Results

Software refers to programs designed to perform mechanical functions of the instruments as well as to manage the calculating of results from raw data and storage of results. This is a set of electronic instructions contained on a computer program for performing specific functions as needed for the laboratory and the facility as a whole. Applications programs are often composed of separate functions and serve to integrate the various computer tasks. A large variety of software packages can be tailored to the specific laboratory and its needs.

Administrative Functions and Related Personnel Tasks

Organization of the laboratory schedules, which may require staffing of various departments for 24 hours per day, is often managed through computer systems; these systems may also include payroll functions. This gives access to other operators for identifying the technical person responsible for following up on random errors and for problems with QC results. This information can also be made available for facility licensure and accreditation site visitors. Other information handled by an information system may include personnel evaluations, continuing and inservice education pertinent to quality assurance and other areas of operation by individuals, and credentials information. Equipment maintenance and budgeting operations for the clinical laboratory are also easily managed through laboratory records stored on computers. Follow-up in problem areas and documentation of actions taken are important components of quality assurance and process improvement.

Specimen Management

Specimen management has become an area in which efficiency and accuracy of specimen collection have been greatly enhanced by computer systems. Identification of specimens is an integral part of specimen management as is providing drawing lists for phlebotomists and technical personnel that itemize amounts and types of specimens, and providing bar code identification of the patient and specimen. Results are often transmitted automatically from the laboratory equipment to the patient's medical records in the hospital or clinic records system. Preanalytical errors have been greatly minimized by systematic handling of patient specimens and record keeping. Preventing errors such as mismatched specimens, requests for the wrong laboratory tests, and posting of laboratory results to the wrong patient's records also plays an important role in avoiding the paper shuffling of previous decades. Efficiency of collection schedules is also accomplished, helping to make collections of specimens more efficient by avoiding the retracing of steps on phlebotomy rounds and the assignment of more than one person to a given area of the hospital.

SUMMARY

While QC is at the center of the laboratory professional's observations when procedures are being performed, this component is just a small portion of a good quality assurance program. Quality assurance programs take into consideration the environment and the physical aspects of the facility and how it is maintained, from adequate lighting to proper ventilation and cleanliness. Just as soldiers must keep their "weapons clean and their powder dry," equipment maintenance is a major component of a smoothly functioning and dependable laboratory. Many breakdowns may be prevented when diligent care is taken of equipment, supplies are properly stored to prevent deterioration, and specimens are correctly handled and identified. Competence of personnel and ensuring adequate staffing of various levels of staff is also of the utmost importance.

REVIEW QUESTIONS

1. Compare *accuracy* versus *precision*.
2. Define *mean, median,* and *mode*.
3. Contrast a *shift* and a *trend* in control values.
4. What is the significance of Westgard rules?
5. Name the types of errors that may occur.

CHAPTER 11

PHLEBOTOMY

LEARNING OBJECTIVES

Upon completion of this chapter, the reader will be able to:

- Demonstrate professional and ethical behavior.

- Understand licensure, registry, and certification.

- Indicate the position of the phlebotomist in the hospital laboratory organization.

- List equipment and basic instrumentation of a hospital laboratory.

- Describe various types of tubes and collection equipment.

- Provide separated blood specimens through use of centrifuges.

- Choose a vein in the correct anatomical region and palpate.

- Perform various types of collection from venipuncture to capillary puncture.

- Process specimens and transport them to the correct departments for testing.

- Input specimen data for record keeping.

- Interact appropriately with patients and visitors.

KEY TERMS

Artery	Cubital vein, medial	Order of draw
Basilic vein	Hematoma	Professionalism
Bevel	Hemoconcentration	Venipuncture
Capillary puncture	Lumen	Vein
Cephalic vein	Needle gauge	

INTRODUCTION

Phlebotomy is an integral part of medical laboratory practice. It is good to remember that no laboratory procedure will be any better than the quality of the specimen that is being tested. Most blood and other body fluid collections in the past were performed by medical laboratory technicians or technologists and in some cases, by nurses and physicians. Today, most blood is collected by trained phlebotomists, but medical laboratory technologists and technicians must nevertheless be somewhat proficient at collecting blood samples. Phlebotomists are responsible for many tasks other than collecting blood and are valuable adjuncts to the medical laboratory technical personnel. Some phlebotomists are trained to perform point-of-care testing at the bedside for tests that are of a waived nature (not covered under CLIA as being of sufficient difficulty that a technical person must perform them). Many phlebotomists are certified by an agency that ensures validity and effectiveness of training and tests the phlebotomist to ensure that skills and knowledge are sufficient for the position. Note that there are several independent agencies that accredit phlebotomists and at least one state (California) requires licensing of phlebotomists.

Critical Reminder
Glossary of Selected Terms

- **Artery**—blood vessel carrying blood away from heart to tissues, cells, and organs
- **Basilic vein**—secondary choice for drawing blood, on inner top portion of arm
- **Bevel**—slanted cut end of needle used to puncture skin
- **Capillary puncture**—procedure where small vessels of finger, toe, or heel are pricked for blood collection
- **Cephalic vein**—superficial vessel just beneath the skin of the arm in middle of inner part of arm
- **Cubital vein, medial**—vein at bend of elbow connecting cephalic and basilic veins
- **Hematoma**—blood leaking from vessel and collecting under skin
- **Lumen**—internal diameter of needle or other tubular cavity of the body
- **Needle gauge**—outer diameter size of needle; a smaller gauge indicates a larger outer diameter
- **Venipuncture**—the collection of blood from a vein
- **Vein**—reverse function of an artery; carries blood from tissues back to heart and lungs

Exposure to Bloodborne and Airborne Pathogens

The phlebotomist must be aware of the risks associated with performing venipunctures for patients who may have a contagious infection. Bloodborne and airborne precautions must be exercised at all times, even if the patient appears healthy. There is also the danger of an accidental needle stick injury after collecting blood from an infected patient. For these reasons, protection against infection requires strict handwashing before and after venipuncture and the wearing of personal protective equipment (PPE). Engineered controls, which include needles that have safety shields on them and the proper disposal of them, serve to protect the phlebotomist or technical laboratory worker. Table 11-1 provides the basics for precautions, PPE and work practice, and the use of engineering controls.

PHLEBOTOMISTS

A person who collects blood, whether a phlebotomist or a medical laboratory worker, must possess skills in communication and have a good grasp of basic psychology and good common sense when working with patients and family members. Manual dexterity is a must and one must be psychologically prepared for inserting needles into sometimes unwilling patients. As demands increase on the medical worker, and health care facilities are downsizing and simplifying their operations, responsibilities for certain duties are being shifted. The venipuncture is the most common method for obtaining sufficient blood for a number of many different laboratory procedures to determine disease states. A number of devices are available for performing a venipuncture, and some are modifications of earlier devices that have been engineered for safety and efficiency. A safety needle containing guards that clamp over the needle after use is the most common engineering device at the phlebotomist's disposal (Figure 11-1).

Professionalism

Professionalism is the first thing a patient will notice about the person who comes to collect his or her blood. Professional behavior is paramount in the person who is collecting blood from a patient who is already at

Table 11-1 Using Infection Control Methods while Performing Venipunctures

Control Method	Mechanism
Standard precautions	Treat all patients and all specimens as infectious.
Personal protective equipment	Wear gloves to handle blood and all body fluids; wear fluid-resistant gown or laboratory coat; wear eye protection if splashes are reasonably anticipated.
Engineering controls	Use containers for contaminated sharps, designated and marked containers for biohazardous waste, biohazard containers for contaminated reusable apparel, biohazard containers for disposable apparel, appropriate surface disinfectants.
Work practice controls	Always wear gloves when working with blood; never recap, remove, cut, or break needles; use safety needles and needle holders; immediately dispose of contaminated sharps in an appropriate receptacle; wash hands with antiseptic after removing gloves or any other time hands are potentially contaminated.

a high level of stress due to illness or perhaps from having the procedure itself performed. The characteristics that make a technician or technologist a professional must come into play during this critical process. Professional behavior would include a calm and confident approach along with an explanation of the procedure being performed. Since the first critical step in completing a laboratory procedure is that of obtaining an adequate specimen and providing the correct handling and proper identification of the samples, the phlebotomist must be professional, competent, and thorough. Always remember that a laboratory procedure is no more accurate than the specimen used for its performance.

QUALITY ASSURANCE IN PHLEBOTOMY

Quality assurance is as much a part of phlebotomy procedures as it is for performing laboratory procedures with proper quality control specimens and equipment maintenance requirements. Laboratory testing is an important part of diagnosis and prognosis for a patient, as the physician relies on results to either diagnose or confirm a diagnosis as well as to follow the effects of a treatment. To ensure consistent quality of specimen collection and handling, policies are implemented and procedures are developed based on specific guidelines. Poor and inaccurate results for laboratory testing due to inadequate collection of samples may delay providing test data to the physician and may be the basis for a misdiagnosis if test results provide faulty clinical information.

The National Accrediting Agency for Clinical Laboratory Science (NAACLS), among other agencies, provides for accreditation of phlebotomy programs. But not all phlebotomy

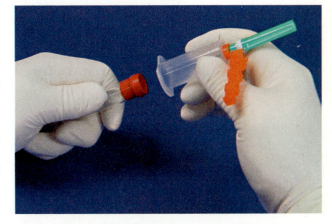

FIGURE 11-1 Vacuum tube system with safety needle, disposable needle holder, and vacuum collection tube. Source: Delmar/Cengage Learning.

programs seek this voluntary accreditation for an institutional phlebotomy program as most states do not require phlebotomists to be certified or licensed, unlike medical laboratory workers. Some certifying agencies, such as the American Society for Clinical Pathologists (ASCP), do require that applicants for medical laboratory registry examinations be graduates of programs accredited by agencies such as NAACLS to qualify for a certification examination.

Statistics are compiled in some facilities that gauge the percentage of acceptable samples and those that require that they be re-collected. Efforts to improve these figures are often a part of the quality assurance or quality improvement programs within a facility. Many of the preanalytical errors that affect laboratory results occur during the phlebotomy procedures for collecting blood samples and entering them into the Laboratory Information System (LIS).

Some of the areas that are a part of patient safety as well as quality control for the phlebotomy section would include monitoring of sharps (needles or lancets) to ensure they are sterile before use. No needle or lancet should be used if the seal guaranteeing sterility has been broken by other than the person collecting the sample. Occasionally a needle may be deficient, and it may be possible to detect this if the needle is visually observed for deformities before use. Used sharps should be discarded in a specially designed sharps container. Disposal of the entire needle assembly is most often the practice following venipuncture, whereas reuse of a syringe and needle were the norm a few decades earlier (Figures 11-2 and 11-3). Commercial disposal companies are hired to pick up these containers when filled, along with other biohazardous wastes, for incineration in specially built furnaces.

Evacuated tubes are used for most collections. If they have expired, it is difficult to collect the proper amount as the amount of vacuum degrades over a period of time, resulting in obtaining too little blood for testing or for problems with the amount of anticoagulant in certain tubes.

STEPS FOR PROPER COLLECTION OF BLOOD SAMPLES BY VENIPUNCTURE

Venous blood is the specimen most often collected by a phlebotomist or medical laboratory technician or technologist. Other specimens that are routinely but less frequently collected are capillary blood from a finger, ear, or toe puncture, or arterial blood for a series of blood tests called blood gases. In most facilities, respiratory therapists collect arterial blood and are also licensed to perform the tests for blood gases. Relatively large amounts of venous, or deoxygenated, blood may be collected for a variety of blood tests by a phlebotomist or a technical laboratory worker.

The proper steps must be followed to minimize the risk of infection to the patient and the person collecting the sample, as well as to ensure that adequate and appropriate samples will be available for testing. There are certain rules that should never be broken. Experiences of each laboratory worker or phlebotomist will help in developing individual manners of greeting patients and the setting up of equipment and supplies. Consistent observation of basic steps will help to avoid mistakes and problems (Table 11-2). One cardinal rule that most facilities observe is that a phlebotomist or technician should perform a venipuncture only

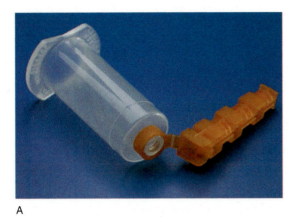
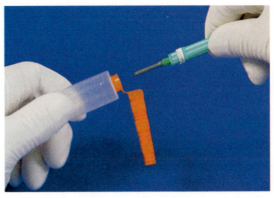

A   B

FIGURE 11-2 Vacuum tube collecting system. (A) Blood collection needle holder with safety shield for used needle. (B) Insertion of multi-sample needle into needle holder.
Source: Delmar/Cengage Learning.

twice on a patient when no blood was obtained on the first "stick." Depending on the confidence and skill of the phlebotomist or technician, a third attempt may be made if the patient is not overtly stressed. Otherwise, another phlebotomist is summoned to perform the collection. This is because a phlebotomist may lose his or her self-confidence and more than likely the patient will question the abilities of the phlebotomist. The general process for preparing to obtain and drawing a sample are presented in the following sections.

SELECTION OF EQUIPMENT

Equipment and supplies used depends on the situation and the condition and anatomy of the patient. A syringe and a Luer-lock needle are used for persons with small veins or for pediatric patients and infants. For adult veins that are not extremely small, a larger needle may be used. When blood is obtained using a needle and needle holder, the blood is collected by pushing the blood collection tubes against the needle inside the blood collection holder. This allows the interior needle to penetrate the rubber stopper on the tube and to allow it to fill fully before being pulled from the needle holder. It is more difficult to obtain large amounts of blood with a syringe, but pediatric-sized tubes are available and will usually provide a sufficient quantity of blood for performing most tests. For most adult normal patients, a 20- or 21-gauge needle is used. Since the smaller the number of needle gauge, the larger is the needle, a person with small veins may require a 22, 23, or 24 gauge. A needle that is too large may cause

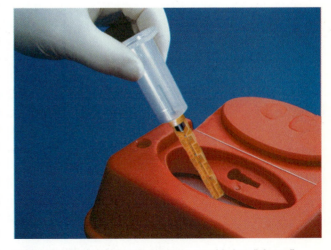

FIGURE 11-3 Disposal of venipuncture assembly into "sharps" container.
Source: Delmar/Cengage Learning.

Table 11-2 Steps That Help to Eliminate Mistakes in Sample Collection

1. Assemble supplies and put them within easy reach. It is difficult to reach for needed supplies while holding the needle apparatus with the needle in the vein. A related precaution is that one should be prepared for the patient to make a sudden move, or to knock the supplies to the floor if the patient is combative or has any dementia.

2. Safety precautions include having alcohol swabs available for cleansing the skin, and ensuring that the needle is sterile. The phlebotomist should have already determined that the tubes are properly selected for size and type and that they are not expired Bar-coded stickers are usually available for affixing to the tubes. If a tube is found to be defective, there are usually additional stickers that can be used if a tube has to be discarded, wasting a label.

3. Varbally prepare the patient for the procedure. If the patient is disoriented, it might be necessary to ask for help from a co-worker or from a nurse or assistant who works with the patient.

4. Place the tourniquet according to the tension taught in the classroom. In addition, the tourniquet should not be left on the arm for more than 30 seconds to 1 minute.

5. Palpate the vein to determine the suitability of the vein or to locate a vein that might not be visible.

6. Cleanse the arm with alcohol swabs, and allow the site to dry for a few seconds. Insert the needle with the bevel up (opening or lumen will be visible).

7. Obtain correct tubes by using pre-selected ones suitable for procedures requested. Allow them to fill fully, as not doing so may cause errors in dilution of anticoagulants if present, or the sample might not be sufficient in volume.

8. Care for the puncture site by loosening the tourniquet after the last tube is collected, and placing a dry gauze sponge or cotton ball over the puncture site. Apply slight pressure on the sponge and withdraw the needle quickly.

9. Maintain pressure on the puncture site for a short period of time. The patient may be able to apply pressure in most instances while the tubes are being safely stored and the waste is discarded properly in the correct receptacles.

10. Remove all used materials for proper disposal. Ensure that no sharp objects are left that might injure the patient. Place wastes in proper containers, e.g. needles in "sharps" container, and routine waste into trash receptacle. Ensure samples are secured properly for transport to the laboratory or other area as applicable.

damage to the red blood cells, causing the plasma to be *hemolyzed*. If a red cell count is being performed, the count may be artificially lowered due to destroyed cells, so this is a consideration in collecting both whole blood samples and where hemolysis will interfere with test results.

In the case of a patient with normal veins, a vacuum tube system—consisting of a barrel and a needle set containing a double-needle that can be screwed into the barrel—is used. While the needle is in the patient's arm, tubes may be exchanged as they fill until all required specimens are obtained. With this system, it is more difficult to know if the needle is in a vein, since there is no *flash* or quick appearance of blood in the hub of the needle as would be the case when using a needle and syringe system. But with experience, a phlebotomist or laboratory technical worker can often feel that the bevel point of the needle is sufficiently into the vein.

Another modified system is used predominantly by many laboratories but is more expensive than the previous systems described. It is the "butterfly" needle, which can be screwed into a barrel as previously described, or the end of the tube may have a needle similar to that of the needle that is screwed into the barrel. This needle may be used to pierce the rubber caps of the tubes; the tubes can then be allowed to fill. Use of the butterfly system may be helpful on extremely difficult veins and a flash of blood will be seen as soon as the needle enters the vein, as occurs with the use of a syringe.

Choosing the correct tube(s) will be critical, as there are a large variety of specialized tubes used in collecting blood. Some tubes contain an anticoagulant and are used to obtain the liquid portion of the blood (plasma), which is commonly used for coagulation tests and some chemistry tests. Other types of tubes without anticoagulant are designed for obtaining serum. Serum is also a liquid component of blood and is derived when the blood collected in the tube is allowed to clot. The tube is then centrifuged to separate the cells of the blood from the liquid portion of the blood. Some types of tubes used to obtain serum contain a barrier device that separates the liquid portion of the blood from the cells or solid components.

PATIENT POSITION AND ORDER OF DRAW

The result of a number of laboratory procedures may be skewed due to the anatomic position assumed by the patient. Results may be altered if the patient is standing, sitting, or lying down, or if the tourniquet is on the arm for more than a half-minute to a minute. Among the many tests that are affected considerably by having a tourniquet on the arm for an extended period, cholesterol determinations and hemoglobin levels are possibly affected the most.

Order of draw refers to the sequence of tubes used in drawing blood. The specific order in which the tubes are used serves to avoid contamination by preventing carryover from tubes containing chemicals, which might result in inaccurate test results. There are several major types of blood collection tubes that have been developed for specific purposes and the color of their tube stoppers may vary by manufacturer. Some tubes are designed to provide preservation of the sample. Others are sterile and are used for determining the presence of bacteria. Several types of tubes allow the blood to clot and serum to be obtained when spun at a high rate of speed in a centrifuge. Some tubes contain a barrier substance that separates liquid and solid portions of blood upon centrifugation, and some of these may include a clot enhancer to speed the clotting process. Several types of anticoagulants are found in some specially designed tubes to preserve the morphology of blood cells or to provide plasma for coagulation studies.

PERFORMANCE OF VENIPUNCTURE

As mentioned previously, phlebotomists are most often responsible for collecting blood samples, particularly in the larger hospitals. Training for phlebotomists includes skills other than the actual process of obtaining blood through venipuncture. Sample transport and separation and logging the sample into the LIS are among the duties of the phlebotomist. The phlebotomist must also have strong skills in dealing with people, such as ill patients and their families and other health care professionals. The following steps take into account the use of many of the attributes the phlebotomist should possess.

Safety Alert

Causes of Injuries to Patient and Phlebotomist

- Phlebotomist sticks himself or herself with a used needle.
- Phlebotomist or laboratory worker leaves used needles and lancets in the bed linen.
- Tube of blood is dropped and broken (more common when glass tubes were used).
- Patient side rails are left down, and patient falls from the bed.
- Patient is combative and injures himself or the phlebotomist.

Assessing the Patient's Mental Status

The phlebotomist or technician should remain calm and professional, regardless of the patient's reactions, which might be fostered by fear, loneliness, or anger. Interacting with patients with cognitive impairments, such as senility, Alzheimer's disease, or mental illness or other cognitive impairments, will require different skills than for those without any of these conditions. The ability to deal well with this type of patient will come with experience and observation of others who have developed an approach that the patient will accept. There will be occasions where the patient speaks by sign language or converses in a language other than the one the phlebotomist speaks, requiring special arrangements for preparing the patient for phlebotomy. If help might be needed, procure aid before beginning the procedure.

Explaining the Procedure to the Patient

Explain to the patient that any detailed questions should be asked of his or her physician. In most facilities, the phlebotomist is allowed to only tell the patient the basics of what is being done. Some facilities do allow a description of the tests, such as routine testing, but the phlebotomist is not to discuss the meaning of the tests or the patient's treatment. Most patients understand that blood tests will be performed to rule out certain conditions and to confirm others. If the patient initially objects to the tests, remind the patient that his or her physician needs the tests to provide treatment. Sometimes a nurse who is dealing with the patient can convince him or her that the tests are absolutely necessary. If the patient is still opposed to having blood taken, the phlebotomist must write on the laboratory request that the patient refused to provide a specimen. The nurse responsible for the patient must be informed of the patient's refusal, and the physician will then be notified.

Identifying the Patient Correctly

Identify the patient by checking the arm band as well as addressing the patient by name. Ensure that a patient who should have been fasting has done so. It is better to ask the patient the last time he or she ate rather than asking if the patient has eaten since some will deny having eaten to try to comply with the requirements for fasting. If the patient should be in a fasting state but is not, it is necessary to consult with the nurse or the physician as to how to proceed.

Assembling the Equipment and Supplies

Depending on the patient's age, condition of the veins, department policy, and amount of blood needed, the decision is made as to what system to use for obtaining the blood. In the example shown in Figure 11-4, the venipuncture supplies arranged for use are appropriate for procedures where a barrel (needle holder) and evacuated tubes will be used. Assemble and label the proper tubes, checking them for expiration date and condition before arranging them in the order in which they should be drawn (see Table 11-3 for a sample order of draw). This sequence largely avoids contaminating specimens from additives in the tubes, which may cause erroneous results. Arrange all of

Table 11-3 Rationale for Order of Draw for Phlebotomy Procedures

Tube Stopper Color	Rationale for Order of Draw
Yellow	Sterile; used for cultures of blood; top must be clean
Red, plain	No additives; used for drug analyses; lack of additives necessary to prevent cross-reactions
Blue	Contains citrate, an anticoagulant; used for coagulation studies; binds calcium and enables other clotting factors to be analyzed; calcium is added for certain procedures
Camouflage ("tiger" or mottled)	Has a barrier gel to separate liquid (serum) and solid components of blood
Red, with gel	Has separator gel to separate liquid (serum) and solid components of blood, but no other additives, in most cases
Gold	Has barrier gel and a clot enhancer; used when it is necessary to separate the blood components quickly
Green	Contains heparin, an effective anticoagulant; most often used in chemistry testing where plasma is used as a sample; some green top tubes contain a lithium gel that also separates plasma from cells and is a barrier additive; small tubes for pediatric patients are available
Pink, purple, lavender	Contain EDTA as an anticoagulant that preserves blood cell anatomy; most often used for blood cell counts as this anticoagulant preserves the morphology of the blood cells, whereas citrate and flouride anticoagulants will not
Gray (grey)	Contains sodium fluoride/potassium; used to preserve glucose values when it is inconvenient to immediately perform a glucose procedure; the sodium flouride/potassium oxalate in the tube preserves the glucose by preventing metabolism by the blood cells, which would consume the glucose and provide a falsely low value

the equipment and supplies you will need within easy reach (Figure 11-4).

Choosing and Using the Appropriate Needle

Choose the correct needle gauge. Usually for the normal patient, a 20- or 21-gauge needle is used (the smaller the gauge, the larger the needle). The 20- or 21-gauge needle allows an adequate flow of blood. Since the smaller-gauge needles may actually damage blood cells, causing morphological changes in the red blood cells and sometimes even lead to destruction, smaller gauges for cell counts should be avoided when and if possible. Screw the needle into the barrel, if reusable barrel/needle devices are used, leaving the cover on the needle outside the tube holder. Seat the first tube in the tube holder but DO NOT push the tube onto the internal needle, as the vacuum will be lost and it will be impossible for blood to enter the tube.

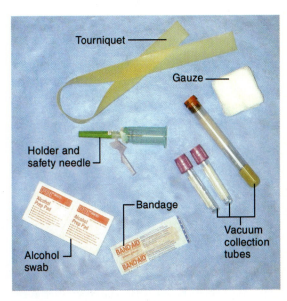

FIGURE 11-4 Venipuncture supplies and equipment. Source: Delmar/Cengage Learning.

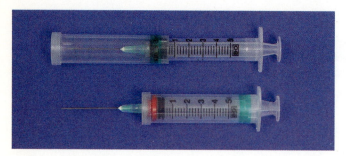

FIGURE 11-5 Safety syringe with sliding plastic sheath covering needle. Source: Delmar/Cengage Learning.

After assembling the materials needed and prior to beginning the procedure, it is necessary for the phlebotomist to find the best site. This gives confidence to the patient and the phlebotomist and is accomplished by visually examining the area and using the tightened tourniquet to evaluate the vein. The phlebotomist then loosens the tourniquet prior to preparing to perform the venipuncture.

Remember that sometimes, in difficult "sticks," it will be necessary to use a syringe (Figure 11-5) or a "butterfly" apparatus (Figure 11-6) to puncture small veins, such as those in young children.

Washing Hands and Gloving

For the phlebotomist's protection, the hands must be thoroughly washed and gloves donned before performing a venipuncture procedure. Nonsterile gloves are used to protect the medical worker. Sterile gloves are worn to protect the patient from infection as well as the surgical worker. Hands should be washed in a circular scrubbing motion with hands in downward position to prevent water and soap from running toward the shoulders. Use friction by vigorously rubbing the hands together; in addition, the cuticles of the nails should be scrubbed against the palms of the hands. After rinsing, dry the hands thoroughly with dry paper towels. On sinks that do not have an automatic shut off, the faucet should be turned off using paper towels. Note that bacteria may travel through wet paper more easily than dry, so the faucet should be turned off with dry towels.

Positioning and Reassuring the Patient

Honestly explain to the patient that there will be slight discomfort but it will be brief. Explain the importance of not moving the arm while blood is being obtained. Patients should preferably be seated or lying down while blood is drawn (it is difficult to collect blood from a standing patient). It is important to remember that certain values are changed by a patient's position, so in some cases it is necessary to place the patient in a certain position. Inpatients in a hospital are almost always in a supine position when blood is being collected. Never allow the patient to stand or to sit on a high stool as it would be difficult to avoid or to control a fall if the patient faints. Special blood-drawing chairs are available for positioning the patient and arranging the supplies in an easy-to-reach fashion. Never restrain the patient or have someone hold a patient against his or her will when drawing blood, as this might constitute the crime of "battery."

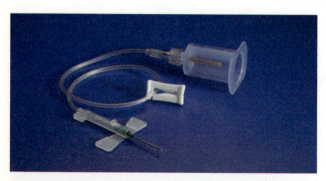

FIGURE 11-6 Butterfly needle for difficult sticks, such as small veins and veins located in difficult-to-reach areas. Source: Delmar/Cengage Learning.

Latex and Bandage Sensitivity

The use of latex tourniquets or gloves should be avoided for patients who indicate they have a latex sensitivity. The phlebotomist or medical worker should have already determined whether he or she has a latex sensitivity. Laboratories provide several varieties of gloves for those who exhibit an allergic reaction to either powder or latex. These reactions may be quite severe, so it is incumbent on the person collecting blood to ask if the patient has such an allergy. In some cases, there might be a warning sticker on any forms used for treating the patient, advising of such a condition. Rarely, some brands of bandages that contain latex or other synthetic materials may cause reactions when placed over the puncture site after the blood is drawn in patients sensitive to certain materials.

Other Precautions

For inpatients, there are other considerations. Bed rails may be let down on the side from which blood will be collected but must be raised again on leaving if they were raised when the phlebotomist or technician entered the room. It is best to avoid collecting blood from limbs with IV (intravenous) lines present. IV solutions may dilute the blood, giving erroneous results. If collecting blood from an arm with an IV is unavoidable, the blood should always be collected from a site BELOW where the IV line enters the vein. Capillary punctures (Figures 11-7, 11-8, and 11-9) are not usually affected by IV solutions and it is possible to collect many samples such as a complete blood count (CBC) by finger stick. However, specimens such as coagulation tests must be drawn from a vein.

Patients with chronic diseases or who have been hospitalized for a period of time often have bruises and sites where they have been stuck for blood tests and other procedures on a number of occasions. Repeat punctures of the skin and subsequent drawing of blood from the same sites may give erroneous results. Upon discontinuation of IV fluid administration, blood should not be drawn from the site for 1 to 2 days following

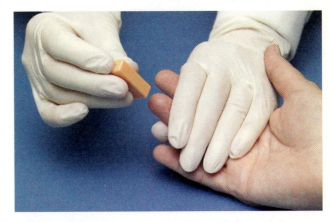

FIGURE 11-7 Positioning of hand and holding of a lancet before capillary puncture.
Source: Delmar/Cengage Learning.

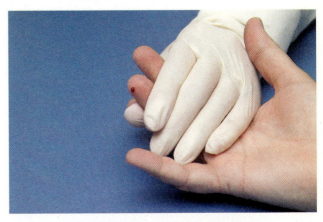

FIGURE 11-8 Well-rounded drop of free-flowing blood after adequate puncture.
Source: Delmar/Cengage Learning.

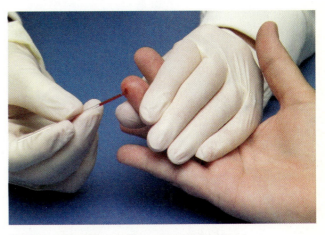

FIGURE 11-9 Obtaining capillary tubes of blood for procedure requiring small volume of sample.
Source: Delmar/Cengage Learning.

removal of the device. If collection of arterial blood is required (this is rare for medical laboratory workers), an arterial line used to measure a patient's blood pressure continuously and accurately may be in place. Blood may be used from this device for blood gas determinations as it would provide arterial blood.

Some patients have *shunts* where a surgical procedure is used to attach an artery and a vein. These can be felt easily by palpating the skin over the site. This vascular rearrangement is often done when a patient is required to undergo kidney dialysis on a regular basis. A tourniquet should never be applied to an arm with a shunt and blood should never be drawn from this arm. Heparin or saline locks are present when a winged or butterfly apparatus is to be left in a patient's vein for up to 48 hours. The heparin and saline are necessary to prevent clotting around the site. Blood may be drawn from this device, but only after removing approximately 5 mL of fluid and discarding it before collecting the sample. This should not be attempted unless one is trained and experienced in the procedure. There are other indwelling lines from which blood may be drawn if necessary, but again, fluid must be removed and discarded before obtaining the testing sample. Only those skilled and experienced in the procedure should perform this task.

Choosing a Puncture Site

Veins are found throughout the body. However, the majority of blood specimens are obtained in the bend of the elbow. It is also possible to obtain venous access in the hands, toes, neck, and elsewhere, but the easiest site and the one with the least trauma and potential for causing harm to the patient is the inside of the elbow region. Figure 11-10 depicts the most favorable sites where blood can be easily obtained from the majority of patients. They include the median cubital, the basilic, and the cephalic vein in each arm. Obese patients, burn patients, and those with amputations pose additional challenges to obtaining an adequate sample of blood.

INITIATING THE VENIPUNCTURE

After gaining experience, the phlebotomist or laboratory worker will become comfortable with the procedure. Many of the following steps will become automatic, and the worker will adopt his or her own particular manner of performing a phlebotomy procedure.

Applying the Tourniquet

The tourniquet should be properly placed on the patient's arm while selecting a site for venipuncture.

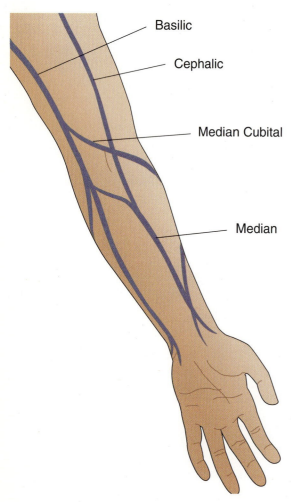

Basilic

Cephalic

Median Cubital

Median

FIGURE 11-10 Veins commonly used for venipuncture.
Source: Delmar/Cengage Learning.

The tourniquet should never be so tight as to arrest the flow of blood in the artery, which lies deeper than the vein. Serious damage may occur if this is done, even for a relatively short period of time.

A tourniquet may be of several varieties. Some patients may be aware of a latex sensitivity and this type of tourniquet would be avoided in these patients. Some medical facilities avoid the problem by using only latex-free tourniquets, or a cloth barrier that is used along with the tourniquet. Some tourniquets are designed with Velcro strips for closure, while others are flat latex tubing or strips. The latter type is placed on the arm as a simple loop tucked or looped under so as to allow pulling on one end to loosen the entire tourniquet with a minimum of movement.

If the patient has large, visible veins, the tourniquet will not need to be placed on the arm and the vein checked by palpation before the final application of the tourniquet.

Apply the tourniquet 3 or 4 inches above the intended puncture site. When the tourniquet is applied with the right tightness, the vein should protrude slightly and enable a pool of blood to collect in the vein for withdrawal, as more blood can flow into the area than is able to leave. If the tourniquet is too tight, the arteries may be constricted and blood cannot flow into the area. If the tourniquet is too loose, it is ineffective for "pumping up" the vein. A tourniquet should feel only slightly tight for the donor and should not be twisted or pinch the skin of the person. Do not apply the tourniquet over areas with chafing, a rash, or an open sore. The tourniquet is placed as shown in Figures 11-11, 11-12, and 11-13.

The site should be cleaned quickly with 70% isopropyl alcohol, using circular motions while moving gradually farther from the center, leaving a 2-inch square area that has been cleansed of surface contaminants and loose cells.

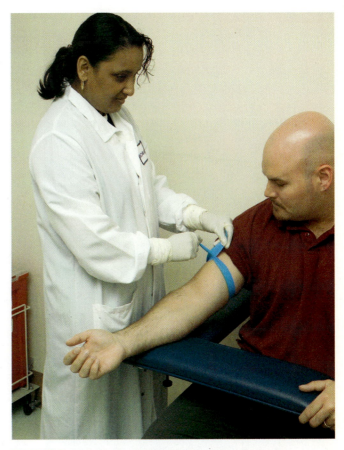

FIGURE 11-11 Patient in donor chair with arm supports in place.
Source: Delmar/Cengage Learning.

Palpating for the Vein

After the tourniquet is properly placed and the skin is cleansed, the patient is asked to make a fist, which serves to make the vein even more prominent. Vigorously squeezing and loosening the fist may cause hemoconcentration (higher density of blood cells) for some tests, so pumping of the fist should be avoided. Veins will usually be more easily visualized in the dominant arm. Phlebotomy procedures

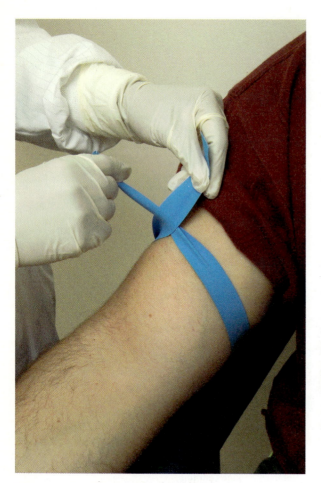

FIGURE 11-12 **Tying the tourniquet around the arm.**
Source: Delmar/Cengage Learning.

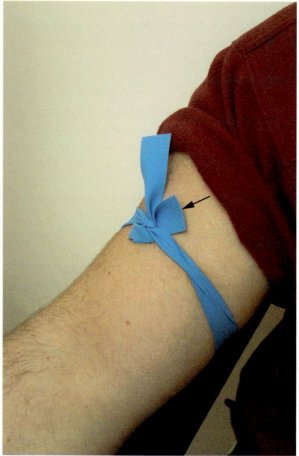

FIGURE 11-13 **To release the tourniquet, pull on the end (marked by an arrow).**
Source: Delmar/Cengage Learning.

are performed where the median cubital, cephalic, and basilica veins are all found close to the surface of the skin. Some veins are visible while others are prominent but can only be felt by palpation with the index finger. Palpation also gives clues as to the direction the vein travels and the size and depth of the vessel (Figure 11-14).

An artery has a detectable pulse and should not be used for ordinary purposes of drawing blood. A vein that feels quite hard should be avoided since it may be sclerosed (hardened) or thrombosed (contain a clot). Tendons are also found in the joint region and are extremely hard. It would be painful for the patient if the phlebotomist inadvertently punctured a tendon; as well, no blood would be obtained. Hard veins "roll" more easily, and rotating the hand and wrist slightly will sometimes place the vein in a more advantageous position for collecting blood.

Once all of these conditions have been considered, the venipuncture should proceed.

Entering the Vein

Unsheath (remove the cover from) the needle just before performing the actual entry through the skin. Leave the tube that should be drawn first lying loosely in the barrel (tube holder). The bevel or flattened open side of the needle should be visible from above as one looks down toward the patient's arm (Figure 11-15). Anchor and pull the skin tight at approximately 1 inch below the intended puncture site. Hold the barrel (tube holder, syringe, etc.) with the thumb and forefingers of the dominant hand. Enter the skin at a 30- to 45-degree angle. The angle can be adjusted to better accommodate the patient's anatomy as the phlebotomist gains experience. In those patients who are normal in weight with little fatty tissue beneath the skin, an insertion of the needle for only a few millimeters will be sufficient to be properly positioned in the vein.

Make sure the barrel does not move by anchoring the barrel with the fingers of the nondominant hand, then push the first tube onto the inner needle of the barrel. When the tube stops filling and if the draw is without problem, there will be sufficient blood in the tube, including the amount designed for the level of an anticoagulant, if required, for the test. If more than one tube is needed, remove the first and insert the second prepositioned tube, allowing it to also fill completely. When all needed tubes are filled, remove the last tube and lay it aside with the previous one(s).

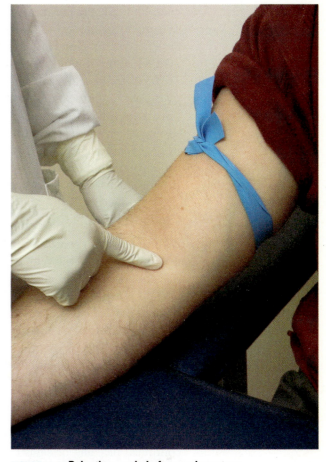

FIGURE 11-14 Palpating a vein before venipuncture. Source: Delmar/Cengage Learning.

Loosen the tourniquet appropriately depending on the type of tourniquet used and leave it lying flat on the support surface beneath the arm. Continue to maintain support of the barrel while loosening the tourniquet. NEVER remove the needle while the tourniquet is still in place! Place moderate pressure with a gauze sponge or cotton ball over the puncture site and over the needle before smoothly withdrawing the needle. Carefully lay the needle and barrel in a safe place while maintaining pressure on the site. Maintain pressure for a minute or so but if the patient is alert and

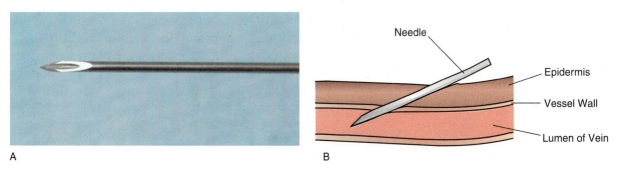

A   B

FIGURE 11-15 (A) View of the needle's bevel, and (B) Illustration of proper position in lumen (open area) of the vein. Source: Delmar/Cengage Learning.

compliant, the patient may be asked to hold the gauze or cotton ball for a couple of minutes or more. Discard used needles and any bloody materials in properly designed receptacles. Place needles in sharps containers. Alcohol swabs and wrappers, along with wrappers for sponges, may go into regular trash. Ensure tubes of blood are properly labeled and placed in racks for transport. Place a bandage over the puncture site and over the sponge to maintain pressure. Patients who have a sensitivity to adhesive bandages should have paper tape placed over the sponge covering the puncture site. After removing the gloves in an aseptic manner to avoid contact with the outside of the gloves, discard the gloves in the ordinary trash receptacle. The hands should again be washed thoroughly before the specimens are transported to the proper location in a timely fashion.

Postphlebotomy Care at Site of Puncture

Again, and it bears repeating, the tourniquet should be released BEFORE the needle is withdrawn from the vein. In some cases, the phlebotomist may release the tourniquet immediately after entering the vein, if the vein is large enough to allow sufficient flow of blood to fill the required tube(s). Failure to release the tourniquet before pulling the needle from the vein is a common error by the beginner, and often results in the formation of a hematoma. A hematoma may also appear while the sample is being drawn if the skin of the patient is thin and fragile, as in the elderly. It is best to remove the needle as quickly as possible to avoid unwarranted stress on the vein.

Following the procedure, the patient should be instructed to maintain firm pressure directly on the site while the technician or phlebotomist places labels, prepares blood, or identifies the samples. After several minutes of pressure, the phlebotomist should remove the pressure materials (cotton or gauze) and examine the site for continued bleeding or signs of a hematoma. If the needle transfixed the vein and entered the tissue below the vein, bruising will almost certainly result. It may be necessary to apply cold packs that are wrapped in cloths to avoid freezing of the skin. The patient, if mentally alert and oriented, may be instructed to use a cold pack for a day or so, for a few minutes at a time. Warm wet cloths will also help to remove dead blood cells from beneath the skin following a day or two of cold treatment.

Completion of Procedure

Clean the area of used needles and any material that may have become bloodstained. Do not leave any trash in the patient's room. Patients have been injured by forgotten hypodermic needles and lancets used for capillary punctures. If any blood was spilled or dripped onto surfaces in the patient's room or on the patient, this matter should be properly taken care of before leaving the room.

Perform any documentation such as logging of specimens in the laboratory. If the patient is fasting, as in an outpatient clinic, and there are no other dietary restrictions, the patient may be informed that he or she may eat.

INABILITY TO OBTAIN SPECIMEN

If, on the first try, the phlebotomist or medical laboratory worker is unable to obtain a specimen, a second attempt may be made. If the patient is overly anxious or questions the phlebotomist's qualifications or competency, it is best to ask another phlebotomist to make the second attempt. A second attempt should be in the opposite arm or on another vein such as one in the hand or wrist. Small or fragile veins may require a butterfly apparatus, which includes a small gauge of needle, or a syringe with a small gauge of needle. If the second attempt is fruitless, the same phlebotomist should not try for a third time. Solicit another phlebotomist or laboratory worker for the third attempt. Often the patient or the venipuncturist will become frustrated and emotional, which further exacerbates the problem. Sometimes it is best, unless the results are needed on an emergency basis, to allow the patient to relax for a few hours before subsequent attempts are made.

Other reasons for failure to obtain a specimen would be a refusal by the patient to allow his blood to be taken, or the patient may be out of his room and undergoing another procedure in another department of the hospital. In the case of an outpatient, the clinic staff or the physician should be notified of the failure to obtain a blood specimen. For inpatients, the nurse with responsibility for the patient should be notified, and the nurse will in turn contact the physician if necessary.

PROBLEMS ENCOUNTERED WHEN COLLECTING AND PROCESSING SPECIMENS

The quality of the specimen is of paramount importance in avoiding erroneous results. With proper training, practices can be avoided that could cause results that are at variance with the patient's condition, which could lead to delays in treatment, the wrong treatment, or no treatment at all.

1. The most common error is that of *hemolysis* of the sample. This occurs when the red blood cells are destroyed or *lysed*, imparting a reddish color, partly from the release of hemoglobin, to the plasma or serum. Some tests are affected dramatically by hemolysis, while others are altered little. Potassium (K^+) and certain cardiac enzymes are affected to a great extent, and would lead the physician to draw the wrong conclusions if the condition is not noted or if a repeat collection is not made to obtain a proper specimen. Other conditions that will destroy red cells and cause hemolysis include the use of a needle that is too small for collecting blood, freezing of the whole sample rather than just the plasma or serum, vigorous shaking of the sample, nearby high heat sources, and poor phlebotomy techniques resulting in tissue trauma to veins, skin, and muscles.

2. *Hemoconcentration* and *evaporation* are related conditions. A sample will be hemoconcentrated if the tourniquet remains on the limb for more than one-half to one minute. The liquid portion of the blood is able to flow more easily under the tourniquet while the blood cells may remain trapped, especially when there is a higher concentration in the ratio of blood cells to the liquid portion. If a sample is left uncapped, some of the water in the plasma or serum will easily evaporate, leaving the analytes in greater concentrations. Exchanges of gases in the sample and those in the air may also cause changes in the acidity or alkalinity of the sample.

3. *Centrifugation* and *separation of blood components* are areas in which errors may occur. Before centrifugation (where centrifugal force is used to

force components of the blood to assume certain levels based on density of the constituents), the specimen must be allowed to clot undisturbed for up to 30 minutes. Centrifugation before a complete clot is achieved will result in a fibrin clot that requires removal before use of the specimen. Small fibrin clots may cause blockages in the small lines that carry the specimen in an automated instrument. Separation of serum and plasma from the cells should be performed immediately. This avoids consumption of some materials from the liquid portion by the blood cells and slight mixing of red cells with the plasma or serum, resulting in erroneous results.

4. *Contamination by bacteria* is a common occurrence that will render results invalid for treating patients. Often the serum or plasma will become cloudy if contaminated by bacteria, since some bacteria multiply rapidly and may completely cloud the sample within a few hours. These bacteria, depending on their species, use materials from the blood for their own metabolism, thereby lowering the levels of certain components, particularly glucose. Byproducts of bacterial metabolism may also cause falsely elevated or lowered results for certain tests.

5. *Chemical contamination* may occur for several reasons. The tubes themselves may have somehow become contaminated, or if samples are transferred to other tubes, contamination may occur during the transfer through use of unclean syringes or pipette tips. Chemical contamination of test reagents will create the same problem results as that of specimen contamination.

The phlebotomist and the laboratory professional must become familiar with the wide variety of vacuum collection tubes. Tubes intended for similar purposes may vary in appearance depending on their manufacturer. Figure 11-16 shows a representative sample of the variety of collection tubes available.

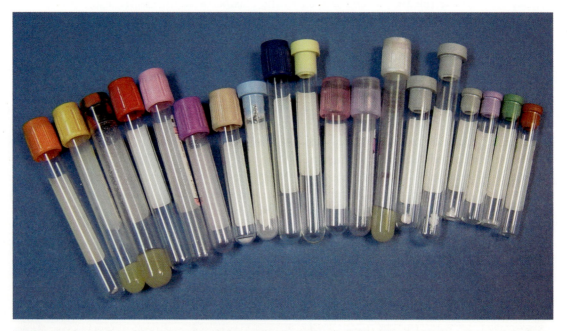

FIGURE 11-16 **A sampling of the many types of blood collection tubes available. Note the barrier substances in three of the tubes.**
Source: Delmar/Cengage Learning.

EVALUATING PHLEBOTOMY PRACTICAL PERFORMANCE

Two forms are presented in Tables 11-4 and 11-5 for evaluating a student's performance in collecting blood. These forms are flexible by nature and can be modified to ascribe points for proper performance and to record a grade if desired. All of the essential steps in sequence are provided on these forms.

The students should review the entire pictorial presentation of Figure 11-17 before attempting a venipuncture, or use the photographs to assess any prior attempt and to troubleshoot any problems encountered.

Table 11-4 Evaluation Chart for Clinical Performance of a Phlebotomy Procedure

Phlebotomy Clinical Practicum Progress Chart

Student _____

Facility_____ Clinical Instructor _____

For each of the following tasks, the student will demonstrate an understanding of background theory and perform each task accordingly. Place a check in the column marked "C" for *complete,* "I" for *incomplete,* or "N" for *not performed in your facility.* Space is provided for additional tasks you may add at your facility. A student evaluation form will be completed at the end of this rotation.

Assigned Tasks	C	I	N	Date
Collection of Blood Specimens				
1. identified patient				
2. established rapport with patient				
3. selected correct tubes according to prescribed tests				
4. labeled tubes correctly				
5. used correct technique for assembling supplies				
6. used aseptic technique				
7. disposed of used equipment properly				
8. performed 6–10 complete procedures per hour				
Processing of Samples				
1. logged specimens correctly				
2. handled specimens carefully				
3. centrifuged specimens as needed				
4. diluted samples properly				
5. delivered specimens to correct department in a timely manner				
Collection of Blood Cultures				
1. used sterile technique				
2. cleaned area adequately with iodine				
3. followed procedure as demonstrated				
Additional Tasks (list below)				

Instructor's Signature _____ Evaluation _____

Table 11-5 Grading Sheet for Performance of Phlebotomy Procedure in Class

Phlebotomy Class Evaluation Form

Student _____ Date _____

OBJECTIVE: Upon completion of the introduction for performing a venipuncture, the student will:

- Utilize proper tourniquet application and vein selection.
- Properly and successfully obtain blood samples from a patient.

EVALUATION: Rating system is as follows:

Each area has a maximum of 2 points that may be assigned. A perfect score would yield a total of 30. A score below 24 is unacceptable and is not a passing grade. For scores below 23, the procedure must be repeated, correcting mistakes and omissions.

2	All steps satisfactorily performed	A = 26 + points
1	Acceptable, improvement necessary	B = 24–25 points
0	Incorrect or did not perform	C = 22–23 points

1. Positions arm correctly for vein selection.
2. Assembles equipment and supplies properly, within reach.
3. Selects appropriate tourniquet application site.
4. Places tourniquet in flat position behind arm.
5. Smoothly positions hands when crossing and tucking or using Velcro closure.
6. Fastens tourniquet at appropriate tightness.
7. Tourniquet is not folded into arm or pinching arm.
8. Loop and loose end do not interfere with puncture site.
9. Asks patient to clench fist.
10. Selects antecubital area if appropriate to palpate for vein.
11. Performs palpation using correct fingers.
12. Palpates entire area of both arms if necessary.
13. Checks depth and direction of veins.
14. Performs procedure accurately (insertion of needle, insertion of tubes, removal of needle), and discards wastes properly.
15. Removes tourniquet smoothly and in a timely manner (no more than 1 minute).

	1st Attempt	2nd Attempt	3rd Attempt
Total points earned	_____	_____	_____
Letter grade assigned	_____	_____	_____

Comments _____

_____

_____

_____

_____

Instructor's Signature _____ Date _____

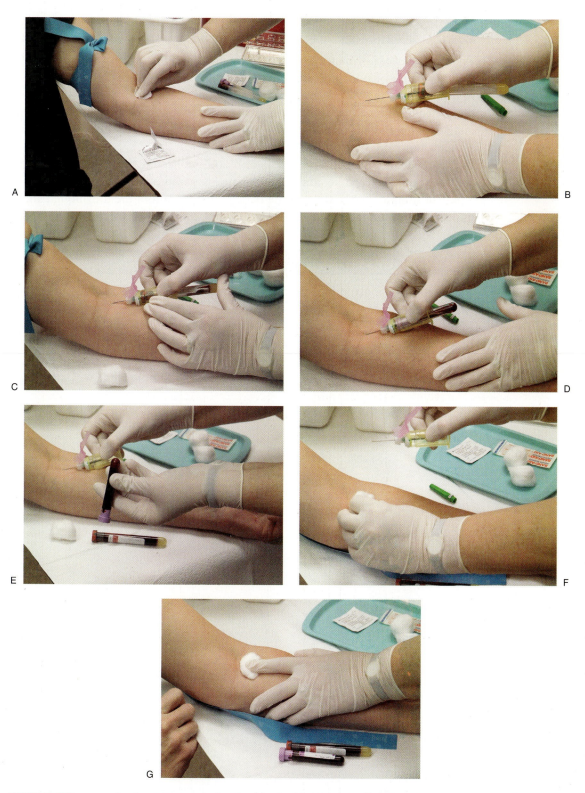

FIGURE 11-17 Sequence for the correct procedure for drawing blood samples. **(A)** Cleansing puncture site with alcohol swab. **(B)** Inserting needle into vein. **(C)** Placing initial collection tube into needle holder. **(D)** Allowing vacuum tube to completely fill with blood. **(E)** Completing the filling and removal of the last tube collected from needle holder. **(F)** Removing needle from vein. **(G)** Placing pressure over the puncture site with cotton ball.
Source: Delmar/Cengage Learning.

SUMMARY

The improper performance of phlebotomy procedures is often overlooked as the primary cause of poor and inaccurate test results. Remember, no test is better in quality than the specimen on which it was performed. Most errors, either in the collection procedure itself or in proper documentation of the procedure to include patient identification and identification of the sample, occur during this primary function of testing a patient's blood.

The sequence for collecting tubes of blood—collecting the right type of sample based on timing, tube, and preservative—is paramount for proper testing of a patient sample. The posture of the patient, application of the tourniquet, and a multitude of other factors all come to play in the process of specimen collection.

REVIEW QUESTIONS

1. What is the most important first step necessary to provide for accurate laboratory testing?
2. In addition to proper collection techniques, why is the job of the phlebotomist so important?
3. What is the significance of the *order of draw*?
4. Name the most common problems with blood samples that will affect test results.
5. What is the purpose for using a vacuum tube with an anticoagulant?

CHAPTER 12

PROCEDURES FOR URINALYSIS AND BODY FLUIDS

LEARNING OBJECTIVES

Upon completion of this chapter, the reader will be able to:

- List the equipment and basic instrumentation of a urinalysis department that is not automated.

- Discuss the differences between the microscopic and macroscopic components when performing a complete evaluation of a urine sample.

- Relate the reasons for performing confirmatory tests when certain screening tests results are significant.

- Perform the physical and rapid chemical examinations within ± 20% accuracy after demonstration by instructor or preceptor.

- Complete the macroscopic, chemical, and microscopic examination of urine sediment, and record the results accurately.

- Ascertain the need for confirmatory tests for certain positive chemistry results.

- Perform basic confirmatory tests.

KEY TERMS

Acetest
Acetoacetic acid
Acetone
Acid-fast bacilli (AFB) stain
Albuminuria
Antispermatic preparations
Bilirubin
Biuret pipette
Caustic
Cerebrospinal fluid (CSF)
Clinitest
Coagulation
Crenated
Cryptococcus
Dipstick
False positive paradox
Fecal materials
Fiber fragments

Ghost cells
Giardia lamblia
Glomerular permeability
Gram stains
High-power field (HPF)
Hypertonic
Hypotonic
Ictotest
India ink prep
Ketoacidosis
Ketones
Leukocyte esterase (leukoesterase)
Leukocytes
Low-power field (LPF)
Macroscopic
Microscopic
Multistix
Necrotic

Nitrites
Parameters
pH
Protozoan
Quantity not sufficient (QNS)
Screening tests
Sodium nitroferricyanide
Subarachnoid hemorrhage
Sulfosalicylic acid (SSA)
Trichloroacetic acid (TCA)
Too numerous to count (TNTC)
Trichomonas
TS (total solids) meter
Tubular reabsorption
Turbidity
Urinometer
Urobilinogen

INTRODUCTION

Several different types of fluids are described as body fluids. Blood is actually a body fluid but is treated separately from urine and other miscellaneous fluids. All of the body fluids, which include CSF, urine, synovial (joint) fluids, exudates and transudates, and tissue fluids, are ultrafiltrates from blood plasma. The levels of certain constituents in the blood are different from those found in other body fluids, and these levels are important in providing nurture and protection to the body. For instance, protein and glucose in the CSF are important in providing the protection and energy needed by the central nervous system. The same is true for synovial fluids, which cushion and nourish cartilage found in the joints of the body.

Changes in urine and body fluids can signal malfunctions in the body ranging from minor to extremely serious conditions. This chapter is not intended to be a definitive "how-to" set of materials to teach procedures in urine and body fluids analyses, but rather is designed to orient the student to the basics of this important segment of laboratory medicine. It is not intended to teach anatomy and physiology, although a diagram of the functional unit of the kidney is presented. Students enrolled in a clinical laboratory program would most likely have already completed or will be concurrently enrolled in courses in chemistry, anatomy, and physiology. Separate courses for teaching each major component of the clinical laboratory program (e.g., urinalysis and body fluids, clinical chemistry, hematology and coagulation, microbiology, and blood banking) should logically follow the information in this book.

The material presented in this chapter includes the basics of laboratory medicine, safety, and pathological conditions for the testing of urine samples and other body fluids. Some of the figures show equipment the student will be using in this chapter's procedures.

RATIONALE FOR A COMPLETE URINALYSIS

The kidneys perform many vital roles in the metabolism of the human body. That of maintaining the pH (alkalinity or acidity) of the body within a narrow range is of utmost importance. Kidney failure where this is not achieved may lead to an almost immediate death.

The kidneys rid the body of waste products and excess water. If certain products of metabolism are unable to be cleared from the body due to various disease processes, their levels may rise until the patient's life is threatened. If the nephrons (the functioning units of the kidneys) are damaged or malfunctioning, they may be unable to do their job. In extreme cases, the patient may require dialysis with a machine designed to rid the blood of wastes on a regular basis, sometimes until a kidney is available for transplant. Kidney damage may result from bacterial infection or trauma where an injury may have cut off the blood supply to the kidneys and the tissue became necrotic (dead).

Basic laboratory examinations are performed on almost all patients who have a medical appointment or an emergency visit for treatment, regardless of the symptoms and signs the patient exhibits. The complete urinalysis is one of these basic tests that are performed at one time or another on almost all patients. A urinalysis gives the physician or other medical practitioner, such as a nurse practitioner or physician's assistant, a screening test that may immediately indicate a disease process. An abnormal positive finding on a random urine specimen will necessitate further testing and evaluation to rule out a number of diseases that cause changes in the various body systems that rid the body of excess water and waste products. Sometimes, testing for metabolic end-point products that indicate genetic disorders may be required, and while these tests are usually sent to a reference laboratory, certain clues may be found in the urinalysis to indicate a need for referring the sample to a specialized laboratory. It would be advisable to review the urinary (renal) system from anatomy and physiology course books to ensure a thorough understanding of the role the kidneys play in health (Figure 12-1). Body fluids other than blood and urine that are candidates for laboratory testing include cerebrospinal fluid (CSF), synovial fluid from joints, gastric contents from the stomach, and fluids that may accumulate in body compartments.

Urine samples are relatively easy to collect. Several basic tests using urine as the sample will yield much important information regarding the anatomy and physiology of the renal system. Although a large number of tests are possible, only the most basic will be presented here. Specimens may be "random," giving a snapshot of the current condition of the patient. Because a more dilute sample may give erroneous results, it is sometimes necessary to collect an early morning sample that is concentrated. This would give a more accurate picture of a medical condition where there is normally a small amount of certain components and these levels would be increased in an unhealthy patient. For some laboratory procedures and certain quantitative tests, the entire volume of urine excreted in a 24-hour period may be required. For other laboratory examinations, specimens may need to be collected at timed intervals, such as at 2 hours following the administration of food or medication. Certain hormones control blood formation and help to retain or excrete various ions (chemical components), so damage to the kidneys can affect the body in many ways. Some specimens may require preservatives (Table 12-1) to prevent growth of bacteria or a change in the pH, which might destroy some analytes (components being tested for). All of these conditions would be discussed in a course textbook that specifically covers urinalysis and body fluids.

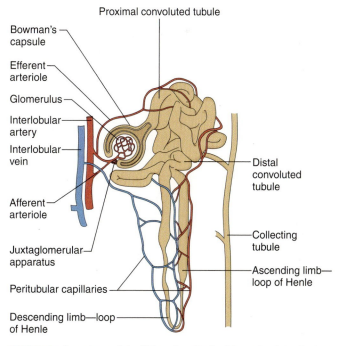

FIGURE 12-1 **A nephron of the kidney involved with production of urine. Source: Delmar/Cengage Learning.**

Table 12-1 Common Urine Preservatives and Their Uses

Preservative	Use
Sulfuric acid	Preserves calcium
Hydrochloric acid	Preserves calcium, magnesium, and phosphorus
Sodium carbonate	Preserves porphyrins, urobilinogen
Sodium hydroxide	Preserves myoglobin
Boric acid	Preserves creatinine, uric acid, protein, steroids, and glucose
Refrigeration	Used for tests for protein, barbiturates, and drug abuse screen

In using the procedure of the urinalysis, it is also a simple matter to perform screening tests on large populations in an economic fashion to determine certain diseases that cause abnormal results in random urine samples.

EXAMINATION OF URINE SAMPLE

A great deal can be determined by an initial examination of a urine sample. The color and clarity of the sample may provide important information. A scant specimen of only a few drops or milliliters could indicate a medical problem and might be noted as quantity not sufficient (QNS) on the laboratory report.

Usually, large automated analyzers are found in the largest laboratories with high volumes of urine examinations. Functions of these machines include chemical analyses as well as gross macroscopic (visible to the naked eye) and microscopic evaluations. A macroscopic examination refers to the observation of physical properties of the urine, including color, clarity, sufficient volume for analysis, and odor. Significantly abnormal samples examined by these complex instruments may require that these samples be examined manually by a technician or technologist-level laboratory professional before releasing the report to the physician.

There are three separate types of examinations, made up of 10 components, that comprise a complete urinalysis. Sometimes the physician will request only one of these components of a urinalysis.

Macroscopic
1. Color
2. Volume
3. Character (turbidity or cloudiness)

Chemical
4. Specific gravity (by TS [total solids] meter) and/or dipstick as a screen only
5. Urine chemical concentrations of protein, glucose, ketones, bilirubin, blood, nitrites, urobilinogen, leukocytes, leukocyte esterase (leukoesterase), and pH using a reagent strip method (chemically impregnated reactive strips)
6. Confirmation of protein by sulfosalicylic acid (SSA)
7. Ketones by Acetest tablet method
8. Bilirubin by Ictotest tablet method
9. Reducing substances by Clinitest tablet method

Microscopic
10. Examination for microscopic components

Table 12-2 Common Causes of Abnormal Urine Colors

Color	Causative Factors
Abnormal Colors Due to Foods	
Red	Ingestion of beets, rhubarb (especially in alkaline urine)
Yellow to orange	Carrots and other vegetables containing carotene, vitamins Some antibiotics
Abnormal Colors Due to Medications	
Orange-red	Pyridium
Green or blue-green	Amitryptiline, some other drugs
Brown to brown-black	Methyldopa, metronidazole (Flagyl)
Abnormal Colors Due to Conditions of Disease	
Clear red	Muscle-wasting diseases where myoglobin is excreted
	Autoimmune disease that destroys fresh red blood cells
Wine red	Porphyria (excess precursors to hemoglobin production)
Cloudy red	Hematuria due to presence of intact red blood cells
Cloudy brown	Hematuria due to old red blood cells
Dark yellow or green-brown	Liver disease causing excess bilirubin in urine
Dark brown to black	Metabolic diseases producing melanin, homogentisic acid
	Hematuria with hemoglobin in acid urine
	Protozoal diseases such as some types of malaria

Conditions That Affect Urinalysis Values

Pathological (disease) conditions and environmental conditions will both affect urinalysis findings. Proper education and training about handling specimens and supplies, and an awareness of conditions that may affect results which should be taken into account, are presented in Table 12-2. Colors other than pale to moderately clear may indicate pathology or may be due to ingestion of any number of foods and medications, including over-the-counter preparations. The beginning laboratory technician or technologist should refer to this table until the principles are understood and remembered.

SUPPLIES AND EQUIPMENT FOR URINALYSIS AND OTHER BODY FLUID PROCEDURES

Some representative simple urinalysis procedures are provided in the remainder of this chapter. Completion of these procedures for the list of 10 standard urinalysis components will require specific supplies and equipment. The tests are performed with the use of kits for each of the procedures, and these kits will contain many of the supply items needed. The instructor will provide urine samples procured from a medical facility or will have students produce their own specimens.

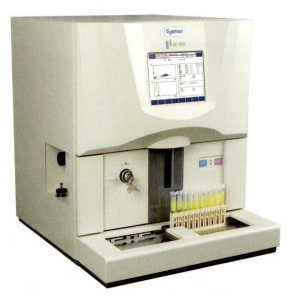

FIGURE 12-2 The Sysmex UF 100i is a fully automated urinalysis analyzer.
Source: Delmar/Cengage Learning.

Supply List

AO Spencer TS Meter or **urinometer**
Centrifuges and centrifuge tubes
Multistix reagent strips
Urine controls for performing quality control procedures
Color charts of urine chemistries
Reagents for remainder of tests
Transfer pipettes, 5¾-inch size
3% sulfosalicylic acid
Acetest tablets and product insert
Ictotest tablets, absorbent pads, and product insert
Clinitest tablets, tubes, and product insert
Sediment system or microscope slides and cover slips

Equipment Commonly Used for Complete Urinalysis

Completely automated urinalysis can be performed by an instrument such as the Yellow IRIS or any of a range of instruments (Figure 12-2). Manual urinalysis requires several pieces of equipment. Specific gravity levels are performed by three basic methods, which, though similar, each use a different methodology with dissimilar results (Figures 12-3, 12-4, and 12-5). Another method is a screening method by a chemical reaction on a dipstick containing chemical pads where the reaction occurs.

Stem

Meniscus (read at bottom)

1.000
1.010
1.020
1.030
1.040
1.050
1.060
1.070

Solution

Urinometer

Cylinder

Mercury weight

FIGURE 12-3 A urinometer is used for specific gravity measurement.
Source: Delmar/Cengage Learning.

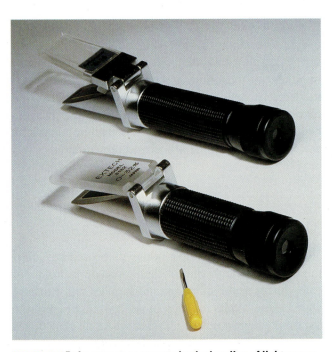

FIGURE 12-4 Refractometers operate by the bending of light waves by dissolved particles.
Source: Delmar/Cengage Learning.

PERFORMING THE URINALYSIS

Urine samples will be tested for chemical and microscopic components in a complete urine analysis. Only in cases where it is indicated will a urinalysis be carried further than the basic components listed.

Macroscopic or Physical Exam

The initial examination for the physical properties of a urine sample (color, volume, and clarity) has been greatly facilitated by the use of standard collection procedures.

Chemical Urinalysis

The chemical components are chiefly tested by a chemical-coated **dipstick** (also called a reagent strip) that contains pads that will change colors in the presence of certain materials in the urine (Figures 12-6 and 12-7). Confirmatory tests may necessary when the protein or bilirubin is positive with the dipstick method.

Chemical results from urine samples may be read by an instrument (Figure 12-8) that scans the dipstick. The chemicals are designed to react in the presence of specific analytes to calculate the semiquantitative value for a number of components. Strips are available that read as few as 2 results and up to 12 different chemistry determinations. These strips are used for screening urine samples. If certain tests are positive, confirmatory testing may be necessary to rule out false positive results and to quantitate some positive findings, such as those of protein and bilirubin. These tests are discussed later in this chapter. There are also specialized strips for diabetics, in which the microalbumin and the creatinine are compared to determine if early renal disease has occurred.

For manual reading of the reagent strips, care must be taken to dip an uncontaminated and fresh strip into the urine, and one edge of the strip should be blotted against a piece of gauze or a paper towel. Using a stopwatch, the times for reaction

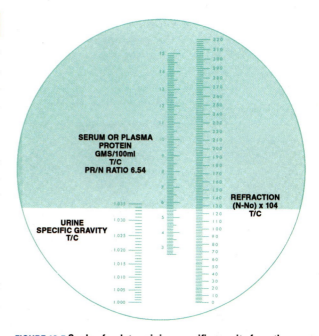

FIGURE 12-5 Scales for determining specific gravity from the refractometer. Note the section for total protein in plasma or serum.
Source: Delmar/Cengage Learning.

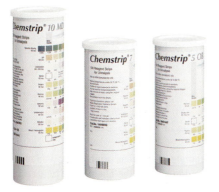

FIGURE 12-6 Urine reagent strips for chemistry determination.
Source: Delmar/Cengage Learning.

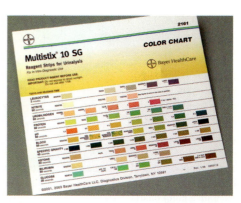

FIGURE 12-7 Color graph for Bayer Multistix 10 SG.
Source: Delmar/Cengage Learning.

on the container must be observed. Some results are available immediately, but the leukoesterase portion requires a 2-minute wait, all of which are accounted for when using a strip reader. Manual reading of the strip is shown in Figure 12-9.

Microscopic Urinalysis

After completing the examination of the urine sample for physical characteristics and performing the dipstick chemistry component of the urinalysis, an aliquot of the sample is centrifuged for microscopic analysis for the formed elements of urine.

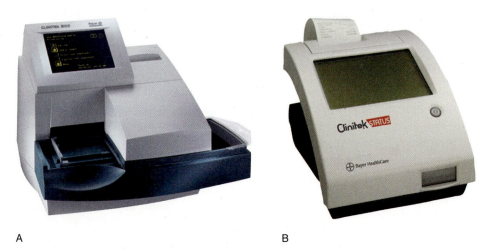

A   B

FIGURE 12-8 (A) The CLINITEK® 500 Urine Chemistry Analyzer is a semi-automated, benchtop analyzer that is capable of processing high volumes of samples; a urine chemistry dispstick may be processed every 7 seconds. **(B)** The Clinitek® Status is used for lower volume testing and handles one urine chemistry dispstick at a time.
Source: Delmar/Cengage Learning.

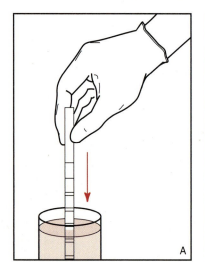
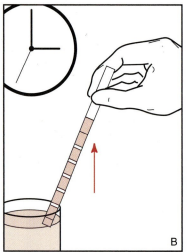
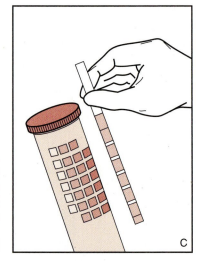

FIGURE 12-9 Manual reading of urine dipstick. **(A)** Reagent strip is inserted into sample. **(B)** Excess urine is allowed to drain from reagent strip; edge of strip should also be blotted using paper towel. **(C)** The reaction color of the chemically treated pads is compared with a color chart.
Source: Delmar/Cengage Learning.

Findings in the urinary sediment commonly include red and white blood cells, epithelial cells, and sometimes crystals, depending on the patient's medical condition. Microscopic examination requires a great deal of care in preparing the sample and in conducting the visual analysis of the sediment. A number of standardized systems are available for preparing a systematic microscopic examination and analysis of a urine sample (Figure 12-10). These systems quantify the amount of urine that is used for centrifuging and preparing sediment from the sample for microscopic evaluation.

FIGURE 12-10 StatSpin CenSlide standardized urinalysis system. Source: Delmar/Cengage Learning.

In Figure 12-11, the steps required for preparing the specimen for microscopic analysis are presented. There are several varieties of systems for systematizing the microscopic examination, where a set volume of urine is centrifuged and a certain volume of the resuspended sediment is stained and examined by microscope.

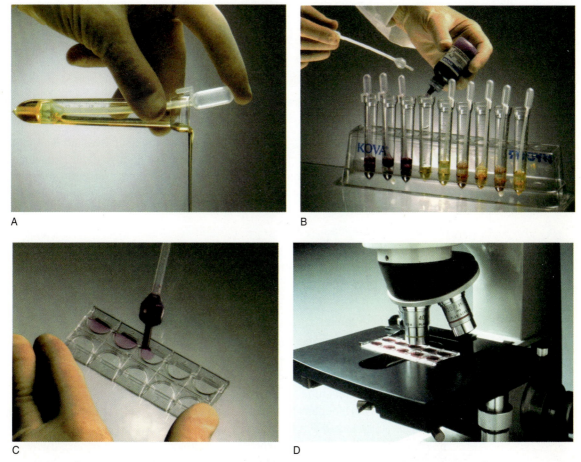

A

B

C

D

FIGURE 12-11 Preparing specimens for microscopic analysis. **(A)** Pouring off supernatant from centrifuge tube. **(B)** Staining urine sediment in preparation for microscopic examination. **(C)** Loading chambers of a specially designed slide. **(D)** Placing samples on the stage of the microscope.
Source: Delmar/Cengage Learning.

IN THE LAB

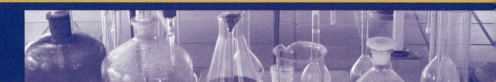

BASIC URINALYSIS AND BODY FLUIDS ANALYSIS PROCEDURES

Urinalysis is a useful indicator of health or disease, especially in the areas of metabolic and renal disorders. Urine undergoes many changes during states of disease or body dysfunction. These changes may be evident even before blood composition is altered to a significant extent. In addition, laboratory procedures for some of the other body fluids are performed in the same manner as for urine samples, so cerebrospinal fluid (CSF) is included in this chapter.

Patients for whom urinalysis is needed should be instructed in how to properly collect a urine specimen for testing. The testing procedures should be performed as quickly as possible following the collection of a sample to avoid bacterial growth and breakdown of formed elements in the sample. If necessary, the specimen should be refrigerated until it can be tested. A urine sample is stable at room temperature for 1 hour or refrigerated for 4 hours. If refrigerated, allow urine to sit at room temperature for at least 15 minutes before testing.

URINALYSIS AND BODY FLUIDS ANALYSIS PROCEDURE #1

Physical and Biochemical Testing of Urine

Principles

Urine dipstick testing is a screening test performed on fresh urine. A chemical-impregnated reagent strip is dipped in fresh urine to determine glucose, bilirubin, ketones, specific gravity, blood, pH, protein, urobilinogen, nitrites, and leukoesterase.

Interfering Substances

Abnormal urine color may affect the readability of the reagent areas on the urinalysis reagent test strip. Such urine specimens should be sent to the urinalysis department of the clinical laboratory.

Equipment and Supplies

1. Gloves, disposable paper towels, and disinfectant or other cleaning solution
2. Report form for urinalysis results (Procedure Report Form)
3. Fresh urine sample, preferably clean catch or catheterized, of at least 10 mL
4. Test tubes and test tube rack
5. Container with biochemical dipsticks and chart for manual reading (urine strip reader may be used if available)
6. AO TS Meter or urinometer to confirm reagent strip results if necessary
7. Normal and abnormal urine controls
8. Electronic timing device or clock/watch with second hand
9. Procedures #3 through #6 are used for confirming biochemical results

Procedural Alert

Critical Specimen Requirements for Accurate Testing

1. Collect a random fresh urine sample and a control specimen to insure accurate results.
2. Perform test as soon as possible.
3. Urine sample is stable at room temperature for 1 hour and refrigerated for 4 hours. *If refrigerated, allow urine to sit at room temperature for 15 minutes before testing.*
4. Minimum volume needed is 1 mL.

Procedure Report Form: Urinalysis Report Form

Patient Name: _____   Pt. ID _____   Date: _____

Age: _____   Gender (Circle One) M   F   Physician: _____

Time Requested: _____   Time Performed: _____   Time Reported: _____

Examination Requested: ☐ UA with Microscopic   ☐ Dipstick UA Only
☐ Culture and Sensitivity   ☐ Other

Physical Examination

Color: ☐ Colorless   ☐ Straw   ☐ Yellow   ☐ Amber   ☐ Red   ☐ Brown
☐ Blue   ☐ Green

Character (appearance):   ☐ Clear   ☐ Hazy   ☐ Cloudy   ☐ Turbid

Chemical Examination by Manual Dipstick [Multistix 10 SG (Bayer)]
(Circle the appropriate responses)

Glucose	Negative	100	250	500	1000	>2000 mg/dL
Bilirubin	Negative	+ (Small)		++ (Moderate)	+++ (Large)	
Ketones	Negative	Trace		Small	Moderate	Large
Specific gravity	1.000	1.005	1.010	1.015	1.020	1.025 1.030
Blood (hemolyzed)		Negative Trace Small		Moderate	Large	
Blood (intact/non-hemolyzed)	Negative Trace Moderate					
pH	5.0	6.0	6.5	7.0 7.5	8.0	8.5
Protein	Negative	Trace	+/30 (1+)	++/100 (2+)	+++/500 (3+)	>2000 (4+)
Urobilinogen	Normal	2	4	6		
Nitrites	Negative	Positive				
Leukocytes	Negative	Trace Small Moderate Large				

Confirmatory Test Results (Circle the appropriate responses)

Specific Gravity (Urinometer/ TS Meter)	1.000	1.005	1.010	1.015	1.020	1.025	1.030
Acetone	Negative, 1+ (small), 2+ (moderate), or 3+ (large)						
Protein	Trace 1+ 2+ 3+ 4+						
Bilirubin	Weak positive Strong positive						
Clinitest	0 Trace ½% 1% 2% 3% 5%						

Microscopic Examination

Constituent	Reported Values	Reference Values
White blood cells	_____	0–4/high-power field (HPF)*
Red blood cells	_____	0–4/high-power field
Squamous epithelial	_____	Occasional; higher in females
Renal/tubular epithelial	_____	0

(continued)

IN THE LAB

Microscopic Examination (continued)

Constituent	Reported Values	Reference Values
Casts (identify type)	_____	0/low-power field (LPF)**
Yeasts (1–4+)	_____	Negative
Bacteria (1–4+)	_____	Negative
Mucus (1–4+)	_____	Negative
Crystals (identify type)	_____	Negative
Amorphous sediment	_____	Negative
Miscellaneous	_____	
Artifacts	_____	
Comments (unusual findings)	_____	

Performed by: _____   **Date Reported** _____

*HPF or high-power field refers to use of the microscope objective of 40X or higher.
**LPF or Low-power field refers to use of the microscope objective of 10X or 20X.

Procedure

1. Wash hands and don gloves.
2. Assemble necessary equipment and supplies.
3. If the specimen has been refrigerated, allow it to reach room temperature before proceeding with further testing.
4. Pour a small sample of urine into a clear test tube. Observe and note the color, odor, and clarity of the urine sample.
5. Perform the reagent dipstick test.
   a. Mix the sample well by swirling.
   b. Quickly dip the strip into the urine (Figure 12-12A), ensuring that all test pads have been saturated.
   c. Remove the strip from the urine and tap or draw the edge of the strip along the rim of the container to remove excess urine from the strip. Blot the edge of the strip on a paper towel (Figure 12-12B). Never blot the pads of the test strip.
   d. Note the time. Reading the color at the indicated time is critical for optimal results.
6. Compare the color on the dipstick pads to the reaction chart on the dipstick container (Figure 12-12C).
   a. Each color pad must be read at the designated time printed on the color chart on the dipstick container.
   b. Any color change that occurs after 2 minutes is of no diagnostic value.
   c. Read the values that require the least amount of time first, then progress to the results that require a longer period of time for the reaction to be completed.
   d. If an automated strip reader is available, follow directions provided by the manufacturer for performing and recording test results.

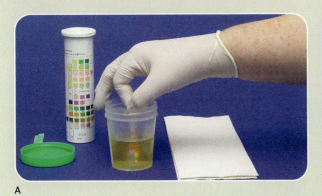
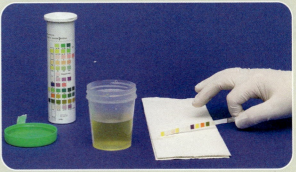

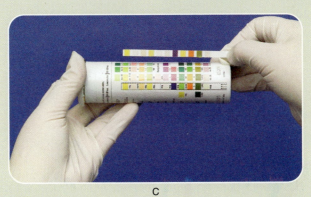

**FIGURE 12-12 Chemical testing of urine by reagent strip. (A) Saturating chemical pads of dipstick. (B) Draining and blotting edge of dipstick. (C) Comparing for color reactions using reaction chart.
Source: Delmar/Cengage Learning.**

7. Variations in an individual's urine color may cause the patient test strip to have a slightly different color than the color chart on the bottle. In addition, differing brands of chemical strips may have different reporting values. If the test strip color does not match a particular color square on the color chart, then match the test strip to a color square of equal intensity. If the color development is slightly uneven, then match the average color on the test pad.

8. Record results on the appropriate form and dispose of the dipstick in the proper waste receptacle

9. If necessary for confirmation, the estimate of the specific gravity provided by the dipstick may require the use of instruments for confirming the results before they are reported. When required, perform a specific gravity for the urine sample using a urinometer (Figure 12-3) or a refractometer (Figure 12-4).

10. Perform confirmatory tests for protein, reducing substances, ketones, and bilirubin if the dipstick indicates positive results for these (see Procedures #3 through #6).

11. Discard all supplies used for the procedure in appropriate containers. A disinfectant should be used to clean work surfaces, and equipment should be cleaned and restored to its former position. Discard gloves appropriately and wash hands thoroughly in accordance with established policies.

IN THE LAB

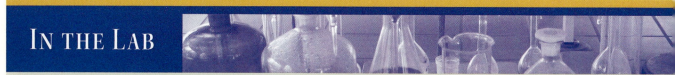

Table 12-3 Urine Chemistry Report with Normal Values

Analyte	Normal
Glucose	Negative to trace*
Bilirubin	Negative*
Ketone	Negative*
Specific gravity	1.005 to 1.030*
Blood	Negative*
pH	5.0 to 6.0*
Protein	Negative to trace*
Urobilinogen	0.2 to 1.0 mg/dL*
Nitrite	Negative*
Leukocytes	Negative*

*Range that is found in most normal individuals.

Reporting of Results

1. Using the laboratory report form provided (Procedure Report Form*) or other appropriate form, record the biochemical test results. Use the following terms in your report. Note that "normal" values are shown in Table 12-3.

Urine color	colorless, straw, yellow, amber, red, brown, blue, or green
Urine appearance	clear, hazy, cloudy, or turbid
Glucose	negative, 100, 250, 500, 1000, or ~2000 mg/dL
Bilirubin	negative, + (Small), ++ (Moderate), +++ (Large)
Ketone	negative, trace, small, moderate, or large
Specific gravity	1.000, 1.005, 1.010, 1.015, 1.020, 1.025, or 1.030
Blood	present as intact RBCs or non-hemolyzed (negative, trace, moderate), and as hemolyzed (negative, trace, small, moderate, large)
pH	5.0, 6.0, 6.5, 7.0, 7.5, 8.0, or 8.5
Protein	negative, trace, +/30 (1+), ++/100 (2+), +++/500 (3+), >2000 (4+) in mg/dL
Urobilinogen	normal, 2, 4, or 6 Ehrlich units
Nitrites	negative or positive
Leukocytes (white blood cells)	negative, trace, small, moderate, or large

2. Perform confirmatory tests (see Procedures #3 through #6) if indicated and report the results in the appropriate portion of the report form or on a separate form.

*Note: Some sections of the Procedure Report Form will not be completed until after you have undertaken additional procedures in this chapter. Confirmatory test results for acetone (Acetest) will be obtained in Procedure #3, for bilirubin (Icotest) in Procedure #4, for glucose (Clinitest) in Procedure #5, and for protein in Procedure #6. Procedure #2 addresses microscopic examination.

URINALYSIS AND BODY FLUIDS ANALYSIS PROCEDURE #2

Microscopic Examination of Urine

Principles

Microscopic examination of urine sediment is a noninvasive procedure that provides information useful in the diagnosis and prognosis of certain diseases. For example, in renal parenchymal disease, the urine usually contains increased numbers of cells and casts discharged from an organ that might otherwise be accessible only by an invasive procedure.

An aliquot (portion) of a urine sample is centrifuged, and the sediment is examined using a brightfield microscope to detect cells and other formed elements such as crystals and casts.

Charts may be used to assist in identifying and defining the sediment elements various crystals, and unidentifiable artifacts obtained after centrifuging the sample.

Optimally, microscopic examination of a specimen require a sample of more than 10 to 12 mL of fresh urine. In some conditions, the patient is unable to void more than a very small amount of specimen. Although the microscopic examination may be performed with less than 10 mL of urine, the minimum volume is 1 mL. Very small samples should be evaluated without centrifugation and by slide and cover glass. Perform the procedure as soon as possible after collection.

Equipment and Supplies

1. Gloves, disposable paper towels, and disinfectant or other cleaning solution
2. Report form for urinalysis results (Procedure Report Form)
3. Fresh urine sample, preferably clean catch or catheterized, of at least 10 mL. (minimum of 1 mL required)
4. Centrifuge and centrifuge tubes
5. Microscope slides with cover slips or an engineered system for performing microscopic analysis (e.g., Kova)
6. Test tubes, test tube rack, and disposable transfer pipettes (may be part of some standardized systems for urine microscopic examinations)
7. Brightfield microscope
8. 2% acetic acid and dropper
9. Normal saline solution and dropper
10. Biological stain for enabling easier identification of cells (optional)

Procedure

1. Wash hands and don gloves.
2. Assemble necessary equipment and supplies.

Procedural Alert

Interfering Substances That May Cause Misleading Results.

It is essential that the laboratory worker become aware of and account for the following:

1. Hyaline casts and other partially transparent elements may be obscured by excessively bright light. Always use subdued light.
2. Vaginal secretions may contaminate the urine with epithelial cells, bacteria, or *Trichomonas* (a sexually transmitted **protozoan**).
3. Urine may be contaminated with **fecal materials** or **Giardia lamblia** (a parasite).
4. Starch granules, oil droplets from lubricants, **antispermatic preparations**, **fiber fragments**, or bacteria and yeast from contaminated urine containers may be present.

IN THE LAB

3. Pour the urine sample into a disposable 12-mL centrifuge tube (Figure 12-13).
   a. If less than 1 mL urine is collected, do not centrifuge the sample.
   b. If the microscopic exam is performed on uncentrifuged urine, note it on the report.
4. Centrifuge tubes for 5 minutes at 400 RCF*.
5. Pour off the supernatant (Figure 12-11A) and resuspend the sediment with urine remaining in the centrifuge tube designed for concentrating urine sediment. Approximately 0.8 mL urine supernatant and 0.1 mL of urine sediment will remain in the bottom of the tube. If graduated tubes or pipetters are used, follow the directions provided by the manufacturer.

   The use of a stain for the urinary sediment is optional. After the supernatant is poured off, a drop of stain is added to the remaining 0.8 mL of concentrated sample, and it is mixed by aspirating and emptying the pipette bulb repeatedly several times.
6. Place a drop of the resuspended urine sediment onto a glass slide and place a cover slip over the suspension. Or, follow the instructions for using an engineered system (e.g., Kova) for examining urinary sediment (see Figure 12-11C).
7. Place the sample on the stage of the microscope (Figure 12-11D and Figure 12-14)
8. Adjust the microscope condenser down and close the diaphragm so that light is subdued to provide better visualization of sometimes colorless constituents.
9. Scan at least 10 fields using the low-power objective and subdued light. (Hyaline casts and other partially transparent solid elements may be obscured by excessively bright light.) Count the number of casts seen per **low-power field (LPF)** and record the average number casts/LPF in the Procedure Report Form.
10. Scan at least 10 fields using the high-power objective. Count and record the average range of red blood cells (RBCs) per **high-power field (HPF)**. If more than 100 RBCs are present, record 100/HPF in the Procedure Report Form.
11. If the field is obscured by more than 100 RBCs/HPF, add a drop of 2% acetic acid to 2 drops of urine sediment to lyse the RBCs so that other cells and elements may be counted. RBCs may be confused with yeast, fat droplets, and degenerated epithelial cells.
12. Observe and note RBC morphology. If the RBCs were lysed in Step #11, it may be advisable to dilute a small portion of the unlysed sample before performing a microscopic evaluation of the morphology of the RBCs.
    a. Normal, unstained RBCs in wet preparations sometimes appear as pale yellow-orange discs. They vary in size, but are usually about 8 microns in diameter.

Note: *RCF is the acronym for relative centrifugal force and is a method of comparing the force generated by various centrifuges on the basis of the speeds of rotation and distances from the center of rotation. For clinical laboratory procedures, the RCF required is quite low.

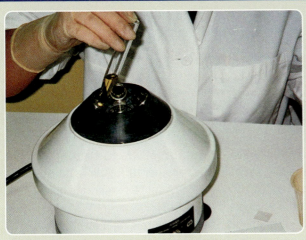

FIGURE 12-13 Approximately 10 mL urine is centrifuged in preparation for staining and a microscopic examination of sediment.
Source: Delmar/Cengage Learning.

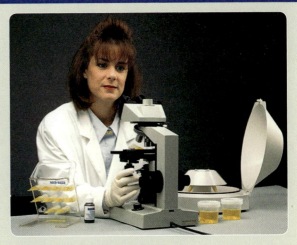

FIGURE 12-14 Technologist performing microscopic exams using StatSpin CenSlide urinalysis system.
Source: Delmar/Cengage Learning.

b. With dissolution of hemoglobin in old or **hypotonic** urine specimens, RBCs may appear as faint, colorless circles or **ghost cells**.

c. With **hypertonic** urine specimens, RBCs may appear **crenated** with irregular edges and surfaces.

13. Scan at least 10 to 15 fields using the high-power objective. Count and record the average number of white blood cells (WBCs). If more than 100 WBCs are present, record >100/HPF in the Procedure Report Form. Note: The oil immersion objective is NOT used for the microscopic examination of urine specimens.

14. If the microscopic field is obscured by more than 100 WBCs/HPF, dilute the sample with saline so all cells and other elements may be counted. Add 2 drops of saline to 1 drop of mixed urine sediment and place a drop of this mixture on the slide. If the sample is diluted, see Step #13 for correcting the values obtained for elements of the sediment that are enumerated.

15. When a dilution with saline is required due to an extremely high concentration of certain constituents, the clinical laboratory personnel must multiply the average number of elements counted by the dilution factor (e.g., 12 yeast seen/LPF × 3 (dilution factor) = 36 yeasts/HPF).

16. Using the high-power objective, continue scanning for crystals, yeast, bacteria, epithelial cells, mucus, and other formed elements. Count and record in the Procedure Report Form the elements seen per HPF.

17. Discard all contaminated supplies used for this procedure. If microscope slides with sharp corners were used, place in appropriate sharps containers. A disinfectant should be used to clean work surfaces and equipment should be cleaned and restored to its former position. Discard gloves appropriately and wash hands thoroughly in accordance with departmental policies.

IN THE LAB

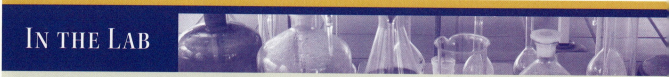

Reporting of Results

1. Report casts as the average number of casts seen per LPF. Differentiate and quantify the various different types of casts as hyaline, cellular, fatty, or waxy.
2. Report RBCs as the average number of RBCs seen per HPF. If more than 100 RBCs/ HPF are seen, report as >100/HPF or **too numerous to count (TNTC)**.
3. Report WBCs as the average number of WBCs seen per HPF. If more than100 WBCs/HPF are seen, report as >100/HPF or TNTC. A range is reported but should never be wider than 5 cells (for example, 7–10 cells/HPF).
4. Report other cellular or formed elements as few, moderate, or many. Use Tables 12-4 and 12-5 as the protocol for estimating microscopic components and enumeration of them. Values are provided for the majority of formed elements that may be encountered in the typical urinalysis department.

Table 12-4 Urine Sediment Microscopic Report

Element	Few	Moderate	Many
Crystals	0–4/HPF	5–10/HPF	>10/HPF
Bacteria	0–25/HPF	25–50/HPF	>50/HPF
Yeast	0–25/HPF	25–50/HPF	>50/HPF
Epithelial Cells	0–4/HPF	5–10/HPF	>10/HPF
Casts†	Number/HPF	Number/HPF	Number/HPF

†**The absence of casts is normal.** Under certain conditions, hyaline casts may be present for a short time.

Table 12-5 Normal (Reference) Levels and Conditions for Cellular Microscopic Elements

Components	Reference Values	Conditions	Interferences
RBCs	0–4/HPF	Normal concentration of urine	Hypotonic urine will cause RBC breakdown
WBCs	0–4/HPF	May be broken down	Yields positive leukoesterase values in chemistry (dipstick) evaluation
Squamous epithelial cells	Rare to few	Higher in females	
Renal and tubular epithelial cells	Negative	May indicate kidney involvement	
Bacteria	Negative	May indicate urinary tract infection	Contaminated containers and non–clean-catch or catheterized samples
Yeasts	Negative	Antibiotics use, diabetes, compromised immune system	
Trichomonas	None	Sexually transmitted protozoa	
Ova of parasites	None	Fecal contamination	
Spermatazoa	None	Prostatitis in males	Never reported in females except in cases of possible sexual assault

Components of Urine Sediment Most Frequently Found

Only a few types of microscopic elements are ordinarily found in normal urine specimens. A standardized system such as KOVA enables the technician or technologist to provide a quick and simple analysis of centrifuged urine sediment. Examples of commonly found formed elements are provided in Figures 12-15 through 12-21. Figures 12-15 through 12-18 reveal types of cells that are found in low numbers in normal urine samples. Figure 12-19 shows an increased level of WBCs (1–2 would be normal) and Figures 12-20 and 12-21 depict more unusual findings, the latter of which may be significant when found in males with prostatitis (inflammation or disease of the prostate glands).

Significance of Cells Found in Urine Sediment

The beginning laboratory student is often confused over what is normal and what is abnormal, including the average numbers of various cell types found routinely in the urine of normal persons. See Table 12-5 for normal levels of the cells shown in Figures 12-15 through 12-18.

Casts—Formed Elements in Kidney Tubules

Casts form in kidney tubules where small amounts of mucoprotein are secreted. Sluggish flow of urine for a number of reasons, such as acidotic conditions, and increased levels of certain solutes cause a gelling of the dissolved materials

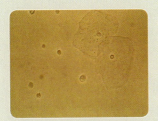
FIGURE 12-15 Mixed cell types, including squamous epithelial, red, and white cells. Source: Delmar/Cengage Learning.

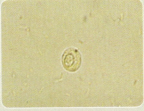
FIGURE 12-16 Renal tubular cell. Source: Delmar/Cengage Learning.

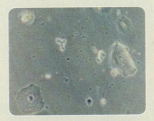
FIGURE 12-17 Squamous epithelial cells and yeasts. Source: Delmar/Cengage Learning.

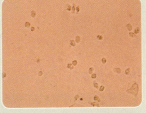
FIGURE 12-18 Leukocytes, or white blood cells. Source: Delmar/Cengage Learning.

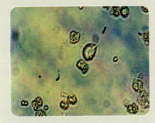
FIGURE 12-19 A protozoan called *trichomonas*. Source: Delmar/Cengage Learning.

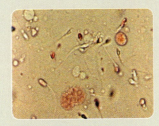
FIGURE 12-20 Spermatozoa among other types of sediment. Source: Delmar/Cengage Learning.

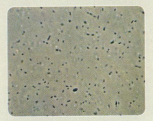
FIGURE 12-21 Bacteria (may result from contaminated specimen or from an infection). Source: Delmar/Cengage Learning.

IN THE LAB

(including but not limited to mucoprotein), forming casts shaped by the walls of the tubules. When increased numbers of red and white cells are also present in the tubules, they may become trapped in the protein. The protein and the cells may then decompose and form a variety of casts identified by their appearances. Casts are categorized as shown in Table 12-6. Images of the casts are shown in Figures 12-22 through 12-25.

Normal Crystals—Formed Elements in Urine

Figures 12-26 through 12-29 show crystals that are found in normal urine samples. Calcium carbonate and ammonium biurate crystals are found predominantly in alkaline urine. Crystals that form in alkaline urine may be dissolved by the use of strong acids such as hydrogen chloride. Amorphous (without shape) phosphate and triple phosphate crystals are common in alkaline urine, and sometimes calcium carbonate crystals will be found in neutral or slightly alkaline urine samples. Uric acid and calcium oxalate crystals will be chiefly found in acid urine, along with amorphous urates (Table 12-7). Urine specimens that have been refrigerated or for which testing has otherwise been delayed will often form crystals called amorphous sediment from the dissolved chemicals present in the sample. This may cause the urine sample to become completely cloudy, but the phenomenon can be reversed by warming of the sample through immersing the specimen tube in warm water for a few minutes. Acid urine specimens, a normal condition as most urine samples will be pH 5.0 to 6.0, will yield amorphous urates, while alkaline specimens will provide amorphous phosphates.

Table 12-6 Examples of Casts with Descriptions and Conditions under Which Formed

Cast Classification	Descriptions	Conditions Associated with Casts
Hyaline	Transparent and colorless, visible under low light levels in microscopic examination	Occasional hyaline cast is normal; increased in extreme exercise and stress, but also found in chronic renal disease, congestive heart failure (poor circulation), glomerulonephritis, and pyelonephritis
Granular	Granules from breakdown of cells and metabolic components	Previously classified as finely and coarsely granular casts, but this terminology seldom used today
RBC	Glycoprotein entraps intact RBCs; cast appears often as bright red	Blood transfusion incompatibility, trauma and strenuous exercise, glomerulonephritis
WBC	Outline of transparent material with visible WBCs within the cast	Pyelonephritis chiefly from bacterial ascension from bladder infection
Epithelial cell	Cylindrical form of epithelial cells where nuclei may be visualized	Damage to renal tubules; renal epithelial cells may be visualized within the cast
Waxy	Appearance is consistent in appearance with a broken and splintered wax tube and contains few or no inclusions	Broken areas with sharp ends appear much as a broken piece of glass

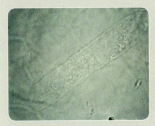

FIGURE 12-22 Hyaline cast (may be nonpathological). Source: Delmar/Cengage Learning.

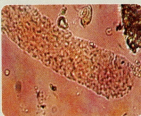

FIGURE 12-23 Granular cast. Source: Delmar/Cengage Learning.

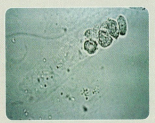

FIGURE 12-24 Cellular cast. Source: Delmar/Cengage Learning.

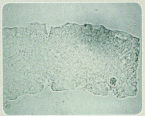

FIGURE 12-25 Waxy cast. Source: Delmar/Cengage Learning.

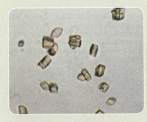

FIGURE 12-26 Uric acid crystals. Source: Delmar/Cengage Learning.

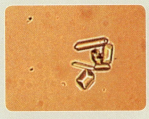

FIGURE 12-27 Triple phosphate crystals. Source: Delmar/Cengage Learning.

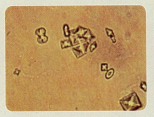

FIGURE 12-28 Calcium oxalate crystals. Source: Delmar/Cengage Learning.

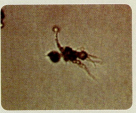

FIGURE 12-29 Ammonium biurate crystals. Source: Delmar/Cengage Learning.

Abnormal Crystals—Formed Elements in Urine

Figures 12-30 through 12-32 and Table 12-8 explain and show crystals that are found in patients with metabolic diseases and in some cases in the urine of those who are being administered certain medications. Samples containing cystine crystals indicate a condition where the amino acid crystal cystine is not reabsorbed by the kidney, as

Table 12-7 Crystals Found in Normal Urine Specimen

Crystal	Urine pH		
	Acid	Neutral	Alkaline
Uric acid	+		
Amorphous urates	+		
Calcium oxalate	+	+	
Amorphous phosphates		+	+
Calcium phosphate		+	+
Triple phosphate		+	+
Ammonium biurate			+
Calcium carbonate			+

IN THE LAB

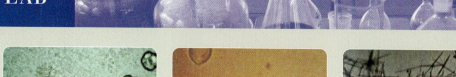

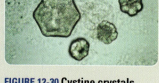

FIGURE 12-30 **Cystine crystals.**
Source: Delmar/Cengage
Learning.

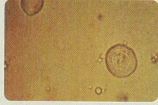

FIGURE 12-31 **Leucine crystals.**
Source: Delmar/Cengage
Learning.

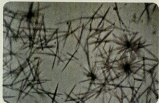

FIGURE 12-32 **Tyrosine crystals.**
Source: Delmar/Cengage
Learning.

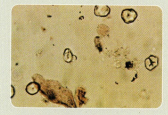

FIGURE 12-33 **Starch granules.**
Source: Delmar/Cengage
Learning.

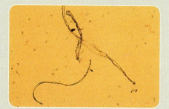

FIGURE 12-34 **Cotton or other
plant fibers.**
Source: Delmar/Cengage
Learning.

are most amino acids. Leucine crystals are present in some liver conditions, as well as the amino acid tyrosine. Cholesterol crystals are sometimes seen, while sulfa crystals are less common due to the newer sulfa drugs in use today.

Artifacts and Other Formed Elements Found in Urine Sediment

A number of microscopically visible elements may be found when examining urine sediment (Figured 12-33 and 12-34). Most of these are due to diet and/or environment and are not to be confused with substances that are clinically significant. One thing that is important for the beginning laboratory student to remember is that the finding of a single unusual component of the urine is not clinically significant. The clinically significant elements will be found in considerable numbers in most instances. If a urine sediment is allowed to dry in the system used for enumerating elements from the urine, the results can be quite distracting. Artifacts are to be recognized but are not to be reported. Mucus is not a clinically significant finding, but is reported as 1 through 4+.

Confirmatory Tests for Positive Urinary Chemistry Findings

A multitude of factors may be involved in yielding a positive protein in a urine sample that is not truly an excretion of protein from the kidneys. Lysed red blood cells, mucus (mucin), myoglobin, and others will give a false-positive result. It is necessary to follow up on a

Table 12-8 Abnormal Crystals in Urine Sediment

Crystal	Microscopic Appearance
Cholesterol	Colorless flat plates with notched or broken corners
Cystine	Colorless, hexagonal plates
Hippuric acid	Colorless to yellow needles or prism-like structures
Leucine	Yellow-brown spherical crystals showing concentric circles
Sulfa	Yellow to brown-green rosettes or bundles of needles
Tyrosine	Colorless to pale yellow sheaves of needles

positive protein, as the clinical ramifications of protein being lost through the kidneys are significant. Certain medications will also cause color changes or odor changes and may interfere with the reading of the chemistry results by dipstick. Confirmatory tests are necessary when these conditions are present. Several of these tests are presented on the following pages.

URINALYSIS AND BODY FLUIDS ANALYSIS PROCEDURE #3

Acetest—Semiquantitative Test for the Presence of Acetone in Urine

Principles

A positive test for acetone indicates that fatty tissue is being broken down, which is a common manifestation of diabetes when a patient may be suffering from a condition known as **ketoacidosis**. **Acetone** is an example of a simple ketone. Testing for the presence of acetone can help determine the extent of the patient's medical condition. The determination for the presence of ketones by Acetest reagent tablets may be performed on urine, or on blood serum or plasma. The test is based on the development of a purple color when **acetoacetic acid** or acetone reacts with **sodium nitroferricyanide**. Acetoacetic acid or acetone in urine or blood forms a purple-colored complex with nitroferricyanide in the presence of glycine.

Equipment and Supplies

1. Gloves, disposable paper towels and disinfectant or other cleaning solution
2. Report form for urinalysis results (Procedure Report Form)
3. Fresh urine sample that has tested positive for acetone by dipstick (see Procedure #1)
4. Disposable pipettes such as Pasteur or plastic bulb pipettes
5. Filter paper disc or other white absorbent paper
6. Stoppered dark container of Acetest tablets (examine for color changes or deterioration)
7. Electronic timing device or clock/watch with second hand

Procedure

1. Wash hands and don gloves.
2. Assemble necessary equipment and supplies.

IN THE LAB

3. Place an Acetest tablet on a filter paper disc or other white absorbent paper.
4. Place 1 drop of urine directly on the Acetest tablet (Figure 12-35).
5. At 30 seconds, compare the color of the tablet with that on the chart provided by the manufacturer.
6. Discard all supplies used for the procedure in the appropriate containers. A disinfectant should be used to clean the work surfaces and equipment should be cleaned and restored to its former position. Gloves should be discarded appropriately and the hands washed thoroughly in accordance with established policies.

Reporting of Results

Report on the Procedure Report Form or other appropriate form the semiquantitative amounts of acetone present as follows:

Negative   1+ (small)   2+ (moderate)   3+ (large)

URINALYSIS AND BODY FLUIDS ANALYSIS PROCEDURE #4

Ictotest—Semiquantitative Test for Bilirubin in Urine

Principles

Bilirubin is a product derived from the breakdown of red blood cells. Extremely high levels of bilirubin may be found in liver disease, where the liver is unable to form other products from the excess hemoglobin, and in cases of high destruction of red blood cells. Testing for the presence of abnormal levels of bilirubin in the urine is most often performed by using Ictotest reagent tablets. When exposed to clinically significant levels of bilirubin in the urine, these tablets react based on the coupling of a unique solid diazonium salt with bilirubin in an acid medium, resulting in a blue or purple reaction product. Mild colors, including pink, are not to be reported as positive bilirubin findings.

Pyridium is a medication sometimes used in cystitis (bladder infections) that will mask positive results when small amounts of bilirubin are present. Other drugs (e.g., chlorpromazine or etodolac) may also cause a false positive result or atypical results.

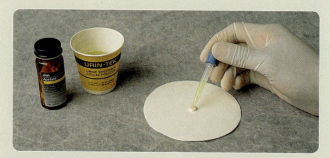

FIGURE 12-35 Acetest for the presence of urinary ketones. Source: Delmar/Cengage Learning.

Equipment and Supplies

1. Gloves, disposable paper towels and disinfectant or other cleaning solution
2. Report form for urinalysis results (Procedure Report Form)
3. Fresh urine sample that has tested positive for bilirubin by dipstick (see Procedure #1)
4. Disposable droppers
5. Deionized or distilled water

6. Absorbent square pads (test mats) upon which the tablet will be placed and the reaction will occur (provided with the kit containing tablets)
7. Stoppered dark container of Ictotest tablets (examine for color changes or deterioration)
8. Electronic timing device or clock/watch with second hand

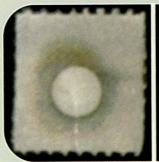 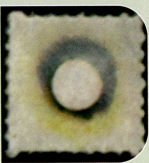

Weak positive   Strong positive

FIGURE 12-36 Ictotest for bilirubin, performed on test mat. Source: Delmar/Cengage Learning.

Procedure

1. Wash hands and don gloves.
2. Assemble necessary equipment and supplies.
3. Place a square of the absorbent test mat onto a sheet of white paper.
4. Place 10 drops of urine on the center of the test mat.
5. Place 1 Ictotest tablet on the moistened mat.
6. Carefully place 1 drop of deionized or distilled water on the top of the tablet (Figure 12-36). Wait 5 seconds. Add a second drop of water to the tablet so that the water runs off the tablet and onto the mat.
7. The presence of a blue or purple color on the mat indicates a positive test for bilirubin. A slight pink or red color should be ignored.
8. The test is subjectively graded as either negative or positive. See manufacturer's product insert with images of positive results.
9. Discard all supplies used for the procedure in the appropriate containers. A disinfectant should be used to clean the work surfaces and equipment should be cleaned and restored to its former position. Gloves should be discarded appropriately and the hands washed thoroughly in accordance with established policies.

Reporting of Results

Report on the Procedure Report Form or other appropriate form the amounts of bilirubin present as either positive or negative only. There is no semiquantitative determination for this procedure.

URINALYSIS AND BODY FLUIDS ANALYSIS PROCEDURE #5

Clinitest—Semiquantitative Test for Glucose and Other Reducing Substances

Principles

The presence of a number of reducing substances may be determined by the Clinitest method even when a negative result has been found with the use of dipsticks, as most dipstick brands are specific for glucose by using the glucohexokinase method. The Clinitest will provide a positive result for any of the reducing substances,

IN THE LAB

including cellulose from undigested vegetable matter, and may also be performed on fecal matter. It is an important test for determining digestive problems in infants. Originally, the Clinitest was used for determining glucose levels in the urine of diabetics, but was abandoned for this purpose due to false positive results from other reducing substances present in the urine of diabetic patients.

The Clinitest is based on Benedict's copper reduction reaction. Copper sulfate reacts with reducing substances, converting cupric sulfate to cuprous oxide. Colors range from blue through green to orange. Sugars other than glucose may be detected with this test.

The Clinitest procedure may be performed on the feces of infants to determine the presence of undigested foods. When malabsorption conditions are present, the stool will often be liquid in consistency. When collecting a fecal sample from an infant, use nonabsorbent diapers for the specimen collection. The solid and liquid portions of the stool MUST be combined. It is possible to aspirate the liquid portion of the stool from the diaper using a syringe or the sample can be squeezed from the diaper into a cup. A large cotton swab may also be necessary for collecting the liquid portion of a stool from a gel absorption diaper. It is critical to avoid mixing urine with the fecal specimen as urine may contain components that will interfere with the results.

Equipment and Supplies

1. Gloves, disposable paper towels and disinfectant or other cleaning solution
2. Report form for urinalysis results (Procedure Report Form)
3. Fresh urine sample in clean urine container (The sample may have yielded a negative result when tested by the dipstick method. Note the requirements for obtaining a fecal specimen listed under the principles for this procedure.)
4. Disposable dropper pipettes such as Pasteur or disposable bulb pipettes for dispensing drops of water and urine
5. Deionized or distilled water
6. Stoppered dark container of Clinitest tablets (examine for color changes or deterioration)
7. Flat-bottomed test tubes and test tube holder (enclosed in the kit containing the test tablets)
8. Color chart from the test kit for use in interpreting results

Procedure

1. Wash hands and don gloves.
2. Assemble necessary equipment and supplies.
3. Place 5 drops of urine into a clean glass test tube that is provided with the kit (Figure 12-37).
4. Using a clean dropper the same size as that used in Step #3, add 10 drops of deionized water.

5. Drop 1 Clinitest tablet into the test tube containing the water and urine (or fecal) sample. When a fecal sample is used, refer to the collection procedures described under the principles section for this procedure.

   a. Watch for a boiling reaction.

   b. Do not shake the tube during the reaction or for 15 seconds after the boiling stops.

   c. Remember to watch for what is called the "pass-through phenomenon." This action is defined as a series of color reactions over a period of time until the end-point occurs.

6. Determine results of the procedure from the chart provided with the manufacturer's kit.

7. Discard all supplies used for the procedure in the appropriate containers. A disinfectant should be used to clean the work surfaces and equipment should be cleaned and restored to its former position. Gloves should be discarded appropriately and the hands washed thoroughly in accordance with established policies.

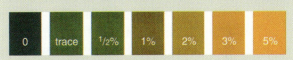

FIGURE 12-37 Performing Clinitest by placing 5 drops of urine into test tube.
Source: Delmar/Cengage Learning.

Reporting of Results

Record the semiquantitative results on the Procedure Report Form or other appropriate form as follows:

0   Trace   ½%   1%   2%   3%   5%

URINALYSIS AND BODY FLUIDS ANALYSIS PROCEDURE #6

Confirmatory Semiquantitative Test for Total Protein in Urine

Principles

Measurement of urinary proteins is becoming increasingly important in the detection of renal pathology. Proteinuria (increased amounts of protein in urine) can occur in increased **glomerular permeability**, defective **tubular reabsorption**, and abnormal secretion of protein into the urinary tract. Proteinuria can also be transient, during cases of urinary tract infection or severe stress. **Albuminuria** (increased albumin in urine) has been implicated as an early indicator of renal damage in diabetes that can be reversed if identified and treated sufficiently early. Measurement of total protein and specific proteins in cerebrospinal fl uid (CSF) is used to detect increased permeability of the blood–brain barrier.

Often it is necessary to measure components of urine that may be positive when screened by a dipstick, as certain conditions may yield a false positive. These confirmatory tests can be time consuming but should be performed to avoid unnecessary

IN THE LAB

expense and problems for a patient whose results may be due to factors other than disease. When a urine sample shows a positive total protein by chemical dipstick, the supernatant and not the original noncentrifuged sample should be used to confirm the presence of protein. This includes confirmation of albumin and globulin, which are fractions of the total protein. Remember that the dipstick method is only positive for amounts of protein at or above 10 mg/dL. Normal disease-free individuals will excrete a small amount of protein that does not exceed 10 mg/dL.

Total protein will precipitate and form turbidity when exposed to sulfosalicylic acid (SSA) or **trichloroacetic acid (TCA)** as the reagent. Centrifuged aliquots of urine are treated with SSA or TCA for turbidity. The greater the amount of total protein, the more turbidity is observed. The results are reported in a range from a trace (mild turbidity) to one in which there is almost total coagulation (Figure 12-38).

The procedure for semiquantitative protein using SSA or TCA can also be modified to perform a quantitative protein procedure on a 24-hour urine specimen.

Equipment and Supplies

1. Gloves, disposable paper towels and disinfectant or other cleaning solution
2. Report form for urinalysis results (Procedure Report Form)

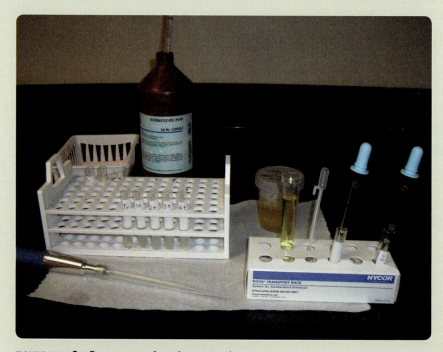

FIGURE 12-38 Confirmatory test for urinary protein.
Source: Delmar/Cengage Learning.

3. Fresh urine sample that has tested positive for protein by dipstick (see Procedure #1)
4. Disposable dropper pipettes such as Pasteur or disposable bulb pipettes
5. Deionized or distilled water
6. Centrifuge and centrifuge tubes
7. Normal and abnormal urine controls (see following note)

    Some urine controls contain different levels of protein, such as a low level for normal controls and a high level for abnormal controls. These levels can be then be graded as either negative or 1– 4+. If the controls are not suitable for this procedure, semiquantitative controls can be made by using a sample of protein that may be obtained from serum and that is diluted to obtain various amounts of protein, from a low level to a high level.

8. 13 × 100 mm test tubes and test tube rack
9. Trichloroacetic acid (TCA) or sulfosalicylic acid (SSA)
10. Black background (helpful for observing the white-colored turbidity that results from a positive reaction as the precipitate is white)
11. Electronic timing device or clock/watch with second hand

Procedure

1. Wash hands and don gloves.
2. Assemble necessary equipment and supplies.
3. Pour 5 mL of urine sample into a disposable centrifuge tube (Figure 12-13).
4. Centrifuge tubes for 5 minutes at 400 RCF. This removes cellular components and other solid substances that may affect the turbidity of a positive test result.
5. Separate the supernatant from the sediment by use of a serological or other mechanical pipette, placing 2 mL of the supernatant into a 13 × 100 mm test tube.
6. Add 2 mL SSA or TCA and mix thoroughly. Exercise care in handling SSA, as it can be caustic if it comes into contact with the skin.
7. After 10 minutes, observe for the amount of turbidity using the following scale.

Negative	No turbidity (clear)
Trace	Barely visible turbidity
1+	Noticeable turbidity
2+	Significant turbidity with granulation
3+	Granulation with clumps
4+	Completely opaque and chiefly clumps

8. Discard all supplies used for the procedure in the appropriate containers. A disinfectant should be used to clean the work surfaces and equipment should be cleaned and restored to its former position. Gloves should be discarded appropriately and the hands washed thoroughly in accordance with established policies.

Critical Reminders

False Positives

The **false positive paradox** is a situation where the incidence of a condition is lower than the false positive rate of a test and therefore when the test shows that a condition exists, it is probable that the result is a false positive.

Conditions That May Lead to a False Positive Test for Urinary Protein by Dipstick

- Highly alkaline urine samples
- Some pigmented (colored) medications
- Disinfectants (quaternary ammonium compounds)
- Antiseptics such as chlorhexidine
- High specific gravity
- Loss of reagent strip buffer by increased contact with specimen

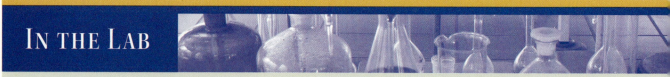

IN THE LAB

Reporting of Results

The interpretation of the presence of urinary protein in a turbidimetric specimen is somewhat subjective. Grade and record the semiquantitative results for the presence of urinary protein using the scale provided in step #7.

URINALYSIS AND BODY FLUIDS ANALYSIS PROCEDURE #7

Total Protein, Quantitative, for CSF, Urine, and Miscellaneous Body Fluids

Principles

Measurement of urinary proteins is becoming increasingly important in the detection of renal pathology. Proteinuria (increased amounts of protein in urine) can occur in increased glomerular permeability, defective tubular reabsorption, and abnormal secretion of protein into the urinary tract. Albuminuria (increased albumin in urine) has been implicated as an early indicator of renal damage in diabetes that can be reversed if identified and treated sufficiently early.

Laboratory personnel should ensure that total protein is confirmed before reporting a positive total protein, as a positive total protein may lead the physician to order a needless 24-hour specimen for total protein. Total protein will precipitate and form turbidity when exposed to SSA or TCA; it will form a blue color when tested similarly with Coomassie blue instead of SSA or TCA as the reagent. Turbidity may also be measured for calculation of the total protein by determining absorbance (Abs) using a spectrophotometer.

Measurement of CSF total protein and specific proteins is used to detect increased permeability of the blood–brain barrier. The same procedure may be used for measuring total protein in both CSF and urine. As the color of the urine sample may vary widely, a urine specimen blank may be used to negate the normal color of the urine. Proteins in CSF and urine are precipitated in finely dispersed form by TCA. The absorbance of a sample is read at 420 nm. Protein in blood serum is measured in grams per deciliter (g/dL), while that of other body fluids is measured in milligrams per deciliter (mg/dL). The process is otherwise the same.

The following parameters may be used for manual methods or programmed into an analyzer for automated systems.

Test Parameters (Acceptable Ranges)

Wavelength (TCA method)	340 nm
Wavelength (dye method)	600 nm
Sample/reagent ratio	3:100
Reaction type	Not applicable
End-point equilibration time	5 sec
Reaction direction	Not applicable
Increasing reaction time	5 min
Reaction temperature	Room temperature
Standard	166 mg/dL (may vary by manufacturer)

Specimen Collection and Preparation

For urine specimens, a random or 24-hour specimen may be used, depending on the clinical situation.

For CSF measurements, great care must be exercised in handling CSF samples. CSF samples are difficult to collect and some are highly infectious. CSF should be free from hemolysis for the protein performance. Centrifuge all specimens containing RBCs or particulate matter.

Equipment and Supplies

1. Gloves, disposable paper towels and disinfectant or other cleaning solution
2. Report form for recording results
3. Fresh urine sample that has tested positive for protein by dipstick (see Procedure #1)
   a. Other body fluids will be collected by a physician and should be appropriate for testing.
   b. CSF sample divided among 3 test tubes. The first tube should be centrifuged to remove RBCs or particular matter and the supernatant is used in testing for protein.
4. Serological pipettes for measuring reagents. A Burette pipette with graduated markings similar to that of a serological pipette may be used.
5. Micropipetters and disposable tips
6. 13 × 100 mm test tubes (one for each control sample and one for each sample to be tested) and test tube rack.
7. Trichloroacetic acid (TCA), sulfosalicylic acid (SSA), or Coomassie blue dye
8. Standards appropriate for fluid being tested, i.e., in g/dL for serum and in mg/dL for other body fluids
9. Prepared normal and abnormal control samples
10. Cuvettes for determining absorbance of each tube containing reagent, standards, controls, and samples (patient or unknown samples)
11. Spectrophotometer capable of reading turbidity or color, depending on methodology chosen
12. Vortex mixer (optional) or "parafilm," a waxy paraffin sheet from which small areas can be cut to use on the various tubes
13. Electronic timing device or clock/watch with second hand
14. Sharp permanent marker

Procedure

1. Wash hands and don gloves.
2. Assemble necessary equipment and supplies.
3. Label the 13 × 100 mm test tubes as follows for proper identification of blanks, standards, controls, and unknowns: label one tube "B" for the blank specimen, one tube "S" for the standard sample, and one or more tubes "C (number)" for the control samples (e.g., C-1 and C-2 to differentiate between normal and abnormal controls).

Critical Reminders

Units of Measurement

Protein in blood serum is measured in grams per deciliter (g/dL), while that of other body fluids is measured in milligrams per deciliter (mg/dL). Protein that is found in body fluids outside the vascular system is derived from protein in the blood that has passed through barriers such as cell membranes and has entered into other body fluids. It is imperative that the appropriate standard is used for determining protein in blood or in other body fluids. It is important to remember that protein in body fluids other than blood is never higher or as high as that found in the serum from the blood.

IN THE LAB

The unknown samples should be labeled by patient name or other identifier such as a patient number.

4. Using a Burette pipette or a 5 or 10 mL serological pipette, place the following volumes into the labeled 13 × 100 mm tubes and mix well:

	Reagent Blank (RB)	Standard (S)	Controls (C)	Unknowns (U)
Reagent	2 mL	2 mL	2 mL	2 mL
Standard	-	20 µL	-	-
Controls	-	-	20 µL	-
Unknowns	-	-	-	20 µL

5. Mix well using a vortex mixer or by covering each tube with parafilm and inverting several times before allowing the tubes to stand for at least 5 minutes.
6. Read the absorbance of the standard and unknowns at 340 nm for SSA method and 600 nm for the Coomassie blue dye method.
7. Record the absorbance (Abs) reading for each tube, including the standard (see Example 12-1).
8. Calculate results by dividing the absorbance of the unknown samples by the absorbance of the known standard. Then multiply the result obtained by the value of the standard (See Example 12-1).

Calculation

$$\text{Total Protein (mg/dL)} = \frac{\text{Absorbance of unknown (Au)}}{\text{Absorbance of standard (As)}} \times \frac{\text{Concentration}}{\text{of Standard}}$$

Example 12-1

A 24-hour urine sample of 1850 mL was mixed and tested for protein.
The result of the protein was 240 mg/dL.

1850 mL / 100 mL × 240 mg/dL = 18.5 × 240 = 4440 mg / 24 hours

Since there are 1000 mg in 1 gram (g), 4440 / 1000 = 4.44 g / 24 hours

9. Discard all supplies used for the procedure in the appropriate containers. A disinfectant should be used to clean the work surfaces and equipment should be cleaned and restored to its former position. Gloves should be discarded appropriately and the hands washed thoroughly in accordance with established policies.

Reporting of Results

Record the results on an appropriate form. Report results for CSF and other body fluids in mg/dL. For a 24-hour urine sample, the value is obtained for the total volume of the sample obtained. Results obtained are in mg/dL. A dL is 0.1 of a liter (L). The total volume is divided by 100 to obtain the number of dLs in a 24-hour sample.

URINALYSIS AND BODY FLUIDS ANALYSIS PROCEDURE #8

Cerebrospinal Fluid Examination and Cell Counts

Principles

The presence of RBCs and WBCs above minimal levels in CSF is significant. CSF levels of protein and glucose are indicative of bacterial and viral infections, based on which constituent is elevated or decreased. Both protein and glucose levels in CSF are slightly lower than the levels found in the blood under normal circumstances. Normal CSF values are as follows:

Cell counts	$<5 \times 10^6$/L for mononuclear WBCs and RBCs
Glucose	60% to 70% of plasma levels (usually at 50–80 mg/dL or 2.8–4.4 mmol/L) but may vary slightly with methodology used for measurement
Protein	Infant = 0.1–1.2 g/L; adult = 0.15–0.45 g/L
IgG/albumin ratio	<0.2

CSF analysis procedures are useful in diagnosing bacterial, viral, or fungal meningitis; encephalitis; malignant infiltrates such as acute leukemias and lymphomas; multiple sclerosis; and subarachnoid hemorrhage.

Specimen Collection and Preparation

A 5 mL to 15 mL specimen of CSF divided between three plain sterile tubes should be used. A minimum of 2 mL is required for immunoglobulin analysis if it is to be performed. Centrifuge all specimens containing RBCs or particulate matter.

Red and White Cell Enumerations

Unless the counts are extremely elevated for RBCs and WBCs, these counts are performed undiluted on a hemacytometer (Figures 12-39, 12-40, and 12-41).

Equipment and Supplies

1. Gloves, disposable paper towels and disinfectant or other cleaning solution
2. Report form for recording results

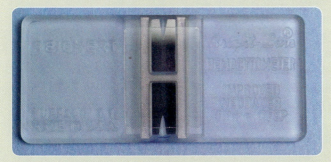

FIGURE 12-39 Top view of hemacytometer with cover slip in place.
Source: Delmar/Cengage Learning.

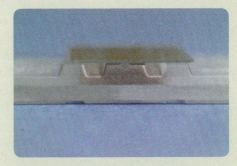

FIGURE 12-40 Side view of hemacytometer.
Source: Delmar/Cengage Learning.

IN THE LAB

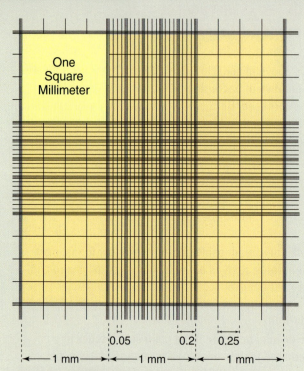

One
Square
Millimeter

0.05   0.2   0.25

←— 1 mm —→ ←— 1 mm —→ ←— 1 mm —→

FIGURE 12-41 Ruled area of hemacytometer showing grid squares for counting RBCs and WBCs.
Source: Delmar/Cengage Learning.

3. CSF sample divided among 3 test tubes (The first tube should be centrifuged to remove RBCs or particular matter and the supernatant is used for testing for protein.)
4. Hemacytometer with cover glass
5. Microscope slides
6. Gram stain kit for bacterial pathogens
7. Acid-fast bacillus (AFB) stain for TB organisms if required
8. India ink for prep to screen for Cryptococcus
9. Normal saline solution

Procedure

1. Wash hands and don gloves.
2. Assemble necessary equipment and supplies.
3. Perform the cell counts for the CSF in the number 3 tube as quickly as possible since the WBCs and RBCs may disintegrate quite rapidly in dilute (hypotonic) fluid.
4. When the CSF sample is clear, perform the cell count as follows:
   a. Transfer well-mixed CSF to a hemacytometer chamber. The sample should remain undiluted when clear.
   b. Count the WBCs and RBCs in all nine of the large squares (these large squares are subdivided) on both sides of the hemacytometer.
   c. Average the two sides by dividing by 2.
   d. Multiply the results by 1.11, to compensate for the fact that 9 squares or 0.9 mm surface area are counted, which is less than 1 mm.
5. When the spinal fluid is hazy or slightly cloudy (may be red if RBCs are present), perform the cell count as follows:
   a. Mix the CSF sample carefully by inverting or swirling to avoid breaking down the RBCs.
   b. Dilute one volume of CSF with 9 volumes of normal saline (to preserve the cells), creating a 1:10 dilution.
   c. Transfer well-mixed CSF to a hemacytometer chamber.

     d. As with the undiluted specimen, count the WBCs and RBCs in all nine of the large squares on both sides of the hemacytometer.

     e. Average the two sides and multiply the results by 1.11.

     f. Multiply the final result by 10 to account for the dilution.

6. Discard all supplies used for the procedure in the appropriate containers. A disinfectant should be used to clean the work surfaces and equipment should be cleaned and restored to its former position. Gloves should be discarded appropriately and the hands washed thoroughly in accordance with established policies.

Reporting of Results

Report the cell count as cells/µL for both WBCs and RBCs.

URINALYSIS AND BODY FLUIDS ANALYSIS PROCEDURE #9

Determining Glucose in Cerebrospinal Fluid

Principles

CSF levels of protein and glucose are indicative of bacterial and viral infections, based on which constituent is elevated or decreased. Both protein and glucose levels in CSF are slightly lower than the levels found in the blood under normal circumstances.

    Abnormal results include increased and decreased glucose levels. Abnormal results may be due to infection (bacterial or fungal), inflammation of the central nervous system, or tumor.

    The following procedure is adapted from the glucose kits available from Stanbio Laboratory, Boerne, TX. Any reliable glucose procedure that employs either enzymatic or end-point colorimetric methodology may be used for CSF glucose determinations.

Specimen Collection and Preparation

CSF glucose procedures may be performed on any of the 3 tubes normally collected from a lumbar puncture. Centrifuge all specimens containing RBCs or particulate matter.

Equipment and Supplies

1. Gloves, disposable paper towels and disinfectant or other cleaning solution
2. Report form for recording results
3. CSF sample (Centrifuge to remove RBCs or particular matter and use the supernatant for testing for glucose.)
4. Reagents for the quantitative enzymatic or colorimetric determination of glucose in CSF. These are the same as those used for serum or plasma testing.
5. Glucose reagents and standards
6. Cuvettes for determining absorbance of protein or glucose
7. Spectrophotometer capable of reading turbidity or color, depending on methodology chosen
8. Micropipetter

IN THE LAB

9. Serological pipettes
10. Electronic timing device or clock/watch with second hand

Procedure

1. Wash hands and don gloves.
2. Assemble necessary equipment and supplies.
3. Using a serological pipette, place into cuvettes the following volumes (mL) and mix well. The volumes may be increased if the instrument requires volumes greater than 1.0 mL.

	Reagent Blank (RB)	Standard (S)	Controls (C)	Unknowns (U)
Reagent	1.0 mL	1.0 mL	1.0 mL	1.0 mL
Standard	-	10 µL	-	-
Controls	-	-	10 µL	-
Unknowns	-	-	-	10 µL

4. Incubate all cuvettes at 37°C for 10 minutes, or incubate at room temperature for 20 minutes.
5. Read S (standard) and RB (reagent blank) at 500 nm within 15 minutes.
6. Discard all supplies used for the procedure in the appropriate containers. A disinfectant should be used to clean the work surfaces and equipment should be cleaned and restored to its former position. Gloves should be discarded appropriately and the hands washed thoroughly in accordance with established policies.

Quality Control

Two levels of control material, including both a normal and an abnormal value, with known glucose levels, should be analyzed by this method on each day of testing.

Reporting of Results

Results are obtained using the following equation:

Calculation

$$\text{Glucose (mg/dL)} = \frac{\text{Absorbance of unknown (Au)}}{\text{Absorbance of standard (As)}} \times 100$$

where Au is the absorbance value of the unknown, As is the absorbance value of the standard, and 100 is the concentration of the standard in milligrams per deciliter (mg/dL).

Results are reported in milligrams per deciliter (mg/dL). In some countries, they are reported in SI (International System) units that are derived from the metric system. Conversion to SI units is often performed by the instrument upon which the test is performed. Some health care facilities report values in both SI and metric units of measurement.

SUMMARY

The kidneys are arguably the most important organs of the body as they maintain the equilibrium between water and dissolved particles of the blood and also maintain the pH of the body at a slightly alkaline state in order for metabolism to occur. Urine is the body fluid most easily available for assessing the health of an individual, and urinalysis is one of the most common procedures performed in the clinical laboratory.

Normal urine samples should be clear and light yellow. Any departure from these characteristics may be evidence of disease. Although chemical testing at one time was performed as a single procedure for each analyte, advances have allowed for screening for as many as ten separate entities by the use of a single dipstick with a chemically reactive pad.

A microscopic exam is performed after the macroscopic (physical) and dipstick exams, and often confirms what has been determined through those procedures. The presence of abnormal crystals and significant levels of red blood cells and/or white blood cells in the urine are indicative of medical conditions that require treatment.

Other body fluids may yield clinical findings of disease through the presentation of entities similar to those found in urine. Glucose and protein levels in the CSF provide clues as to whether bleeding is or has occurred and if a viral or bacterial infection is present. The presence of white blood cells, and the types that predominate, are significant in the spinal fluid as well as in the synovial fluid. In the synovial fluid, crystals such as those found in urine specimens are an important clinical finding that indicates inflammation. Transudates and exudates are similar, except that transudates indicate a disruption of fluid production and dispersion between the serous membranes, and exudates are fluids that are produced by serous membranes in response to injury or infection. Learning the important clinical tests for one of these fluids provides the techniques for performing examinations for other types of fluids.

REVIEW QUESTIONS

1. Besides blood, what are some other body fluids that may require laboratory testing?
2. In your opinion, how has testing of body fluids improved in accuracy and ease of performance?
3. Why is the testing of CSF so critical?
4. Why are confirmatory tests important?
5. What are some reasons that urine is the most often tested body fluid?
6. How would one determine if bleeding has occurred in the cerebrospinal column?

CHAPTER 13

HEMATOLOGY AND COAGULATION

LEARNING OBJECTIVES

Upon completion of this chapter, the reader will be able to:

- List the types of blood that may be collected for hematological procedures.

- Provide the major functions for white blood cells and red blood cells.

- Name the five types of white blood cells.

- Discuss the reasons for having a well-prepared blood film.

- Describe the relationship between hemoglobin and hematocrit values.

- Discuss the need for an anticoagulated specimen for performing a complete blood count.

KEY TERMS

Autolet device
Basophils
Calcium ions
Capillary pipette
Capillary tube
Coagulation
Complete blood count (CBC)
Cyanmethemoglobin
Direct leukocyte count (DLC)
EDTA
Eosinophils
Extrinsic factor
Factor X
Ferricyanide

Gross lipemia
Hemacytometer
Hematocrit
Hemorrhage
International Normalized
    Ratio (INR)
International Sensitivity Index
Intrinsic factor
Lancets
Leukocytes
Lymphocytes
Macroglobulinemia
Methemoglobin
Microcapillary reader

Monocytes
Neutrophils
Oxyhemoglobin
Polycythemia
Prothrombin
Random error
Reticulocytes
Sealing putty
Sulfhemoglobin
Supernatant
Thromboplastin
Unopette disposable diluting pipette
Warfarin (Coumadin)

INTRODUCTION

The word *hematology* literally means "study of blood." There is not just one test, but a multitude of tests available for all sorts of disease states that may afflict a patient. Hematology provides another basic test, or actually a set of tests, used almost routinely along with a urinalysis to assess a patient's health. Changes in body fluids signal malfunctions in the body ranging from minor to extremely serious conditions. As is possible with a complete urinalysis, a number of conditions can be easily determined by a **complete blood count (CBC)**. The basic tests determine if an infection is present or if a state of anemia is present. **Coagulation** is the process that leads to clotting of the blood. Usually, a coagulation study is included in the hematology section to determine if a person is likely to bleed spontaneously (**hemorrhage**) of if the blood clots too readily, which might lead to a stroke or heart attack.

Students of clinical laboratory medicine should already have a basic knowledge of the formation of blood and its functions from anatomy, physiology, and other academic courses. The material presented is not intended to be a "how to" for procedures in urine and body fluids analyses. However, this chapter's "In the Lab" activities will serve to combine the theory of the laboratory department with the practice of several basic procedures.

Exploration of the basics in the background of laboratory medicine and safety, and an overall orientation into the field of clinical laboratory medicine, will help the student to become well-equipped to meet the challenge of this demanding profession and achieve a meaningful level of knowledge required for advancement and for improving skills. This chapter is designed to facilitate practical classroom laboratory experience. The graphics show some of the equipment the medical laboratory student will be using. It is important that the student possess sufficient knowledge regarding safety in handling of human specimens and a respect for the care that must be exercised to compile accurate reports used in the treatment of patients.

Hematology

Hematological tests for routine purposes require a CBC. Several tests for anemia are included in the CBC and provide a basic means for determining the type of anemia. Most of these tests are done on automated instruments, which provide a complete picture in just seconds. For practical training, it is important for a student to be able to perform these tests manually to understand the functions of the equipment and to know when a malfunction has occurred or if the results do not match, as with a **random error**. Certain conditions of the blood may also provide less-than-accurate results and lead to mistreatment or no treatment in a patient needing medical attention.

A CBC contains a red blood cell (RBC) count, a white blood cell (WBC) count, a hemoglobin (Hgb), and a **hematocrit** (Hct). Both the RBCs and the WBCs are made into a thin smear and stained for examination under a microscope. All the individual tests that make up a CBC should correlate with each other, so in a case of either the RBCs or WBCs being normal or abnormal, the results will fit together in a pattern that the technician or technologist will understand following completion of a course in hematology.

Coagulation

Some patients receive medications that prevent the blood from clotting at a normal rate, creating a prolonged coagulation time. This treatment helps to prevent clots from occurring in the blood vessels, which might lead to stroke, heart attack, or a dangerous condition where clots occur in the lungs. These tests require accuracy and are usually performed on semiautomated instruments, but it is important that the technician or technologist be able to perform emergency tests manually if the instrument malfunctions. The two most important coagulation tests (prothrombin time, or PT, and the activated partial thromboplastin time, or APTT) will be described as manual procedures in this chapter. The extremely complex study for all of the clotting factors that might be deficient or absent in a patient will be covered in the academic portion of your program in hematology and coagulation, or coagulation studies may be presented as a separate course.

HEMATOLOGY AND COAGULATION PROCEDURES

Hematology and coagulation procedures are most frequently performed in the same area of the laboratory. Equipment chosen for the basic procedures would be based upon the volume of testing performed in the department. Instruments range in cost from the low thousands of dollars for semiautomated instruments to more than $100,000 for highly automated versions. Many brands and levels of instruments are available for performing an automated CBC.

Hematology Procedures

One of the mainstays of the production of automated hematology analyzers has been Coulter Electronics, which merged with Beckman and now produces a significant number of the hematology instruments used throughout the world. Other widely used blood cell counters are manufactured by Abbott (the Cell-Dyne) and Sysmex. Some of these instruments are capable of analyzing animal blood, which for some species is quite different from that of humans. The hematology analyzer originated from a basic industrial particle counter, which analyzed solutions for crystals and bits of contaminants in the solution. A solution passes through an almost microscopic opening called an aperture that has an electrical current passing from outside the tube housing the aperture, while bathed in a saline solution to allow a current to flow through it. This saline solution also keeps the blood cells normal in size and shape. As cells are pulled through the opening by a vacuum, electronic counters enumerate the number of "blips" caused by cells as they interrupt the current flow.

A blood cell counter require only a small amount of anticoagulated blood but produces a considerable number of measurements. Samples should be collected in EDTA tubes. EDTA is an anticoagulant used when blood cells are required to be unaltered, so abnormal results will not be produced on blood from normal individuals. Blood cell counters, regardless of the manufacturer, generally perform the following measurements:

- White blood cell (leukocyte) count (WBC)
- Red blood cell (erythrocyte) count (RBC)
- Hemoglobin concentration (Hgb) (g/L)

- Hematocrit (relative volume of erythrocytes) (Hct)
- Mean corpuscular (erythrocyte) volume (MCV)
- Mean corpuscular (erythrocyte) Hgb (MCH) (pg)
- Mean corpuscular (erythrocyte) Hgb concentration (MCHC) (g/L)
- Platelet or thrombocyte count (platelets) ($\times 10^9$/L)

The MCV, MCH, and MCHC, which are called the RBC indices, are calculated from the RBC count, along with the Hgb and Hct values.

Because WBCs are normally less than 10,000 per microliter in number, whereas RBCs number in the millions per microliter, counting both WBCs and RBCs makes little difference in the final RBC count. After the RBCs are counted, they are then lysed, or destroyed, so the solution contains intact WBCs, which are counted in the same manner as the RBCs. The resulting solution of lysed RBCs and WBCs can now be used to measure the Hgb, by determining the absorbance* or concentration of the solution of lysed RBCs from which the Hgb went into solution. The automated cell counter efficiently performs all of these processes and calculations in a matter of seconds. However, all of the tests may be performed manually, and most laboratory training programs teach manual methodology for the student to understand the processes, as well as to provide backup for an uninterrupted workflow during emergencies.

Coagulation Procedures

Normally, a person's blood should not coagulate as it passes through the vascular system, as the results would be disastrous if clots spontaneously occurred in the vessels of vital organs of the body. However, sometimes clotting needs to occur to prevent hemorrhage, so the body is constantly juggling anticoagulant factors as well as coagulation factors to maintain homeostasis. To prevent strokes and heart attacks, it is sometimes necessary to manipulate the body's coagulation system to prevent clots and to prolong the time required for a clot to form. The multitude of factors involved in inhibiting or stimulating clotting at the appropriate time are covered at length in courses for hematology and coagulation. This section will provide the student an overview of the most basic tests and their meanings.

Clotting involves **intrinsic factors** found in the plasma of the blood and an **extrinsic factor** from the tissue called **thromboplastin**. When a fibrin clot begins to form when tissue is damaged by injury, platelets also become enmeshed in the clot, to strengthen it and solidify it. It is later necessary for the body to dissolve

---

*Absorbance is determined by an instrument called a spectrophotometer, which measures the amount of light absorbed by a solution of colored molecules; the amount of light absorbed is also known as optical density, or OD. This measurement, which directly determines the concentration of colored molecules within a solution, is widely used for clinical laboratory determinations.

the clot when the wound has healed. Medication is used to prolong the clotting time to prevent the body from forming dangerous clots. These changes must be regularly monitored by the PT (or prothrombin time). The patient is usually anticoagulated initially with a powerful anticoagulant called *heparin,* which is administered by injection; after the desired results are obtained, the medication is switched to warfarin (Coumadin), which may be taken orally. The laboratory test for monitoring the patient prior to switching to Coumadin is the APTT (or activated partial thromboplastin time). The response of the body to the anticoagulant may change over time, so long-term treatment may require periodic changes in the medical regimen prescribed.

Automated and semiautomated instruments are available from a number of sources. These instruments measure and hold the blood plasma containing the various coagulation factors in a stable environment. The reagents are also kept at a temperature conducive to clotting through the formation of a fibrin clot. For performing the most basic of coagulation tests, the APTT and the PT along with decalcified plasma are required. A citrated specimen, which is preferred, binds the calcium and prevents the clotting of the whole blood specimen. Plasma is removed from the whole blood sample via centrifugation. This process is best accomplished at the body's temperature of 37°C, and the automated systems maintain a constant temperature while the reaction is taking place. Prothrombin is a plasma protein coagulation factor that is synthesized from vitamin K. Prothrombin is converted to thrombin by activated factor X (1 of 13 coagulation factors) in the presence of calcium ions. The laboratory procedure known as the PT is the most frequently ordered coagulation test in a clinical laboratory. The procedure measures the amount of time that elapses before clotting of the plasma occurs upon the addition of *thromboplastin* and calcium to a sample of the anticoagulated plasma.

When a medical need exists to prevent clotting by inhibiting the quick coagulation of the blood, the PT test is used for monitoring the effects of warfarin (Coumadin). After the patient is stabilized on warfarin, the APTT test is used. Most automated and semiautomated instruments provide both of these tests on the same instrument, with the use of different reagents. Extremely accurate pipetting and measurement of the first vestiges of clotting by light interruption, a very sensitive process, are used by these instruments. A calculated result using the actual clotting time divided by the normal control run with the sample(s) is called the International Normalized Ratio (INR). When different instruments and reagents are used, both the patient results and the normal control will be different, for either a longer or shorter period. This will result in the same ratio when both results change to an equal extent.

DIFFERENTIAL WHITE BLOOD CELL COUNT

An important component of a complete blood count (CBC) is that of enumerating the white blood cells (WBCs) and differentiating among the several types to provide clues as to a patient's disease condition. A white blood cell evaluation is the most important tool used to determine the presence of infection and the severity of a condition, as well as whether an infection is of a viral or bacterial nature.

White blood cells are also called **leukocytes**. They are a vital component of the immune system that is important in responding to infections and other conditions that might require an immune response, such as an allergic condition. The total WBC count may be indicative of a medical condition if it is either above or below the normal or average count for humans. An increase or decrease in the number of or changes in the morphology (physical characteristics) of certain types of WBCs may be critical in establishing a diagnosis of certain illnesses and may lend clues as to the presence of a disease and general information that might lead to a diagnosis with further testing.

A total WBC count is not necessarily indicative of the severity of a disease, since some serious ailments may show either a low or an elevated white cell count and counts may vary widely among individuals. Following the determination of the total WBC count, a differential count from a stained smear is necessary to determine any changes in the physical characteristics of the WBCs and the percentages of the several types normally in the circulating blood. A WBC differential consists of an examination of a thin smear to determine the percentages of a number of different types of WBCs. White cells may also invade other body fluids outside the blood system, so it is sometimes necessary to perform a WBC count and differential of the various types of cells from fluids other than blood. Some of these fluids include specimens such as urine, cerebrospinal fluid (CSF) and synovial fluids (fluids present around the joints of the body). Increased percentages of certain WBCs may indicate either a viral or bacterial infection. An overall decrease in total WBCs may also be indicative of overwhelming infections, among other conditions or extreme increases in the total numbers of WBCs may indicate a serious disease such as one of the forms of leukemia. White cells and the percentage of the types found in both the blood system and other fluids of the body are significant, as indicated in Table 13-1.

Table 13-1 Significance of Increases in Types of Leukocytes

Cell Type	Significance
Neutrophils (polys)	Increased in bacterial infections
Eosinophils	Increased in allergic reactions and parasitic infections
Basophils	Reactive to inflammation of a nonspecific origin, such as toxins
Lymphocytes	Increased in viral infections
Monocytes	Increased in respiratory viral infections and, after undergoing morphological and physiological changes, phagocytize (eat) foreign bodies during immune responses

Preparation and Staining of Blood Smear for Differential

The blood smear or "film" is made from a drop of blood spread evenly on a slide and stained. While blood cell film preparation is a simple and straightforward procedure, the quality of blood films in many laboratories is often poor. It is important to ensure that the film is well made and stained with a valid and effective stain. A properly made and stained blood smear should be demonstrated by the instructor. The student should duplicate the streaking and staining of the film, and sufficient practice should be provided for the student to become familiar with identifying the various WBCs.

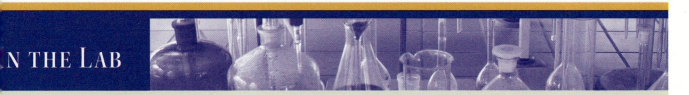

IN THE LAB

BASIC HEMATOLOGY AND COAGULATION PROCEDURES
HEMATOLOGY AND COAGULATION PROCEDURE #1
Preparing a Stained Blood Smear (Film)
Principles

Preparing a blood smear that can be stained adequately and viewed for accuracy is the most important step in producing a complete blood count. The cells must be distributed properly to avoid distortion of shapes by adjacent cells. Visual examination by microscope should confirm the results of the complete count obtained from an autoanalyzer. Such examination is often necessary when the autoanalyzer finds an irreconcilable discrepancy in the results obtained.

Wright's or a combination of Wright's-Giemsa stain is most often used for routine blood smear examinations; other special stains are used for determining certain pathological conditions of the blood. It is paramount that the blood be spread properly over the slide or it is impossible to accurately and thoroughly examine the sample. Blood smears may be prepared directly from a finger "stick" or from an anticoagulated (non-clottable) specimen within 1 hour of collection. Specimens in an anticoagulated tube must be mixed adequately before using them to prepare a blood smear.

Equipment and Supplies

1. Gloves, disposable paper towels, and disinfectant or other cleaning solution
2. Sample from a finger "stick" or from an anticoagulated (non-clottable) specimen examined within 1 hour of collection
3. Microscope slides

Safety Alert

It is quite easy to break the slide used to draw blood across the surface of another slide if too much pressure is placed on the slide, or if the slide is not held correctly. Please observe the instructor's demonstration and avoid a nasty cut that would require an incident report being filed, and possible medical treatment and follow-up to prevent complications or to determine if the student has been exposed to infected blood.

IN THE LAB

4. Alcohol prep pad
5. Lint-free material such as a gauze square or lens paper for drying the slide prior to making the film
6. Unheparinized (plain) **capillary tube** or safety blood dispensers (DIFF-SAFE) designed to puncture the cap of a tube and to deliver a small drop of blood onto the slide
7. Staining rack
8. Wright's or Wright's-Giemsa stain kit (The instructor will determine whether a quick-stain procedure or a traditional method will be used.)
9. Prepared fixative or absolute methanol
10. Forceps for handling stained slides
11. Electronic timing device or clock/watch with second hand
12. Sharps container for disposal of used slides and blood dispensers, and other appropriate waste disposal containers

Procedure

1. Wash hands and don gloves.
2. Assemble necessary equipment and supplies.
3. Prepare the slide for the blood film.
   a. Select a glass microscope slide with at least one smooth end. Unfrosted slides are the best for blood films. The slide should be free of oils, fingerprints, and even powdered glass that may be found on some slides.
   b. Clean the slides with an alcohol prep pad and then wipe dry completely with a lint-free material such as a gauze square or lens paper before attempting to make the smear.
4. Either directly from a finger "stick" or using an unheparinized (plain) capillary tube or safety blood dispensers (DIFF-SAFE), place one drop of blood approximately 1 cm from one end of the slide.
5. Without delay (the platelets will begin to clump and the blood drop will begin to dry if too much time elapses), place a "spreader" slide at a 30- to 40-degree angle in front of the drop of blood. Move the slide backward toward the drop until contact is made with the blood drop (Figure 13-1).
6. Allow the blood to run along the contact line of the two slides.
7. Without lifting it, move the spreader slide along the blood film slide until it hits a finger placed at the far edge of the slide or some other means of preventing the slide from moving. It takes practice before acceptable slides are made consistently.
8. Allow the blood on the slide to dry, in preparation for performing a staining procedure as demonstrated by the instructor. The instructor will choose one of several different methods (Figure 13-2).

9. Assess the blood film on the slide before proceeding with the staining steps.
   a. After the film has dried, check the film macroscopically to assess its quality as to consistency (Table 13-2). Note that in actual laboratory practice, each slide should be clearly identified with the patient's name, ID number, etc., and these would be checked as well).
   b. The film should "feather" into a very thin edge when prepared properly (Figure 13-3).
10. Firmly grasp the slide with forceps and "fix" the dried smears in prepared fixative or absolute methanol for 30 seconds.
11. Allow excess fixative to drain from the slide for approximately 15 seconds following removal from the fixative.
12. Stain slides using a quick stain as described here (steps 12a through 12d, below). Quick stains are used by most laboratories. (If a more time-consuming traditional staining method is used, the directions will require timing of each step with a timing device. Follow the directions provided with such stains).
   a. Quick stains will be placed in three specially designed staining containers called Coplin jars and do not require drying between stains.
   b. The "fixed" slide is dipped 5 – 6 times in an eosin solution and is allowed to drain into the jar. The end of the slide is then blotted on a paper towel.
   c. The slide is then immediately immersed in a methylene blue solution by dipping it into the stain 5 – 6 times.
   d. The slide is then rinsed with a slow stream of water and is placed in an upright position in a rack and allowed to dry.
13. Discard all supplies used for the procedure in the appropriate containers. A disinfectant should be used to clean the work surfaces and equipment should be cleaned and restored to its former position. Gloves should be discarded appropriately and the hands washed thoroughly in accordance with established policies.

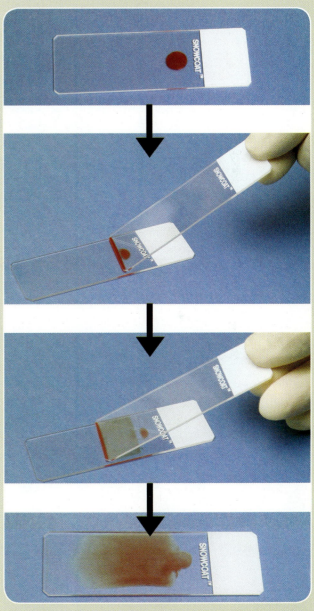

FIGURE 13-1 Preparing a blood smear for staining by making a thin film of blood on a glass slide.
Source: Delmar/Cengage Learning.

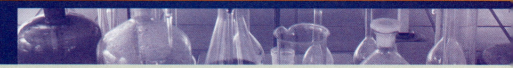

IN THE LAB

Table 13-2 Common Problems in Making Blood Films

Problem	Possible Cause(s)
Smear too thin or too long	Drop of blood too small Spreader slide at too low an angle Improper speed in making smear
Smear too thick or too short	Drop of blood too large Spreader slide at too high an angle Improper speed in making smear
Ridges or waves in smear	Uneven pressure on spreader slide Hesitation in pushing spreader slide
Holes in smear	Slides not clean Uneven or dirty edge of spreader slide
Uneven cell distributions	Uneven pressure during spread of blood Delay in spreading blood Uneven or dirty edge of spreader slide
Artifacts or unusual cell appearance	Smear dried too slowly Smear not fixed within 1 hour after preparation High humidity

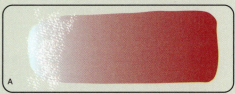

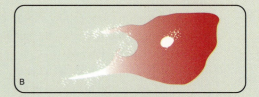

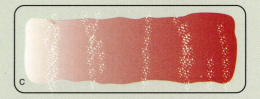

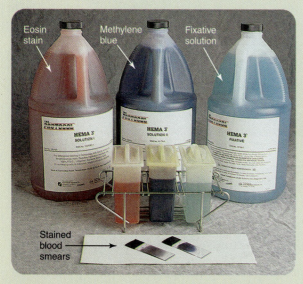

FIGURE 13-2 Quick type of stain for preparing blood films for microscopic examination (modified Wright-Giemsa). **Source: Delmar/Cengage Learning.**

FIGURE 13-3 (A) Properly prepared smear. (B) Smear made on an oily or dirty slide. (C) Improperly prepared smear where blood is not drawn smoothly in one motion across slide. Source: Delmar/Cengage Learning.

Evaluation of Results

A blood smear that has been properly made and stained greatly facilitates the accuracy and efficiency of the hematology department (Figures 13-4).

HEMATOLOGY AND COAGULATION PROCEDURE #2
Practical White Blood Cell Differentiation
Principles

The first step in performing the white blood cell (WBC) differentiation is to examine the slide under low power to look for consistent distribution of both white and red cells. The experienced hematology professional will develop a quick "look-see" evaluation of the blood picture presented. The quality of the film is readily obvious to the trained eye, and increased or decrease WBCs, quality and numbers of platelets, and whether RBCs are normal in color, size and shape are evident. In some cases, a repeat slide may be necessary due to quality of the slide and the staining characteristics.

WBCs are classified into different type. Normally, 100 to 200 cells are counted and a percentage is calculated for each type to determine if the ranges of types of WBCs fall within a normal pattern. In various disease presentations, certain WBC types are either increased or decreased, or may appear as immature stages. The types may be counted using an automated or mechanical counter (Figure 13-5). WBC characteristics are useful in diagnosing and monitoring a variety of diseases such as leukemias and anemias.

Remember that the technical laboratory professional should not merely focus on WBCs during a white blood cell differentiation procedure but should evaluate all cellular components of the smear, including platelet appearance and RBC appearance.

To determine the type of leukocyte (WBC), the student should consider the following characteristics, in conjunction with the illustration of cell types in Figure 13-6:

- Look at the size of the cell. Monocytes are almost always larger than lymphocytes.
- Eosinophils have more granulation than basophils and are coarser than neutrophils.
- Neutrophils are smaller than eosinophils in most cases.

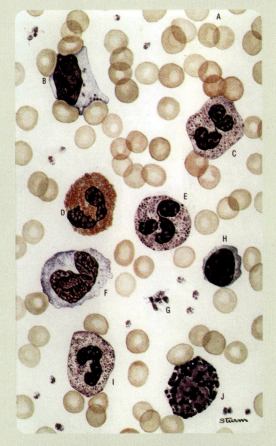

FIGURE 13-4 Normally distributed red and white blood cells on properly made blood smear. (A) Red blood cells. (B) Large lymphocyte. (C) Neutrophil. (D) Eosinophile. (E) Neutrophil. (F) Monocyte. (G) Platelets. (H) Small lymphocyte. (I) Band cell. (J) Basophil. **Source: Delmar/Cengage Learning.**

Critical Reminder

One may count 200 cells if desired, although the standard is 100 for the experienced worker. The higher number will ensure a more accurate percentage of the various WBCs. For this microscopic manual count, a WBC differential counter is used such as the one illustrated in Figure 13-6.

IN THE LAB

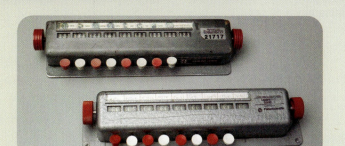

FIGURE 13-5 **Differential white blood cell counter (manual) for determining percentages of the various types of white blood cells. Source: Delmar/Cengage Learning.**

- Look at the color and character of the cytoplasm. Lymphocytes often contain blue cytoplasm, while monocytes reveal a grayish, possible dirty ground-glass appearance.
- Look at the nucleus. The nucleus of neutrophils almost always has three or more lobes. Neutrophils may appear as young cells called bands. The cell line is a band if the narrowest section of the lobed nucleus is wider than one-half of the widest portion of the nucleus.

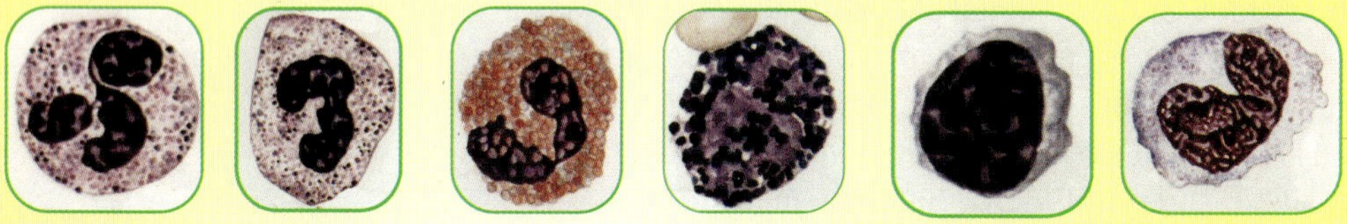

	Neutrophilic Series					
	Segmented (mature)	Band or Stab (immature)	Eosinophil	Basophil	Lymphocyte	Monocyte
Cell Size (μm)	10–15	10–15	10–15	10–15	8–15	12–20
Nucleus						
Shape	2–5 lobes	Sausage or U-shaped	Bilobed	Segmented	Round, oval	Horseshoe
Structure	Coarse	Coarse	Coarse	Difficult to see	Smoothly stained, velvety	Folded, convoluted
Cytoplasm						
Amount	Abundant	Abundant	Abundant	Abundant	Scant	Abundant
Color	Pale pink-tan	Pale pink-tan	Pale pink-tan	Pale pink-tan	Blue	Gray-blue
Inclusions	Small, lilac granules	Small, lilac granules	Coarse, orange-red granules	Coarse, blue-black granules	Occasional red-purple granules	Ground-glass appearance

FIGURE 13-6 **Characteristics of white blood cells. Source: Delmar/Cengage Learning.**

- The nucleus of the monocyte is normally ropy, or less dense than that of the lymphocyte. The nucleus of the lymphocyte is normally more condensed, round, and darker than the nucleus of the monocyte.
- Cytoplasm-to-nuclear ratio is also an important component in differentiation of white blood cells. For instance, the amount of cytoplasm of a monocyte is most often more abundant than that of the lymphocyte.

Equipment and Supplies

1. Gloves, disposable paper towels, and disinfectant or other cleaning solution
2. Report form for Procedure #2
3. Stained blood film (see Procedure #1 for directions on properly preparing and staining a blood film)
4. Brightfield microscope
5. Microscope immersion oil
6. Lens paper
7. Sharps container for disposal of used slides, and other appropriate waste disposal containers

Procedure

1. Wash hands and don gloves.
2. Assemble necessary equipment and supplies.
3. The instructor may choose to provide stained blood films from a normal patient for students to become familiar with the morphology of both RBC and WBCs, or the student may prepare a stained blood film following the steps in Procedure #1.
4. Visually inspect the slide to ensure that the blood film is properly distributed on it and that a feathered edge is present (see Procedure #1).
5. Place the stained blood film on the microscope stage.
6. Focus the microscope using the low-power objective, locating the feathered end of the smear.
   a. Examine the slide under low power to determine the best area(s) in which to count. The RBCs should not be touching each other.
   b. Do not count WBCs in the extreme edge of the feathered area, where WBCs may be congregated.
   c. Use the charts and diagrams in this chapter to identify normal cells.
7. Using the fine adjustment knob of the microscope and adjusting the light source, find an area where the distribution shows RBCs that are not touching but that are close to each other.
8. Place a drop of immersion oil on the smear where the light is brightest from the condenser.
9. Rotate the nosepiece of the microscope until the oil immersion objective comes in contact with the immersion oil.
10. Use the fine adjustment to gain a sharp image of the blood cells.

IN THE LAB

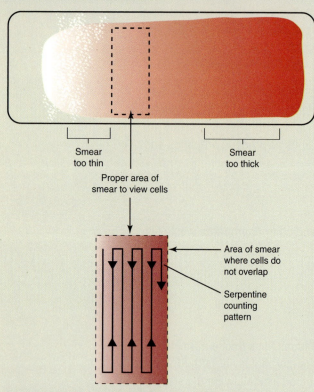

Smear too thin

Smear too thick

Proper area of smear to view cells

Area of smear where cells do not overlap

Serpentine counting pattern

FIGURE 13-7 Finding the proper area of the slide for evaluating red blood cell morphology and counting white blood cells accurately. Source: Delmar/Cengage Learning.

11. Adjust the condenser and the iris diaphragm until a good image of the cells is obtained.

12. Scan the slide from side to side, making sure the focal field is in an area where the cells are not touching. Move the slide along the stage of the microscope in a broad lane running transversely across the body of the film, avoiding the edges completely (Figure 13-7), as cells are sometimes dragged there in greater numbers.

13. Count 100 or 200 cells.

   a. Use the ×40 objective high-power lens to perform a 200 cell count. (The ×100 objective oil immersion lens should be reserved for examining fine intracellular details and when searching for parasites inside the cells.)

   b. Count in multiples of 100 so that you can later calculate the percentage of the various cell types.

   c. Take your time! Count 200 cells to be sure of your results. You should refer to Figure 13-6 to help differentiate the various types of cells.

   d. If 200 WBCs are counted, the total of each type is divided by 2 to obtain a percentage. Some differential counters will perform this task for you.

14. Record the numbers of each type of WBC counted on the report form. If available to you, use a mechanical or electronic differential counter.

15. Remember that the technical laboratory professional should not merely focus on WBCs. RBC evaluation will be covered in Procedure #5. The experienced laboratory professional may assess both WBCs and RBCs simultaneously.

16. Observe at least 10 fields for platelet evaluation under oil immersion (1000X). Observe for size and morphology (shape). Estimate the approximate platelet count by taking the total platelets appearing in 10 fields, and divide by 10 to obtain the average number per microscopic field. Platelets are reported as adequate, increased, or decreased. Record the information on the report form.

17. Return the low-power objective (10X) into place and remove the slide from the stage.

18. Clean the microscope stage with lens paper or tissue. Clean the condenser if necessary.
19. Retain the slide if required.
20. Discard all supplies used for the procedure in the appropriate containers. A disinfectant should be used to clean the work surfaces and equipment should be cleaned and restored to its former position. Gloves should be discarded appropriately and the hands washed thoroughly in accordance with established policies.

Reporting of Results

Calculate the percentage of each of the five basic leukocytes (neutrophils, eosinophils, basophils, lymphocytes, and monocytes). Report the direct leukocyte count (DLC) as a percentage. If the total WBC is known, the count may also be reported in absolute numbers by multiplying the percentages of each type by the actual WBC count. Under "Comments", note the presence of any immature cells, especially blast cells (early immature types), and report these as percentages also.

In addition, the numbers and morphology of platelets can also be evaluated along with the RBCs. Report your findings from the Practical White Blood Cell Differentiation procedure in the Procedure #2 Report Form or other form supplied by your instructor.

Procedure #2 Report Form: Practical White Blood Cell (WBC) Differentiation

Patient Name: _____   Pt. ID _____   Date: _____

Age: _____   Gender (Circle One) M   F   Physician: _____

Time Requested: _____   Time Performed: _____   Time Reported: _____

Examination Requested: ☐ WBC Differential   ☐ Other

White Blood Cells

Neutrophils	_____ %	Lymphocytes	_____ %	Monocytes	_____ %
Eosinophils	_____ %	Basophils	_____ %	Bands	_____ %

Comments (unusual findings) _____

Performed by: _____   **Date Reported** _____

Evaluation of Student Results for Procedure #2

The differentials have been evaluated by counting 200 cells. Grades will be determined as follows:

1. Segmented neutrophils and lymphocytes must come within ±2% of the target value determined by the instructor. In the case that the total percentage is extremely low (i.e., a lymphocyte count of less than 10%), two cells on either side of the target value will be acceptable.
2. One letter grade will be deducted for EACH type of cell that is not within an acceptable range.

IN THE LAB

HEMATOLOGY AND COAGULATION PROCEDURE #3

Determining Hematocrit

Principles

The number of erythrocytes in the blood must be high enough to carry sufficient oxygen to the peripheral tissues. However, if the number of erythrocytes becomes elevated, as occurs in some disease states, the blood viscosity (thickness or stickiness) may be increased. This will adversely affect the heart's ability to circulate the blood throughout the body.

A simple test called the hematocrit (Hct) is used to determine the percent of formed cells in whole blood. Normally, 99% of all the cells in the blood are RBCs; the remaining 1% includes WBCs and platelets. The term "hematocrit" (Hct) comes from the Greek "hemato" meaning "blood" and "crit" meaning "to judge." Another name for the Hct is PCV (packed cell volume), or simply "crit." The test provides an estimate of the adequacy of numbers of RBCs required to carry oxygen to the cells and organs of the body.

For this test, a fresh sample of blood is introduced into a capillary tube coated with heparin to prevent clotting. The end of the tube is sealed with putty, and the tube is spun at a rapid rate in a special centrifuge called a microhematocrit centrifuge (Figure 13-8A) to compact the cells into the end of the tube, where the percentage of RBCs will be determined.

Safety Alert

To reduce the risk of transmission of bloodborne diseases such as AIDS and hepatitis B, wear protective gloves when handling other peoples' blood, dispose of all blood-contaminated materials in the provided containers, and clean up thoroughly when finished.

Hematocrit Calculation

The hematocrit (Hct) determination is actually a separation of solids (blood cells) from the liquid portion (plasma) of the blood. A centrifuge uses centrifugal force to press the RBCs to the bottom of the capillary tube, leaving the liquid part or plasma overlying the RBCs.

Hct values are determined in two ways. They may be performed by calculations from an automated cell counter or by centrifuging a small amount of blood in a capillary tube. The manual method for measuring the Hct requires a reader, of which there are various versions (Figure 13-8B).

The straw-colored supernatant is the plasma, the RBCs sink to the bottom, and the WBCs are seen as a thin buffy coat, if the WBC count is normal, at the top of the RBC column. WBCs are not included in the Hct. (Note that the WBC count might be quite high in a patient with a severe infection or leukemia.) Figure 13-9 shows a centrifuged capillary tube with blood kept from clotting by a thin layer of heparin (an anticoagulant) on the inside of the tube. The percentage of the total RBCs represented by the packed cells is the percentage of RBCs in the whole blood specimen. Normal Hct values for males are 40% to 54%, and those for females, 37% to 47%.

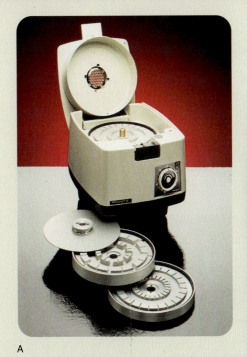

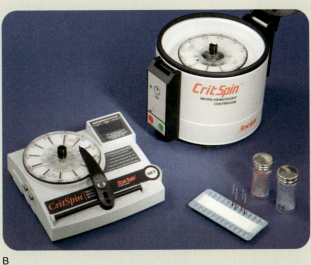

A   B

FIGURE 13-8 (A) Microhematocrit centrifuge with two sizes of centrifuge heads. (B) Crit-Spin centrifuge with microhematocrit reader and capillary tubes with sealant.
Source: Delmar/Cengage Learning.

Anemia is defined as an Hct level lower than "normal" values. Anemia may have a number of causes, including genetic abnormalities, inadequate nutrition, blood loss, hemolytic disease (destruction of RBCs), and exposure to substances such as radiation, certain pesticides, medications, or chemotherapeutic agents that might affect the division of immature RBCs.

Initial and Weekly Quality Control

Microhematocrit centrifuges must periodically be tested for the "maximum packed cell volume," a process that is performed on a monthly basis (or other regular schedule established by the facility's policies) to determine if electrical components of the centrifuge are deteriorating.

To determine the amount of time necessary for obtaining accurate results, a series of measurements are conducted, where paired samples are centrifuged for various lengths of time, (i.e., for 1.0 minute, 1.5 minutes, 2.0 minutes, and so on). When the result reaches a plateau and does not change after the time of centrifugation is increased for another 30 seconds, the first time in which the desired result was achieved is determined as the minimum amount of time in which the Hct should be spun (centrifuged) to achieve complete compaction of the RBCs. Usually a label is placed on the centrifuge indicating the minimum length of time a specimen should be centrifuged.

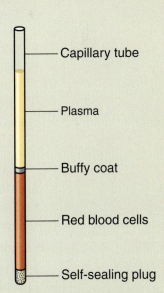

— Capillary tube

— Plasma

— Buffy coat

— Red blood cells

— Self-sealing plug

FIGURE 13-9 Column of blood that has been separated by centrifugation.
Source: Delmar/Cengage Learning.

IN THE LAB

Determining the Maximum Packed Cell Volume

Before beginning the Hct, determine the maximum packed cell volume by following these steps:

1. Use two different samples, one with an Hct of greater than 50%.
2. Prepare two Hct tubes per sample and centrifuge for 2 minutes.
3. Read and record results.
4. Prepare two more Hct tubes per sample and centrifuge for 2.5 minutes.
5. Read and record results.
6. Repeat this procedure, increasing the time by 30-second intervals, until the Hct reading remains the same for two consecutive time periods. Use this time for routine testing.
7. Once per shift, run a duplicate analysis on the microHct and use another analytical procedure for obtaining a microhematocrit.
8. Record your results. The results should be within ±2%. If your results are outside of these limits, repeat with a second sample.
9. If the second analysis is beyond the limits, notify your supervisor, as recalibration of the microhematocrit centrifuge or other centrifuge may be required.

Equipment and Supplies

1. Gloves, disposable paper towels, and disinfectant or other cleaning solution
2. Report form for Procedure #3
3. Sealing putty (Critoseal)
4. Clinical centrifuge fitted with Hct head
5. Microcapillary reader
6. Anticoagulated blood sample and plain hematocrit tubes (if using a supplied sample).
7. If the procedure will include collection of the sample through finger stick and capillary tube, the following supplies will also be needed:
   Alcohol prep pad
   Cotton balls or 2 × 2 gauze pads
   Sterile lancets (or Autolet device)
   Heparinized hematocrit tubes
8. Disinfectant for cleaning work surfaces following procedure
9. Sharps container for disposal of lancets and slides, and other appropriate waste disposal containers

Procedure

1. Wash hands and don gloves.
2. Assemble necessary equipment and supplies, arranging them in a systematic manner where each item may be easily reached. For a microhematocrit, it is simple to lay out necessary supplies in a small area.
3. If an anticoagulated blood sample is available, use it to fill a plain capillary tube (Figure 13-10A), then proceed to step #10. If you will be performing a finger "stick" to obtain the sample, follow steps # 4 through #9 below.

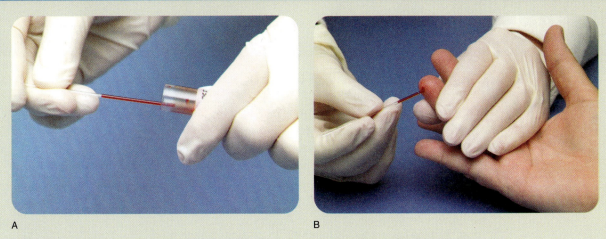

A   B

FIGURE 13-10 Filling a capillary tube from **(A)** a sample of anticoagulated blood and **(B)** a capillary puncture.
Source: Delmar/Cengage Learning.

4. Wash hands properly with soap and water, using friction by rubbing the hands together. After washing hands and before beginning the procedure, put on gloves made with nitrile or other nonallergenic materials.

5. Swab the tip of one of the patient's less-used fingers, such as the ring finger on the nondominant hand, with alcohol.

6. With a lancet, prick the finger tip with a quick firm jab to the side of the fingertip (or use a device such as an Autolet).

7. Immediately discard the lancet in the sharps container.

8. Use a clean dry cotton ball to wipe off the first drop of blood that appears. It is important to wipe the first drop from the finger as fluid from the tissues may create inaccuracies in the reading as well as cause the puncture to stop bleeding prematurely.

9. Fill a *heparinized* capillary tube 75% full with blood by slightly tipping it to allow blood to flow downhill into the tube (Figure 13-10B).
   a. Capillary action will naturally aid in this filling.
   b. Lightly "milk" the finger by placing your index finger around the patient's finger tip, but avoid squeezing. Intense squeezing will cause more rapid clotting and a cessation of the blood flow due to coagulation factors in the skin. Also avoid bubbles, which will appear as skip marks in the tube.

10. Hold the tube horizontally and press the filled end into the sealing putty (Critoseal) to plug the end. Critoseal trays are designed with small holes to store the filled capillary tubes until they are ready to be centrifuged. Collect any additional samples needed for other tests before clotting occurs.

11. Collect and prepare a second tube to be averaged with the result of the first.

12. Lay the tubes in the centrifuge Hct head with the plugged ends to the outside to avoid the blood spinning out of the tube. Record the numbered slots for each sample. A tube should be used as a balancing Hct tube when there is only one tube being spun, or if there is an uneven number of tubes that would leave an empty slot across from a tube to be spun.

IN THE LAB

13. Lock the top of the centrifuge Hct head following the instructions for the instrument you will be using.
14. Start the centrifuge and operate it for 5 minutes, then turn the machine off. Most microhematocrit centrifuges have one speed. For those that are adjustable, refer to the instrument instruction manual to set a proper speed.
15. Wait until the rotor has completely stopped before removing the tube(s). Place each tube in the slots in the Hct reader and determine the percentage of RBCs in the whole blood sample.
16. Record the results.
    a. List the results by the numbers you assigned each tube.
    b. Average the two tubes for each determination. The values of the two should agree to within ±2% of each other.
    c. Repeat the process for any samples that return abnormal results.
17. Discard all supplies used for the procedure in the appropriate containers. A disinfectant should be used to clean the work surfaces and equipment should be cleaned and restored to its former position. Gloves should be discarded appropriately and the hands washed thoroughly in accordance with established policies.

Sources of Error Encountered for the Hematocrit

Improperly mixed specimens that have been allowed to settle in a collection tube will dramatically affect the results. For specimens collected by capillary puncture, tissue fluids and perspiration may contribute to the volume of the liquid portion of the blood. Sometimes an inadequately sealed capillary tube will leak some of the RBCs from the sealed base of the tube and the results will be drastically affected. Other factors leading to errors are inadequate volume of specimen; inadequate or improper centrifugation (e.g., incorrect speed and time); including the buffy coat (WBCs and platelets) in the reading; and improper use of the reader.

Reporting of Results

Report your findings from the Determining Hematocrit procedure in the Procedure #3 Report Form or other form supplied by your instructor. Report the average of the duplicate tests. If the tests are not within ±2% of each other, the sample should be retested. The averaged results are reported as a percentage of red cells in the sample of whole blood. If the hemoglobin result is available, normocytic blood will yield a hemoglobin value that is roughly one-third the value of the hematocrit.

Procedure #3 Report Form: Determining Hematocrit

Patient Name:_____   Pt. ID _____   Date: _____

Age: _____   Gender (Circle One)   M   F   Physician: _____

Time Requested: _____   Time Performed: _____   Time Reported: _____

Examination Requested: ☐ Hematocrit   ☐ Other

Procedure Results

Test Results #1	Test Results #2	Average of #1 and #2 Results

Comments (unusual findings) _____

Performed by: _____   **Date Reported** _____

HEMATOLOGY AND COAGULATION PROCEDURE #4

Manual Hemoglobin Determination by Spectrophotometer

Principles

Hemoglobin is a red-pigmented protein that serves to transport oxygen from the lungs to body tissues and carbon dioxide from the cells of the body back to the heart and to the lungs to be expelled before picking up more oxygen. Oxygen gives blood a characteristic bright red color, and venous blood, a deoxygenated state, is darker in color.

Ferricyanide oxidizes oxyhemoglobin to methemoglobin, and cyanide converts methemoglobin to cyanmethemoglobin. Absorbance measurements are made on a spectrophotometer at 540 nm. The cyanmethemoglobin reagent contains a surfactant to promote rapid hemolysis and to accelerate formation of cyanmethemoglobin. The reaction is completed in less than 3 minutes.

From a clinical perspective, the quantitative determination of cyanmethemoglobin in the blood is an extremely important procedure for determining a number of types of anemia as well as any bleeding that cannot be seen readily (e.g., internal bleeding). In almost all types of anemia, Hgb levels are abnormally low and the condition could give evidence of an underlying disease. Some disease conditions actually have increased Hgb levels, such as polycythemia, which means "many or much blood."

The Hgb should compare with the Hct by a 1:3 ratio. If it does not, this indicates certain abnormalities of the RBCs.

A suitable specimen for a manual hemoglobin determination may be obtained from a capillary puncture in which a heparinized capillary tube is used or from whole blood with EDTA used as an anticoagulant; in the latter case, a plain or nonheparinized capillary tube will be used. Anticoagulants other than EDTA, such as heparin, citrates, and oxalates, do not maintain the RBC morphology to the extent that EDTA does but may be used, taking into account the dilution factor occurring with the use of citrated samples in particular. Hemoglobin in whole blood collected with EDTA remains stable for 1 week at room temperature (15°C to 30°C) and even longer when refrigerated.

Only a few interfering substances affect the hemoglobin measurement. Gross lipemia (fatty materials in the blood) will cause elevated Hgb values. Leukocytosis (abnormally elevated WBC counts) and macroglobulinemia (high levels of large proteins) may also falsely cause high Hgb values. Although most Hgb determinations are performed on automated cell counters, it is necessary to perform a manual Hgb when a sample is lipemic , as the presence of fatty materials in the blood will interfere

Safety Alert

Most of these reagents contain cyanide, an extremely poisonous substance, but it is used in low concentrations for this test. The reagent should not be combined with a number of chemicals, including acids. If the reagent comes in contact with the skin, the cyanide may be absorbed through the skin. If the reagent is ingested, perform gastric lavage (irrigation of the stomach) and call a physician. Reagents for disposal should be discarded by flushing with copious amounts of water.

IN THE LAB

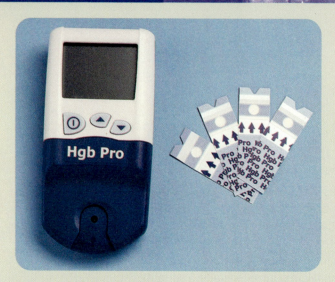

FIGURE 13-11 Hgb Pro instrument.
Source: Delmar/Cengage Learning.

with the spectrophotometer in the cell counter. If it is necessary in a manual procedure to perform the test on a diluted sample, the result should be multiplied by the factor of the dilution (e.g. a 1:2 dilution would require that the result be multiplied by a factor of 2).

In physician office laboratories and for point-of-care testing, the use of a direct read-out device called a hemoglobinometer may be required. A variety of these instruments designed for point-of-care testing are available and may be used in place of the manual procedure outlined below; Hgb determinations can also be made by the automated systems in use in large laboratories. The Hgb Pro (Figure 13-11) provides a quick and accurate Hgb estimate and requires a very small blood sample, such as that available by capillary puncture. For a direct read-out instrument, set the read-out concentration value of the Standard and read the Unknown concentrations directly.

Although the final reaction for hemoglobin values using methods where cyanmethemoglobin is formed appears quite stable, the test samples should be read within 1 hour before evaporation of the reaction solutions becomes significant. Results should be reported as grams per deciliter (g/dL) or in SI units.

Equipment and Supplies

1. Gloves, disposable paper towels, and disinfectant or other cleaning solution
2. Report form for Procedure #4
3. Cyanmethemoglobin reagent
4. Hgb standard
5. Micropipetter capable of measuring small volumes
6. Pipettes or pipetter for measuring reagent
7. Spectrophotometer or colorimeter calibrated at 540 nm
8. Properly drawn blood sample in an anticoagulated tube or microhematocrit tube (clots will cause errors in the determination)
9. 13 × 100 mm test tubes and test tube rack
10. Waterproof sharp marker
11. Electronic timing device or clock/watch with second hand

Procedure

1. Wash hands and don gloves.
2. Assemble necessary equipment and supplies.

3. Label the test tubes as follows for proper identification of blanks, standards, controls, and unknowns: Label one tube "RB" for the reagent blank specimen, one tube "S" for the standard sample, and one or more tubes "C-(number)" for the control samples (e.g., C-1 and C-2 to differentiate between normal and abnormal controls). The unknown samples should be labeled by patient name, patient number, or other identifier.
4. Pipette 5.0 mL cyanmethemoglobin reagent into the tubes labeled "RB" and "S" and into each sample tube.
5. Add by pipette 0.02 mL of the standard specimen to the tube labeled "S." Mix well.
6. Add by pipette 0.02 mL of the controls and unknown specimen to the sample tubes. Mix well.
7. Using a micropipetter, add 0.02 mL of deionized water (in place of a specimen) to the tube labeled "RB." Mix well.
8. Allow the specimens to stand at room temperature (15°C to 30°C) for at least 3 minutes.
9. Use the "RB" specimen to adjust the spectrophotometer or colorimeter to zero absorbance at 540 nm
10. Read the absorbance values for the standard, controls, and unknowns, and record the results
11. Discard all supplies used for the procedure in the appropriate containers. A disinfectant should be used to clean the work surfaces and equipment should be cleaned and restored to its former position. Gloves should be discarded appropriately and the hands washed thoroughly in accordance with established policies.

Reporting of Results

Report your findings from the Manual Hemoglobin Determination by Spectrophotometer procedure in the Procedure #4 Report Form or other form supplied by your instructor. Results should be reported as grams per deciliter (g/dL).

Hemoglobin Calculation (Manual Method)

$$\text{Hemoglobin (g/dL)} = \frac{\text{Abs of unknown (Au)}}{\text{Abs of standard (As)}} \times \text{Standard Value}$$

Example 13-1

The absorbance for a 15.0 g/dL HGB standard is 0.256
The absorbance for the unknown is 0.301.

$$\text{Unknown (g/dL)} = \frac{0.301}{0.256} \times 15.0 \text{ g/dL or } 1.18 \times 15.0 = 17.6 \text{ g/dL}$$

Limitations

Sulfhemoglobin, which forms when hydrogen sulfide and hemoglobin are combined, is toxic when present in excess. It is not measured by the above procedures.

Linearity

Accurate up to 20 g/dL for most reagents, standards, and methodology utilized.

IN THE LAB

Procedure #4 Report Form: Manual Hemoglobin Determination by Spectrophotometer

Patient Name:_____   Pt. ID _____   Date: _____

Age: _____   Gender (Circle One) M   F   Physician: _____

Time Requested: _____   Time Performed: _____   Time Reported: _____

Examination Requested:· ☐ Hemoglobin ☐ Other

Procedure Results

Test Results	Normal Range	Quality Control Values/Acceptable Range

Comments (unusual findings) _____

Performed by: _____   **Date Reported** _____

HEMATOLOGY AND COAGULATION PROCEDURE #5

Red Blood Cell Morphology

Principles

Red blood cells are constantly being produced in the bone marrow. Even under normal circumstances, cells at various stages of development may be released into the vascular system slightly earlier than the majority of RBCs. In serious diseases of the bone marrow, RBCs may be released as primitive cells and may appear similar to early forms of white blood cells. In this early form, some cells may still have a nucleus, which is usually lost prior to the cells entering the blood vessels. Clues as to the morphology of RBCs may be found in the results of the hemoglobin and the hematocrit when a complete blood count is performed prior to a microscopic evaluation.

Red cells are evaluated relative to color, shape, and size. These characteristics are invaluable in discovering various types of anemia. Some changes in the morphology and appearance of RBCs may be due to dietary deficiencies; others occur secondary to medications, infections, or illness; and still others are hereditary (e.g., sickle cell anemia). Most of the cells available to the laboratory student are normal in morphology. The ability to recognize normal cells is critical, for it is the pattern of normal cells against which all other cells are measured (Figure 13-12).

Although the evaluation of red blood cell morphology is one of the most important facets of hematology, it is important as well to concurrently examine the WBCs. RBC size should be approximately the size of the nucleus of a lymphocyte, a white blood cell, when the RBC is normal in size. In addition, some disease conditions (e.g., megaloblastic anemia) affect both the RBCs and WBCs.

Equipment and Supplies

1. Gloves, disposable paper towels, and disinfectant or other cleaning solution
2. Report form for Procedure #5

3. Stained blood film (See Procedure #1 for directions on properly preparing and staining a blood film.)
4. Brightfield microscope
5. Microscope immersion oil
6. Lens paper
7. Sharps container for disposal of used slides, and other appropriate waste disposal containers

Procedure

1. Wash hands and don gloves.
2. Assemble necessary equipment and supplies.
3. The instructor may choose to provide stained blood films from a normal patient for students to become familiar with the morphology of both RBC and WBCs, or the student may prepare a stained blood film following the steps in Procedure #1.
4. Visually inspect the slide to ensure that the blood film is properly distributed on it and that a feathered edge is present (see Procedure #1).
5. Place the stained blood film on the microscope stage.
6. Focus the microscope using the low-power objective, locating the feathered end of the smear.
7. Using the fine adjustment knob of the microscope and adjusting the light source, find an area where the distribution shows RBCs that are not touching but that are close to each other.
8. Place a drop of immersion oil on the smear where the light is brightest from the condenser.
9. Rotate the nosepiece of the microscope until the oil immersion objective comes in contact with the immersion oil.
10. Use the fine adjustment to gain a sharp image of the blood cells.
11. Adjust the condenser and the iris diaphragm until a good image of the cells is obtained.
12. Scan the slide from side to side, making sure the focal field is in an area where the cells are not touching. Move the slide along the stage of the microscope in a broad lane running transversely across the body of the film, avoiding the edges completely (Figure 13-7), as cells are sometimes dragged there in greater numbers.
13. Observe at least 10 fields for RBC morphology.
14. Analyze the size of the RBCs. The size of RBCs should be roughly equivalent to the nucleus of a WBC known as a lymphocyte, one of the five types of WBCs.
15. Analyze the color of the RBCs. A normal RBC will have a "central pallor" surrounded by a darker edge. Central pallor of more than one-half of the RBC would indicate a lack of hemoglobin concentration.

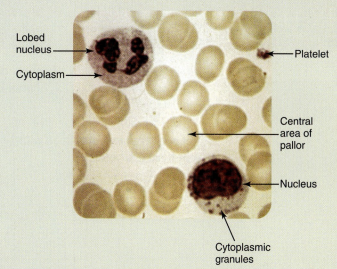

Lobed nucleus
Cytoplasm
Platelet
Central area of pallor
Nucleus
Cytoplasmic granules

FIGURE 13-12 Blood cells normally found in circulation. Source: Delmar/Cengage Learning.

IN THE LAB

16. Analyze the morphology (shape) of the RBCs, an important factor in determining various RBC abnormalities (Figures 13-13, 13-14 and 13-15). Record the information on the report form.
17. Return the low-power objective (10X) into place and remove the slide from the stage.
18. Clean the microscope stage with lens paper or tissue. Clean the condenser if necessary.
19. Retain the slide if required.

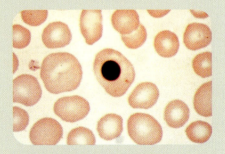

FIGURE 13-13 Nucleated RBCI among other RBCs of varying sizes.
Source: Delmar/Cengage Learning.

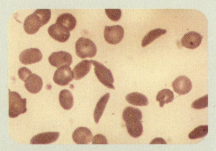

FIGURE 13-14 Sickle-shaped cells from patient with sickle cell anemia.
Source: Delmar/Cengage Learning.

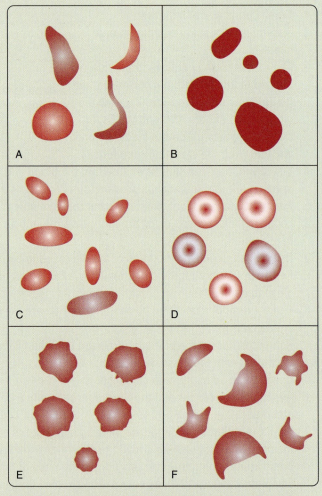

FIGURE 13-15 Morphology of selected abnormal red blood cells. (A) Sickle cells known as drepanocytes. (B) Spherocytes with no central pallor. (C) Elliptocytes with elongated shape. (D) Target cells known as codocytes. (E) Crenated cells often found in dilutional problems such as use of IV fluids. (F) Helmet cells known as keratocytes or schizocytes.
Source: Delmar/Cengage Learning.

20. Discard all supplies used for the procedure in the appropriate containers. A disinfectant should be used to clean the work surfaces and equipment should be cleaned and restored to its former position. Gloves should be discarded appropriately and the hands washed thoroughly in accordance with established policies.

Reporting of Results

Note: Consult figures 13-13, 13-14 and 13-15 when evaluating RBCs. RBCs are reported in a semiquantitative manner, using the terminology in Table 13-3.

Table 13-3 Characteristics for Evaluating RBCs

Size	
Normocytic	Normal size
Microcytic	Smaller than average size
Macrocytic	Larger than average size
Anisocytosis	Cells of Various Sizes Present
Hemoglobin Content	
Normochromic	Normal color, hemoglobin level
Hypochromic	Pale color and lack of adequate hemoglobin
Shape	
Poikilocyte	Abnormally shaped RBC
Ovalocyte, Elliptocyte	Oval red cell
Drepanocyte	Sickle-shaped cells
Tear Drop	Pear-shaped red cell
Schistocyte	Cellular fragment
Keratocyte	Military helmet-shaped ("helmet cell")
Echinocyte	Crenated red cell, regularly spiculated (usually reversible)
Acanthocyte	Irregularly spiculated (irreversible)
Spherocyte	Round red cells with no central pallor (not biconcave)
Stomatocyte	Red cell with mouth shaped area of central pallor
Target Cell	Area of central pallor with dense center ("bulls-eye")

A normal red blood cell should be approximately the same size as a normal lymphocyte nucleus. Two normal-size red blood cells should fit side-by-side across a normal-size poly (not a hypersegmented poly). The presence of abnormal cells is reported as 1+ to 4+ (the most extreme condition). These numbers correlate with the number observed per OIF (oil immersion field), as follows:

IN THE LAB

1+	2+	3+	4+
1–6 per OIF	7–10 per OIF	11–20 per OIF	> 20 per OIF

Report your findings from the Red Blood Cell Morphology procedure in the Procedure #5 Report Form or other form supplied by your instructor.

Procedure #5 Report Form: Red Blood Cell Morphology

Patient Name: _____ Pt. ID _____ Date: _____

Age: _____ Gender (Circle One) M   F   Physician: _____

Time Requested: _____ Time Performed: _____ Time Reported: _____

Examination Requested: ☐ RBC Morphology ☐ Other

Red Blood Cell Morphology

Cell Size ☐ Normocytic   Cell Color ☐ Normochromic
☐ Microcytic   ☐ Hypochromic
☐ Macrocytic

Cell Shape ☐ Anisocytosis (difference in sizes)
☐ Poikilocytosis (various shapes)

Platelet Evaluation

Platelet Numbers ☐ Appear to be adequate
☐ Decreased number (thrombopenia)
☐ Increased number (thrombocytosis)

Platelet Shape ☐ Differences in sizes
☐ Appear to be large
☐ Appear to be small

Comments (unusual findings) _____

Performed by: _____ **Date Reported** _____

HEMATOLOGY AND COAGULATION PROCEDURE #6

Reticulocyte Count

Principles

RBCs undergo a maturation sequence that culminates in a mature RBC. **Reticulocytes** are the last immature stage of RBCs after the intact nucleus has disintegrated. They are just a couple of days or less from being fully mature. It is possible for the RBC to prematurely leave the bone marrow as a reticulocyte yet complete its maturation in the peripheral circulation.

Reticulocytes normally constitute about 1% to 2% of the circulating RBCs. Reticulocyte counts above 3% usually signify increased destruction of RBCs or bleeding episodes that are diminishing the blood supply. A reticulocyte rate that falls below 0.5% indicates a decreased level of blood production. A reticulocyte count also may be used as a tool to determine if a patient is responding to therapy (e.g., iron administration) for anemia. The reticulocyte percentage will increase if the patient is responding to the body's need for increased red blood cells.

Equipment and Supplies

1. Gloves, disposable paper towels, and disinfectant or other cleaning solution
2. Report form for Procedure #6
3. 13 × 100 mm test tubes and test tube rack
4. Capillary tubes
5. Clean glass microscope slides (see Procedure #1)
6. Disposable pipettes
7. Brightfield microscope
8. New methylene blue (reconstitute if necessary)
9. Fresh EDTA anticoagulated blood sample
10. Tally counter for enumerating RBCs and reticulocytes
11. Reticulocyte control slides (optional)
12. Electronic timing device or clock/watch with second hand
13. Sharps container for disposal of used slides, and other appropriate waste disposal containers

Procedure

1. Wash hands and don gloves.
2. Assemble necessary equipment and supplies.
3. Add an equal number of drops of blood and of methylene blue reticulocyte stain in a 13 × 100 mm tube. Mix the blood and stain by tapping gently against the bottom of the tube with a finger.
4. Allow the mixture to stand for 10 minutes at room temperature to completely stain the RBCs. After 10 minutes, mix again by tapping the tube against a finger.
5. Using the pipette, aspirate a drop of the mixture and expel it onto a clean glass slide. Follow the directions in Procedure #1 for properly preparing a blood film. Allow the film to air dry.
6. Place the slide onto the microscope stage and focus on the feathered end of the smear using the low-power (10X) objective.
7. Place a drop of immersion oil on the smear and rotate the nosepiece until the oil-immersion objective comes into contact with the oil drop.
8. Reticulocytes are RBCs showing reticulum. Reticulum will appear as blue dots, filaments, skeins, or wreaths (Figure 13-16).
9. Using the high power oil objective, count the number of erythrocytes (RBCs) in one field and record the number of reticulocytes observed in the same field.

Clinical Alert

Use EDTA anticoagulated whole blood or blood from a capillary puncture that has been collected in an EDTA microtube. Other anticoagulants will distort the RBCs and will lead to erroneous results. Specimens older than 24 hours will give falsely low results.

IN THE LAB

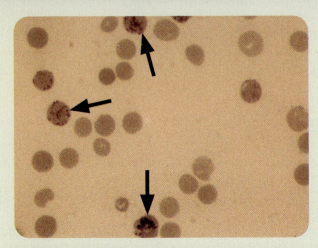

FIGURE 13-16 Image of RBCs with reticulum imbedded in RBCs, stained with new methylene blue.
Source: Delmar/Cengage Learning.

10. Move to the next field until 1000 RBCs and reticulocytes in total (not 1000 of each) are counted for each smear. Usually a low and a high control are analyzed when performing a manual reticulocyte count.

11. Perform a hematocrit (Procedure #3) on the blood for correction. Reticulocyte counts are corrected for anemia by dividing the patient's hematocrit by 45 (normal hematocrit) and then multiplying the result by the calculated value for the reticulocyte count. A gridded square can also be used for enumerating the RBCs. There are also kits that prepare a given dilution of blood with stain included; these are designed to provide a more accurate result for the reticulocyte count.

12. Discard all supplies used for the procedure in the appropriate containers. A disinfectant should be used to clean the work surfaces and equipment should be cleaned and restored to its former position. Gloves should be discarded appropriately and the hands washed thoroughly in accordance with established policies.

Reporting of Results

Report your findings from the Reticulocyte Count procedure in the Procedure #6 Report Form or other form supplied by your instructor. Results are reported as a percentage of the RBCs that are reticulocytes. The results are calculated by the following equation.

$$\% \text{ Reticulocytes} = \frac{\text{Number of Reticulocytes Counted}}{\text{Number of Red Blood Cells Counted}} \times 100$$

Example 13-1

	Erythrocytes Counted	Reticulocytes Observed
Smear 1	521	7
Smear 2	479	5
Totals	1000	12

$$\% \text{ Reticulocytes} = \frac{12}{1000} \times 100 = 1.2\,\%$$

Correction Factor for Reticulocyte Count

A Corrected Reticulocyte Count may be performed to correct for anemia (low RBC count), as shown in the following equation.

$$\frac{\text{Patient's reticulocyte count} \times \text{Patient's Hct}}{\text{Normal Hct (45)}} = \text{Corrected Reticulocyte Count}$$

Example 13-2

Assume the patient's hematocrit = 34%. Using the numbers in Example 13-1:

$$\frac{1.2\% \times 34}{45} \times 0.9\% \text{ (corrected reticulocyte count)}$$

Procedure #6 Report Form: Reticulocyte Count

Patient Name: _____ Pt. ID _____ Date: _____

Age: _____ Gender (Circle One) M F Physician: _____

Time Requested: _____ Time Performed: _____ Time Reported: _____

Examination Requested: ☐ Reticulocyte Count ☐ Other

Procedure Results

Test Results	Normal Range	Correction Factor (Pt. HCT/45 X % Counted)

Comments (unusual findings) _____

Performed by: _____   **Date Reported** _____

HEMATOLOGY AND COAGULATION PROCEDURE #7

Unopette Procedure for WBC Counts

Principles

This method uses a **Unopette disposable diluting pipette system** that provides a convenient, precise, and accurate method for obtaining a WBC count from blood and body fluids. When the Unopette method is used, whole blood is added to a diluent. The diluent lyses (destroys) the RBCs but preserves and slightly stains the WBCs. Once the red cells are completely lysed, the solution will be clear. The diluted blood is then added to a **hemacytometer**. Once the hemacytometer is loaded, the cells should be allowed to settle for 10 minutes before beginning the count.

The Unopette disposable diluting pipette system used to count WBCs is almost identical in shape and application to the Unopette system for RBC counts. The only major difference is that the reservoir contains a different diluent and the capillary pipette capacity differs (RBC = 10 μL and WBC = 20 μL).

Equipment and Supplies

1. Gloves, disposable paper towels, and disinfectant or other cleaning solution
2. Report form for Procedure #7

IN THE LAB

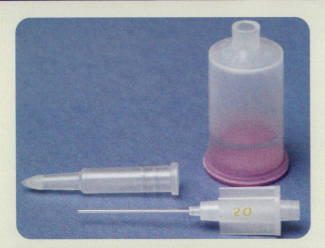

FIGURE 13-17 Parts of Unopette system used to dilute blood sample for WBC and platelet counts.
Source: Delmar/Cengage Learning.

3. Disposable Unopette for WBC counts, which consists of a shielded capillary tube (20 µL capacity), and a plastic reservoir containing a premeasured volume of diluent (1:100 dilution) (Figure 13-17).
4. Clean hemacytometer and cover glass
5. Distilled water and lens paper for cleaning hemacytometer
6. Blood specimens containing an EDTA anticoagulant (or collect a fresh blood sample following the process outlined in Procedure # 3)
7. Brightfield microscope
8. Handheld counter
9. Petri dish with a moist circle of filter paper and two toothpicks or pieces of an applicator
10. Electronic timing device or clock/watch with second hand

Procedure

1. Wash hands and don gloves.
2. Assemble necessary equipment and supplies.
3. Puncture the diaphragm in the neck of the reservoir with the tip of the capillary pipette shield. Your instructor will demonstrate how to do this.
4. Remove the protective plastic shield from the capillary pipette.
5. Hold the capillary pipette apparatus slightly angled over a horizontal plane and gently touch the tip to the blood source. The pipette should fill by capillary action if the device is held at the correct angle. This may take some practice.
6. When blood reaches the end of the capillary bore in the neck of the pipette, the pipette is completely filled and will stop automatically. The amount of blood collected by the capillary pipette is 20 µL. Wipe any excess blood from the outside of the capillary pipette while making sure none of the sample is removed by "wicking" blood from inside the capillary pipette.
7. Between the thumb and forefingers of one hand, gently squeeze the reservoir holding the diluent to force some air out, but do not expel any of the prepared diluent. Maintain pressure on the reservoir. With the other hand, cover the upper opening of the capillary overflow chamber with your index finger and seat the capillary pipette holder in the reservoir neck.
8. Release pressure on the reservoir and remove your finger from the overflow chamber opening. The suction will draw the correct amount of blood into the diluent in the reservoir.

9. Squeeze the reservoir gently two or three times to rinse the capillary pipette, forcing diluent into but not out of the overflow chamber at the end of the pipette. Release the pressure each time to allow adequate mixing of any diluents and blood from the capillary pipette into the large chamber. Close the upper opening with your index finger and invert the unit several times to mix the blood sample and diluent as shown (Figure 13-18).

10. To prevent evaporation when storing a diluted specimen, cover the overflow chamber of the capillary pipette with the capillary shield that was used to puncture the diaphragm of the reservoir.

11. Just before beginning the cell count, again mix the blood and diluent by gently inverting the reservoir several times while taking care to cover the hole with your index finger.

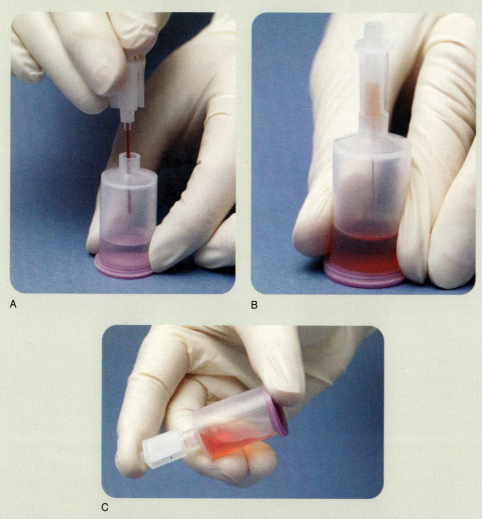

A

B

C

FIGURE 13-18 (A) Inserting the capillary pipette filled with blood into the reservoir. **(B)** Releasing pressure on reservoir to draw blood sample into diluents. **(C)** Insuring mixing of blood and diluents in the reservoir.
Source: Delmar/Cengage Learning.

IN THE LAB

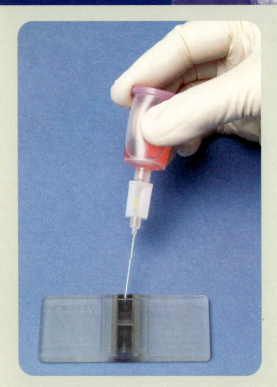

FIGURE 13-19 Filling the hemacytometer using a Unopette capillary system.
Source: Delmar/Cengage Learning.

12. Place a cover glass on a hemacytometer counting chamber, making sure the glass is clean and grease free. Although difficult, removal of fingerprints is essential as they may cause problems with the smooth filling of the chamber.

13. Remove the pipette from the reservoir. Squeeze the reservoir and reseat the pipette in the reverse position. Release pressure to draw any fluid in the capillary pipette into the reservoir. Invert and fill the capillary pipette by gentle pressure on the reservoir. After discarding the first 3 drops in the pipette, load (charge) the counting chamber of the hemacytometer by gently squeezing the reservoir while the tip of the pipette is touched against the edge of the cover glass and the surface of the counting chamber (Figure 13-19). A properly loaded counting chamber should have a thin, even, and consistent depth of fluid under the cover glass.

14. Allow 5 minutes for the cells to settle.
    a. If fluid flows into the grooves (moats) at the edges of the counting chamber or if air bubbles are seen in the field, the chamber is flooded and must be cleaned with distilled water, dried well with lens paper, and refilled.
    b. If the chamber is underfilled, carefully add more fluid until the proper level is obtained.

15. Place the loaded hemacytometer in a petri dish on a moist circle of filter paper and on two toothpicks or pieces of an applicator placed parallel on the paper. This will help prevent the hemacytometer from becoming too wet for the microscope stage. Wait at least 5 minutes for the cells to settle. The count should be initiated no later than 10 minutes after the cells are placed on the counting chamber.

16. Once the cells have settled, ensure that the bottom of the hemacytometer is dry and place the hemacytometer on the microscope stage. Using the low-power objective, count the WBCs in the nine fields of the hemacytometer chamber. Each field is composed of 16 small squares. To count the cells in each field, start in the upper left small square. Count all of the cells within each square, including cells touching the lines at the top and on the left. Do not count any cells that touch the lines on the right or at the bottom. Repeat for each of the other eight fields.

17. When the cells in all nine fields are counted, calculate the result according to Example 13-3, provided in the Reporting of Results section below.

18. Discard all supplies used for the procedure in the appropriate containers. A disinfectant should be used to clean the work surfaces and equipment should be

cleaned and restored to its former position. Gloves should be discarded appropriately and the hands washed thoroughly in accordance with established policies.

Reporting of Results

Report your findings from the Unopette Procedure for WBC Counts in the Procedure #7 Report Form or other form supplied by your instructor. White blood cell counts are reported as the number of WBCs/μL or in SI units as WBCs/L.

Example 13-3

In squares 1–9 of a hemacytometer, the following numbers of WBCs were counted:

Side 1		Side 2	
Square	Cells Counted	Square	Cells Counted
1	6	1	7
2	5	2	7
3	7	3	6
4	8	4	5
5	9	5	6
6	6	6	8
7	7	7	7
8	5	8	8
9	6	9	7
Total	59		61

Find the average number of WBCs.

$$\frac{59 + 61}{2} = 60 \text{ average (number of sides)}$$

Since 9 squares were counted, multiply the total count for all nine squares by 0.1 (10%) and add this number to the total for the nine squares. Multiply this sum by 100, the dilution factor.

$$\text{WBCs/μL} = 60 + 0.1\,(60) = 66 \times 100 = 6,600$$

Procedure #7 Report Form: Unopette Procedure for WBC Counts

Patient Name: _____ Pt. ID _____ Date: _____

Age: _____ Gender (Circle One) M F   Physician: _____

Time Requested: _____ Time Performed: _____ Time Reported: _____

Examination Requested: ☐ Manual WBC Count ☐ Other

Procedure Results

	Square 1	Square 2	Square 3	Square 4	Square 5	Square 6	Square 7	Square 8	Square 9
Side 1									
Side 2									
Totals									

IN THE LAB

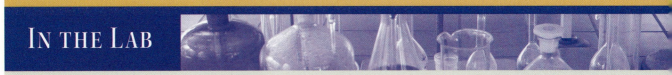

Calculation

> Total of Side 1 + Total of Side 2 divided by 2 = total count average

Average + (average × 0.1) × 100 = _____cells/μL

Average + (average × 0.1) × 10,000 = _____cells/L (SI Units)

Comments (unusual findings) _____

Performed by: _____   **Date Reported** _____

HEMATOLOGY AND COAGULATION PROCEDURE #8

Manual Prothrombin Time (PT)

Principles

Most prothrombin coagulation tests are performed with automated equipment, but it is important for the student to understand the determination of certain clotting factors that affect the formation of a fibrin clot. The beginner can easily visualize the formation of the clot in a glass tube when a patient sample or control is combined with the proper reagent. The one-stage PT measures the clotting time of plasma after adding a source of tissue factor (thromboplastin) and calcium. The recalcification of plasma in the presence of added tissue factors generates activated factor X. This in turn activates prothrombin to thrombin, which converts fibrinogen to an insoluble but visible fibrin clot.

Equipment and Supplies

1. Gloves, disposable paper towels, and disinfectant or other cleaning solution
2. Report form for Procedure #8
3. Citrated blood sample that has been centrifuged. The plasma should be removed from the blood cells for testing
4. Control samples reconstituted with deionized water
5. 13 × 100 test tubes and test tube rack
6. Water bath or heat block set at 37°C
7. Pipetters and tips to measure 0.1 and 0.2 mL
8. Electronic timing device or clock/watch with second hand

Procedure

1. Wash hands and don gloves.
2. Assemble necessary equipment and supplies.
3. Dispense 0.1 mL of citrated plasma into 13 × 100 mm test tubes, one for each sample and control.
4. Prewarm all tubes (samples, controls) and the pool of thromboplastin in the heat block to 37°C.
5. Place 0. 2 mL warmed thromboplastin into a tube containing the citrated plasma sample.

6. Quickly replace the tubes into the heat block for 7 to 8 seconds.
7. Immediately remove the tubes from the heat block. Note the time and gently tilt the tubes slowly back and forth, observing for the appearance of a fibrin clot (Figure 13-20). Record the time elapsed.
8. Discard all supplies used for the procedure in the appropriate containers. A disinfectant should be used to clean the work surfaces and equipment should be cleaned and restored to its former position. Gloves should be discarded appropriately and the hands washed thoroughly in accordance with established policies.

Reporting of Results

Report your findings from the Manual Prothrombin Time procedure in the Procedure #8 Report Form or other form supplied by your instructor. Results are reported in seconds. The prothrombin time is reported as the International Normalized Ratio (INR) value. Since each lot of reagent (thromboplastin) may have a different sensitivity, each lot of reagent is assigned an **International Sensitivity Index** by its manufacturer. There are several equations that may be used for calculating the INR. For this procedure, calculate the INR using the equation below, and as demonstrated in Example 13-4.

Calculation

$$INR = \left(\frac{\text{Measured PT}}{\text{Normal PT}}\right)^{ISI}$$

Example 13-4

Using the equation above and the following sample values, calculate the INR.

Normal control value	= 10.2 sec
Prothrombin time for unknown	= 20.4 sec
ISI	= 1.2

$$INR = \left(\frac{20.4}{10.2}\right) \times 1.2 = 2.4$$

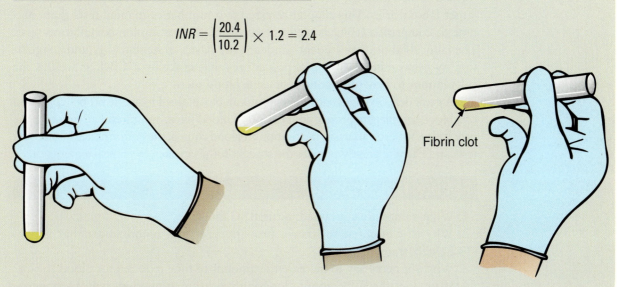

Fibrin clot

FIGURE 13-20 Manual tilt method for prothrombin time test.
Source: Delmar/Cengage Learning.

IN THE LAB

Procedure #8: Manual Prothrombin Time (PT)

Patient Name: _____ Pt. ID _____ Date: _____

Age: _____ Gender (Circle One)   M F   Physician: _____

Time Requested: _____ Time Performed: _____ Time Reported: _____

Examination Requested: ☐ Manual Prothrombin Time   ☐ Other

Tube #1	Tube #2	Average (Tube #1 + Tube #2) / 2	INR Results

INR Calculation

INR = [Patient Result in seconds / Mean normal of the facility in seconds] × ISI*

*ISI supplied by manufacturer of reagents

Comments (unusual findings) _____

Performed by: _____   **Date Reported** _____

SUMMARY

Hematology, the study of blood, is usually incorporated with basic tests for coagulation (hemostasis). Most disease processes will show some sort of changes in the blood picture, depending on the medical condition of the individual being tested. Samples for testing require care in proper collection, processing, and sometimes storage.

A complete blood count (CBC) is the most common set of procedures performed in hematology, but hundreds of specialized tests are also performed in larger laboratories. This chapter referred to a number of manual tests that combine to comprise a CBC, as well as two of the more common coagulation tests. The clinical laboratory student can learn the basics of hematology and coagulation by performing the manual procedures that make up a CBC, as well as the calculations to provide a comprehensive blood picture.

A great deal of diagnostic information can be obtained from the proper collection of a blood sample, the proper preparation of blood films, and careful attention to the procedures for each analysis. In addition to blood counts, the performance of bleeding tests and PTs will greatly prepare the student for a satisfactory clinical experience.

REVIEW QUESTIONS

1. What values are contained in the RBC indices?
2. Why is it essential to have a properly prepared blood smear that is adequately stained?
3. Why is it necessary to increase the amount of time required for blood to clot?
4. How does the WBC count along with a differential count help to diagnose infection?
5. What is the importance of the INR when performing PT measurements?

CHAPTER 14

CLINICAL CHEMISTRY

LEARNING OBJECTIVES

Upon completion of this chapter, the reader will be able to:

- List the most important factors involved in collecting specimens for chemical analysis.

- Describe characteristics of specimens that are inadequate for testing.

- List the major differences between plasma and serum as specimens for testing.

- Discuss the purpose of a standard for the various types of determinations.

- Explain the differences between a kinetic reaction and an end-point reaction.

- List the needs for safety practices in the laboratory, both mechanical and biohazardous.

KEY TERMS

Absorbance
Analytes
Anticoagulants
Colorimetric
Cuvette
Delta change
Discrete analysis
Electrochemistry
End-point reaction
Enzymatic

Fluoride
High-density lipoproteins (HDL)
Kinetic reaction
Linearity
Laboratory Information
    System (LIS)
Low-density lipoproteins (LDL)
Micropipette
Parameters
Plasma

Preanalytical error
Random access
Random error
Sequential analysis
Serum
Short draws
Spectrophotometry
Supernatant
Total cholesterol
Wavelength

INTRODUCTION

Since the earliest attempts to develop procedures for diagnosing diseases—from testing urine for glucose by tasting it or finding it attractive for ants, to boiling and cooling specimens to identify various proteins in body secretions—no aspect of the medical laboratory has become more automated than the chemistry area. A panoply of instruments that are phenomenally accurate, cost-efficient, and fast is commonly used today to perform chemistry procedures that evaluate the physiological functions of cells, tissues, organs, and entire organisms such as the human body.

Many aspects of early testing procedures to measure constituents of the blood are still utilized in the modern clinical chemistry laboratory. The original **end-point reaction** (also called **colorimetric** determination), where a reaction develops to the greatest extent possible, then ceases, is a methodology fashioned more than a century ago. It is still used but is now performed more effectively and in a shorter time frame. A second method now determines many enzymes and even some nonenzymatic **analytes** (constituents being tested for) by **kinetic reaction**, which measures the amount and speed of change occurring in the reagent and sample mixture over a specific period of time. The end-point reaction that required perhaps 30 minutes to reach completion can now be determined by kinetic reaction in only a few seconds. Calculations from basic physics and chemistry principles are also used to provide test results from processes such as **spectrophotometry** (where a reaction is read by the amount of light transmitted or absorbed in a test reagent) and **electrochemistry** (chemical reactions that involve an electron transfer).

In fully automated systems, all the functions and steps are computer driven. The technician or technologist often has little to do except troubleshoot the functions of the instrument after all the preliminary information has been entered and the instrument has been set up to perform a work list of procedures. An automated system is able to move the provided samples about the instrument before, during, and after the procedures are completed.

To provide results from a given sample in an automated system, the sample must first be identified. Following identification, usually from a bar code affixed at the time the sample is collected, the specimen volume is measured to ensure a sufficient sample is available for the number of procedures requested. After making sure there is a sample in the proper position, the system will begin the actual procedures. Samples sometimes require pretreatment for certain procedures (this is fully explained in courses dedicated to clinical chemistry). Reagents and samples will be mixed in the proper proportions and then subjected to certain conditions that may be necessary for the chemical reaction to take place. Some of these conditions include acidity, alkalinity, temperature, and reaction times. The reaction that occurs, for the most part in an instrument called a spectrophotometer, will then be analyzed, results will be calculated, and a valid report will be shown on a visible screen. A printed report can be provided if required. The **Laboratory Information System (LIS)** is often interfaced with the chemistry analyzers and results are then automatically transmitted to the physician's office or to the area of the hospital where the patient is hospitalized.

Methods of Analysis

Most larger chemistry laboratories have a number of instruments that are used for certain groups of tests. When batches of tests are performed only periodically, there may be an instrument dedicated to only that particular set of tests.

Batteries (related groups of tests) may be performed on one type of instrument and another type of panel or profile (other names for batches or batteries of tests) on another. Certain tests may be more efficiently performed on one type of instrument while general testing of broad groups may be more cost effective, accurate, or give a shorter turnaround time on another type of machine. A great deal of thought and organization must go into providing the proper instrument for certain tests, as no one instrument will be the best for all single procedures as well as for a grouping of procedures related to a given disease state.

There are several terms by which the various automated chemistry instruments are known. Some instruments are known as single channel and others as multichannel. The difference between the two lies in the ability of the multichannel instrument to perform a number of calculations simultaneously. This does not always mean that one is faster than another in its analysis of samples. Other types of analytical processes are common. In **discrete analysis**, each test reaction takes place in a separate compartment that requires either cleaning or disposal of an element used in the reaction, before the next procedure begins. **Random access** instruments are able to be programmed to accept samples out of order, even when a large number of tests are already in progress. This is important if a large batch of routine tests is being performed and a "stat" (immediate need) request is made by the physician. **Sequential analysis** means that all tests are performed in the order they were entered into the analyzer, and batteries of tests are performed in a certain order.

History of Analyzer Development

The original multiple analyzers developed in the 1950s and 1960s were either continuous-flow analyzers or used centrifugal analysis to mix the samples and reagents. The first sequential multiple analyzer instruments were developed by Technicon. Over a period of a few years, these instruments were improved until they could perform a larger number of tests in a shorter time. Subsequent chemistry analyzers employed a range of testing methodologies, using built-in computers to handle large volumes of data and store patient results and quality control results.

Micropipettes are also now available to measure very small volumes of patient samples and dispense them into **cuvettes** (reaction chambers) through which spectrophotometers read the reactions. This also nearly eliminates the problem of carryover (new samples being affected by the remnants of previous samples and reagents).

Centrifugal analysis used a wheel-shaped device with two ports—one where the sample, or unknown, was introduced by pipette into a well and another larger port or well where the reagent was placed. When the "wheel" was completed with samples and reagent, the instrument spun the samples and the reagent parcels into the end of the wheel, which was of high-grade, clear plastic. The reading device or spectrophotometer was able to read the reaction in the plastic **cuvette** for each section of the wheel. This system is rarely used today.

Automation in the Chemistry Laboratory

Almost total automation of the clinical chemistry laboratory has now been achieved. Preanalytical steps have been largely automated through use of robotic or other mechanical devices to identify samples by bar code and enter prescribed workloads into the LIS, which in turn generates identification labels for each sample.

The prompt delivery and safe handling of infectious specimens may require protective transportation techniques and containers to ensure personnel safety. Traditionally, specimens are delivered to the laboratory by human transporters and, in some facilities, by a pneumatic tube system. In some areas, robotic tracking and transport systems are available that transport samples from the receiving area to the correct laboratory department. More advanced systems identify the sample, program the analyzers, and even centrifuge the samples to provide serum or plasma for testing. Total automation is designed primarily for larger laboratories as it not feasible or cost effective for smaller laboratories. Commercial laboratories that complete tens of thousands of tests per day all use fully automated systems.

The miniaturization of analyzers has paralleled that of computers. Ion-selective electrodes that are extremely small and perform procedures almost instantaneously are being used for a number of procedures, and others are on the way. Smaller electronic components with microchips use electrophoresis to perform minute separations of proteins into their divisions based on size and weight. *Nanotechnology* is a term used to describe the manipulation of materials that are extremely small and are measured in nanograms (billionths of a gram), such as atoms or molecules, including biochemical components like hormones that are found at very small levels in the human body.

Significance of Specimen Preparation and Testing

Chemistry procedures available for treating diseases or assessing health are many and varied. The sample collection process for chemistry is the first and most important step in performing clinical chemistry tests. Subtle changes or errors in collection will invalidate the results of many procedures, causing delays in treatment or perhaps administration of the wrong treatment. There are also many different types of specimens that are required for certain analyses. Some instruments require a particular type of specimen, such as plasma using only heparin as an **anticoagulant** (a substance to prevent clotting), although there are several other anticoagulants. Others may accept whole blood, plasma, serum, capillary blood, and other body fluids. When drawing lists are provided for specimen collection, the type of tube and any anticoagulant required will sometimes be specified to avoid errors leading to erroneous results from **preanalytical error** (mistakes that occur through mishandling or misidentification of a sample). Remember also that arterial blood is used for blood gases but not for other analyses.

A quick review of specimen requirements for chemistry analysis, covered previously in the phlebotomy section, follows:

1. Specimens must be properly identified according to standard procedures followed by the facility.

2. Specimens containing an anticoagulant must be mixed properly to avoid clots.

3. Hemolysis (the breakdown of red blood cells) may release interfering substances.

4. Lipema, a high level of fatty materials in the serum or plasma, must be noted for proper interpretation of results, or the specimen should be recollected.

5. Specimens must not leak contents onto the outer portion of the tube. Certain specimens may require that they be sealed in leak-proof containers.

6. Timely delivery to the laboratory and proper storage of specimens that will not be analyzed until later is of great importance.

7. **Short draws** are those in which the tube was not completely filled and therefore contains less volume than designed for a given amount of anticoagulant. This will result in an improper dilution ratio and will affect results.

8. Patients being administered IV solutions or who have other implanted devices will require care in the collection of blood. Blood should never be drawn from above an active IV site.

> **Critical Reminder**
> The factors listed here are preanalytical components of performing a laboratory procedure. Errors in any of these steps are capable of providing erroneous results that may harm a patient, hindering a proper diagnosis.

Many safety devices are provided for handling samples, as this process involves the greatest risk when performing clinical chemistry exams. Most of the chemicals utilized in chemistry procedures are quite safe today. However, in the past, many toxic chemicals were used that were carcinogenic (cancer-causing) or could cause serious tissue damage, such as caustics that might "burn" the skin or the mucous membranes. Uncapping tubes (removing the specialized plastic and rubber tops) presents an opportunity for exposure to biohazards. By using a safety shield, this danger is minimized. Some instruments pierce the cap of the tube and aspirate the sample without the medical laboratory worker being required to uncap the tube.

Other considerations in the chemistry laboratory are the collection of timed specimens that either are to be collected at a specific time of day or in a timed sequence to determine a patient's response to medication or food. Fasting specimens are required for some procedures to obtain a baseline or to avoid lipemia (fats in the blood that cause turbidity). Other reasons for requiring samples from fasting patients are to avoid foods containing certain chemicals that may elevate or decrease the values of some laboratory tests. An example of this would be testing for blood glucose level, which may be elevated if a blood sample is taken within an hour of a meal that contains carbohydrates and glucose. But even if due diligence and care are exercised for preanalytical factors and the condition of supplies and operations of equipment are adequate, **random errors** (those whose cause is undetermined) will occur on a statistical basis. Random errors affect precision (reproducibility) and may occur due to a variety of factors, including technique and environmental conditions under which the procedures are performed. As one might recall from the chapter on quality control, roughly 5% of results will be outside an acceptable range.

SERUM AND PLASMA AS CLINICAL SPECIMENS

What is the difference between serum and plasma? A blood tube that contains no anticoagulant may have clot enhancers as well as barrier materials to separate blood cells and platelets from the liquid portion of the blood. When the blood is allowed to clot and is then centrifuged, the resulting liquid portion of the blood that overlays the cells is called **serum**. The barrier gel will move to an area between the cells and the serum, allowing easy separation. Blood collected in a tube containing an anticoagulant will not clot if the blood and anticoagulant are in the proper ratio to each other. When an anticoagulated sample is centrifuged, **plasma** results when the cells and liquid portion are separated. The plasma contains coagulation factors that are absent in serum, which is obtained after the blood has clotted, a process that uses up most of the coagulation factors.

CLNICAL CHEMISTRY PROCEDURES

The following representative laboratory procedures for chemistry determinations demonstrate a variety of manual procedures for several different analytes and for each of the five major departments of the laboratory. For some chemistry procedures, the results will correlate with and confirm the results from other departments. The manual chemistry procedures presented here can be performed with a minimum of equipment and supplies. Basic knowledge of each of these procedures will be valuable to the student of medical laboratory technology as a preparation for working at a clinical site. Even though most clinical sites will perform most of their procedures on automated equipment, there are strong correlations between the manual and automated processes.

Some instructors may wish to have students perform some of these procedures as an introduction to the performance of more comprehensive laboratory procedures in other courses. Programs are often designed where both theory and practice may be taught in specific courses related to each of the major laboratory areas. However, in some medical laboratory programs, the practical portion of your education may be deferred until you are assigned to a clinical site such as a hospital laboratory.

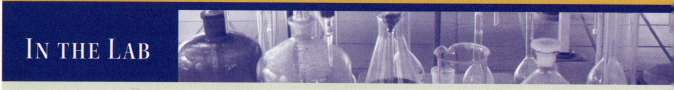

IN THE LAB

BASIC CLINICAL CHEMISTRY PROCEDURES
MANUAL CHEMISTRY PROCEDURE #1
Total Protein
Principles

Abnormal total protein values are most often related to liver disease. Although proteins are found in all body fluids to varying degrees, serum is the best fluid for determining the level of protein. Plasma has an abundance of fibrinogen that will affect the results of a total protein determination.

Total protein determinations test simultaneously for both albumin and globulin through a dye-binding procedure. Albumin, which comprises more than one-half of the total protein value, is often measured in a second and separate test. The difference between the total protein and the albumin is roughly equal to the globulin value. Albumin is important in maintaining fluid balance within the body, while globulin includes antibodies, blood coagulation proteins, and proteins that transport elements such as iron throughout the body. The ratio among these major proteins will be altered in diseases that affect the functions of the liver, where albumin is synthesized.

In this procedure, the student will perform a serum total protein determination by using a simple dye that colors the protein molecules. The intensity of the color is proportional to the level of protein in the sample. This type of reaction is called an end-point colorimetric determination (Figure 14-1). The color development is proportional to the absorbance level.

The Stanbio Total Protein Method is available as a simple test kit that will enable the student to perform a totally manual method for protein. The kit contains both the standards and the reagent for the quantitative colorimetric determination of total protein in serum or plasma. In addition to the reagents provided in the kit, a spectrophotometer capable of absorbance readings at 500 nanometers (nm) is needed.

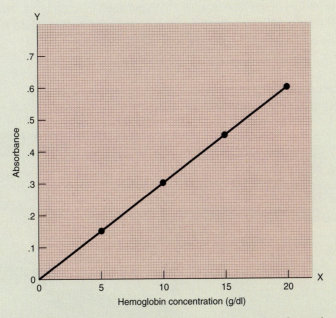

FIGURE 14-1 The graph shows a typical end-point reaction observed in a variety of chemistry procedures.
Source: Delmar/Cengage Learning.

IN THE LAB

Equipment and Supplies

1. Gloves, disposable paper towels, and disinfectant or other cleaning solution
2. Report form provided by your instructor
3. Serum (preferred because fibrinogen is contained in a plasma sample)
   a. For accuracy, the sample must be free of significant hemolysis.
   b. A serum sample that is free from gross hemolysis or lipemia will remain stable for up to one week at room temperature and for 30 days at 2°C–8°C.
   c. When a blood sample is centrifuged immediately after clotting and the serum is removed from the blood cells, hemolysis is greatly reduced.
4. Micropipetter with disposable pipette tips for measuring patient specimen as µLs
5. Serological pipettes
6. Stanbio kit for total protein (contains the reagent copper sulfate pentahydrate in aqueous sodium hydroxide and aqueous protein standard [10 mg/dL])
7. Spectrophotometer capable of absorbance readings at 550 nm (Figure 14-2)
8. Water bath or heat block set at 37°C (optional) (The reaction takes 10 minutes at room temperature, and approximately 3 minutes at 37°C.)
9. Cuvettes
10. 13 × 100 test tubes and test tube rack
11. Waterproof sharp marker for labeling test tubes
12. Vortex mixer (optional) (desirable since the complex of the dye and proteins will fall to the bottom of the tube in which the specimen and reagents are mixed and even in the cuvettes before reading them on the spectrophotometer)
13. Electronic timing device or clock/watch with second hand

Procedure

1. Wash hands and don gloves.
2. Assemble necessary equipment and supplies.

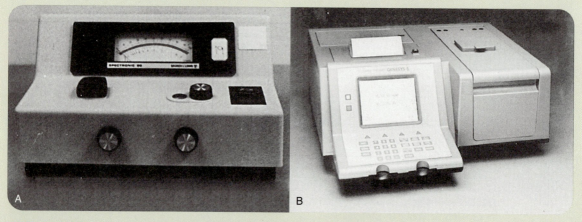

FIGURE 14-2 (A) Spectronic Genesys 5-UV visible spectrophotometer, and (B) with printer.
Source: Delmar/Cengage Learning.

3. Assemble the pipetter with tips for accurate pipetting of the standards, controls, and patient specimens.
   a. The tips should be changed between each sample (including standards and controls) since carryover is possible between specimens.
   b. Accurate pipetting is essential since extremely small amounts of standard, controls, and patient specimens are required for this procedure.
4. Label the test tubes as follows for proper identification of blanks, standards, controls, and unknowns: Label one tube "RB" for the blank specimen and one tube "S" for the standard sample, and one or more tubes "C (number)" for the control samples (e.g., C-1 and C-2 to differentiate between normal and abnormal controls). The unknown samples [Sample (U) in the chart below] should be labeled by patient name or other identifier such as a patient number.
5. Pipette the following volumes into the 13 × 100 tubes and mix well. Note that the reagent is measured in mL and the specimens, standards, and controls are measured in µLs (1000 µLs comprise 1 mL). The volumes indicated below may be increased if the spectrophotometer requires a volume greater than 1.0 mL.

	Reagent Blank (RB)	Standard (S)	Sample (U)	Control (C)
Reagent	1.0	1.0	1.0	
Standard	–	0.01	–	
Sample	–	–	0.01	

6. Use the vortex mixer or gently swirl the mixture to briefly mix the contents of each tube. Take care not to lose any of the sample and reagent mixture.
7. Allow all tubes to stand for 10 minutes.
8. Arrange the cuvettes in the order in which they will be read after filling them from the test tubes.
9. Insert the reagent blank into the well of the spectrophotometer and adjust the absorbance to "0."
10. Within 60 minutes of starting the procedure, read and record the absorbance values for the standard (S), control (C), and the unknowns (U) versus the reagent blank (RB) at 550 nm.
11. Calculate the values for the controls and the patient specimens (unknowns) by the following equation.

Protein Calculation (Manual Method)

$$\text{Protein (g/dL)} = \frac{\text{Abs of unknown (Au)}}{\text{Abs of standard (As)}} \times 10 \text{ (concentration of the standard) (mg/dL)}$$

12. Discard all supplies used for the procedure in the appropriate containers. A disinfectant should be used to clean the work surfaces and equipment should be cleaned and restored to its former position. Gloves should be discarded appropriately and the hands washed thoroughly in accordance with established policies.

IN THE LAB

Quality Control

Two to three levels of control material with known ranges of protein levels determined by this procedure are analyzed each day of testing in a medical laboratory. The total protein value of each specimen can be estimated by using a refractometer where the specific gravity is determined on the appropriate scale (a separate scale is observable for urine samples).

Linearity

When performed as directed this method provides for linearity from 0 to 10 g/dL.

Reporting of Results

Report your findings from the Total Protein procedure in the form supplied by your instructor. Results of the serum total protein are measured in grams per deciliter (g/dL). However, the protein values for some body fluids, including cerebrospinal fluid and urine, are measured in mg/dL.

MANUAL CHEMISTRY PROCEDURE #2

Glucose

Principles

Glucose is the major carbohydrate found in the blood and is used for energy for the organs and tissues of the body. The glucose determination is chiefly used to determine if a person is diabetic or, if the patient has already been diagnosed as diabetic, if he or she is compliant in taking insulin and if the dosage is correct. The test may also determine if a patient is hypoglycemic, a condition in which a low blood glucose is found.

The Stanbio Enzymatic Glucose procedure is specific for glucose and may be used for manual as well as automated systems. It uses an enzymatic procedure for the quantitative enzymatic-colorimetric determination of glucose in serum, plasma, or cerebrospinal fluid.

The reagent for this reaction provides for an enzymatic determination, and is the most common method for determining glucose values. Reagents including enzymatic glucose reagent may require reconstitution with deionized water. The water and a glucose standard (100 mg/dL) are provided with the kit. Other materials required but not provided are control samples to insure reproducibility and validity of the results. Although this reagent may be used on automated and semi-automated systems, the procedure outlined here is that of a manual procedure.

The process of specimen collection and preparation allows for either serum or plasma determinations. If serum is to be used, it must be removed from the clot within 30 minutes of collection to prevent glycolysis (blood glucose will drop significantly after 30 minutes). Plasma obtained by use of a tube with an anticoagulant containing fluoride is recommended, but any of the common anticoagulants may be used if the plasma is separated from the blood cells promptly after centrifugation. This procedure can also be used for the determination of glucose levels in cerebrospinal fluid (CSF). No special preparation is required unless the CSF sample contains blood; in such instance, the sample must be centrifuged and removed from the blood, or glycolysis will occur as it does in blood samples.

Only minimal limitations are incurred when using this procedure where a specific enzyme reacts with glucose. Both serum and plasma samples are processed in the same manner, and the samples, when separated from blood cells, are stable for up to 40 hours if stored in a refrigerator at 2°C–8°C. Excessive levels of ascorbic acid are the chief interfering substance and may result in falsely low glucose values.

Analysis parameters are provided by the manufacturer for procedures using autoanalyzers as well as for adaptations from these parameters than can be used for manual procedures. Manual methods may require the same parameters, but some of them might require manual steps such as manually measuring the samples and timing them. These tasks might otherwise be handled by automated equipment. These procedures will be found on package inserts accompanying the test kits and reagents. Most basic procedures performed in a classroom laboratory, however, will be manual methods.

The Stanbio enzymatic glucose procedure utilizes a quantitative enzymatic determination of glucose in plasma, serum, or cerebrospinal fluid.

Equipment and Supplies

1. Gloves, disposable paper towels, and disinfectant or other cleaning solution
2. Report form provided by your instructor
3. Serum, plasma, or other sample
   a. Serum sample should be free of hemolysis.
   b. Unhemolyzed plasma sample should be from an anticoagulated sample that is separated from blood cells within 30 minutes of collection.
   c. Cerebrospinal fluid sample may be tested by this method.
4. Micropipetter with disposable pipette tips for measuring patient specimen as µLs
5. Serological pipettes
6. Stanbio kit for enzymatic determination of glucose
7. 100 mg/dL standard for calibration; two or three-level control samples depending upon procedure used to ensure precision
8. Spectrophotometer capable of absorbance readings at 550 nm
9. Water bath or heat block set at 37°C (optional) (The reaction takes 10 minutes at room temperature, and approximately 3 minutes at 37°C.)
10. Cuvettes
11. 13×100 mm test tubes and test tube rack
12. Waterproof sharp marker for labeling test tubes
13. Vortex mixer
14. Electronic timing device or clock/watch with second hand

IN THE LAB

Procedure

1. Wash hands and don gloves.
2. Assemble necessary equipment and supplies.
3. Assemble the pipetter with tips for accurate pipetting of the standards, controls, and patient specimens. The tips should be changed between each sample (including standards and controls) since carryover is possible between specimens. Accurate pipetting is essential since extremely small amounts of standard, controls, and patient specimens are required for this procedure.
4. Label the test tubes as follows for proper identification of blanks, standards, controls, and unknowns: Label one tube "RB" for the blank specimen and one tube "S" for the standard sample, and one or more tubes "C (number)" for the control samples (e.g., C-1 and C-2 to differentiate between normal and abnormal controls). The unknown samples [Sample (U) in the chart below] should be labeled by patient name or other identifier such as a patient number.
5. Pipette the following volumes into the 13×100 tubes and mix well. Note that the reagent is measured in mL and the specimens, standards, and controls are measured in µLs (1000 µLs comprises 1 mL). The volumes indicated below may be increased if the spectrophotometer requires a volume greater than 1.0 mL.

	Reagent Blank (RB)	Standard (S)	Sample (U)	Control (C)
Reagent	1.0	1.0	1.0	
Standard	–	0.01	–	
Sample	–	–	0.01	

6. Use the vortex mixer or gently swirl the mixture to briefly mix the contents of each tube. Take care not to lose any of the sample and reagent mixture.
7. Allow all tubes to stand for ten minutes.
8. Arrange the cuvettes in the order in which they will be read after filling them from the test tubes.
9. Insert the reagent blank into the well of the spectrophotometer and adjust the absorbance to "0."
10. Within 15 minutes of starting the procedure, read and record the absorbance values for the standard (S) and the unknowns (U) versus the reagent blank (RB) at 500 nm.
11. Calculate the values for controls and the patient specimens (unknowns) by the following equation.

Glucose Calculation (Manual Method)

$$\text{Glucose (mg/dL)} = \frac{\text{Abs of unknown (Au)}}{\text{Abs of standard (As)}} \times 10 \text{ (concentration of the standard) (mg/dL)}$$

12. Discard all supplies used for the procedure in the appropriate containers. A disinfectant should be used to clean the work surfaces and equipment should be cleaned and restored to its former position. Gloves should be discarded appropriately and the hands washed thoroughly in accordance with established policies.

Quality Control

Two to three levels of control material with known ranges of glucose levels determined by this procedure should be analyzed each day of testing in a medical laboratory.

Linearity

When performed as directed this method provides for linearity from 0 to 500 g/dL.

Reporting of Results

Report your findings from the Glucose procedure in the form supplied by your instructor. Results of serum or plasma glucose are reported in milligrams per deciliter (mg/dL). The glucose determinations for some body fluids, including cerebrospinal fluid (CSF), is always lower than the values found in the blood, but are performed in the same manner as for serum or plasma. The value for CSF fluid is normally only about 60% – 70% of that of the blood.

MANUAL CHEMISTRY PROCEDURE #3

Total Cholesterol and High-Density Lipoprotein (HDL)

Principles

The presence of excess lipids (of which cholesterol is but one type) in the blood has been recognized as a risk factor for cardiovascular disease leading to stroke or heart attack for years. A number of procedures are available for measuring cholesterol. In the manual procedure presented here, total cholesterol is measured first. Low-density lipoproteins (LDL) are then removed from the sample with a precipitating reagent, leaving only the high-density lipoproteins (HDL), and a repeat procedure for cholesterol is performed. The difference between the total cholesterol and the HDL value is the LDL value.

   The Stanbio Cholesterol and HDL Test Kits are intended for the quantitative, colorimetric determination of cholesterol in serum or plasma. Standard laboratory tests for measuring HDL are not usually performed in the clinical laboratory.

Equipment and Supplies

1. Gloves, disposable paper towels, and disinfectant or other cleaning solution
2. Report form provided by your instructor
3. Serum sample (must be free of hemolysis, separated from blood cells within 30 minutes of collection, and tested as soon as possible following collection)
4. Pipetter with disposable pipette tips for measuring 10 and 25 µLs
5. Serological pipettes

IN THE LAB

6. Spectrophotometer capable of absorbance readings at 500 nm
7. Stanbio kit for enzymatic determination of total cholesterol. Total cholesterol standard (200 mg/dL) and HDL standard (50 mg/dL) and HDL precipitating reagent are included in the Stanbio kit.
8. Water bath or heat block set at 37°C (optional) (The reaction takes 10 minutes at room temperature, and approximately 3 minutes at 37°C.)
9. Cuvettes
10. 13 × 100 test tubes and test tube rack
11. Waterproof sharp marker for labeling test tubes
12. Vortex mixer
13. Electronic timing device or clock/watch (exact time is not critical)
14. 2 or 3 levels of control samples to insure precision (recommended)

Procedure

1. Wash hands and don gloves.
2. Assemble necessary equipment and supplies.
3. Assemble the micropipetter with tips for accurate pipetting of the standards, controls, and patient specimens. The tips should be changed between each sample (including standards and controls) since carryover is possible between specimens. Accurate pipetting is essential since extremely small amounts of standard, controls, and patient specimens are required for this procedure.
4. Label the test tubes as follows for proper identification of blanks, standards, controls, and unknowns: the first tube "RB" for the reagent blank; the second tube "TCS" for the total cholesterol standard; the third tube "TCU" for the total cholesterol unknown sample along with the reagent; the fourth tube "HDLS" for the HDL standard; and the fifth tube "HDLU" for the HDL unknown sample taken from the precipitate along with the reagent.
   a. This procedure will require 5 tubes when only one unknown is being tested.
   b. The only difference between HDL determination and total cholesterol is the amount of sample and the standard.
   c. All of the tests may be read using the same wavelength of 500 nm, with only one blank.
5. Performing Precipitate for HDL Cholesterol
   a. This is accomplished by adding an amount of serum, in accordance with the test kit manufacturer's instruction, to a precipitating reagent. This mixture is centrifuged, and after centrifugation the supernatant from which the low density lipoproteins (LDL) have been removed (precipitated out of the serum) is used as the patient sample. If only total cholesterol or only HDL is being performed, use the tables following the one entitled "Total Cholesterol and HDL Procedure."
   b. A vortex mixer is preferable, particularly for mixing the serum for an HDL with the precipitating reagent.

Total Cholesterol and HDL Procedure

Tube 1	Reagent blank
Tube 2	Total cholesterol standard (1 mL reagent and 10 µL standard—200 mg/dL)
Tube 3	Total cholesterol unknown (1 mL reagent and 10 µL serum)
Tube 4	HDL cholesterol standard (1 mL reagent and 25 µL standard—50 mg/dL)
Tube 5	HDL cholesterol unknown (1 mL total cholesterol reagent and 25 µL supernatant from the serum preparation precipitate)

6. Mix well the contents of tubes 1 – 5 by using a vortex mixer if available, or mix by swirling gently or by gently tapping the bottoms of the tubes. Note that volumes may be increased if the instrument requires volumes greater than 1.0 mL, which would require larger volumes of reagent and sample in tubes 1 – 5.

Total Cholesterol

	Reagent Blank (RB)	Standard (S)	Sample (U)
Reagent	1.0	1.0	1.0
Standard	–	0.01	–
Sample	–	–	0.01

HDL Cholesterol

	Reagent Blank (RB)	Standard (S)	Sample (U) from the precipitate
Reagent	1.0	1.0	1.0
Standard	–	0.025	–
Sample	–	–	0.025

7. Allow all tubes to stand for 10 minutes at room temperature.
8. Pipette 1.0 mL color reagent into each tube and again mix by gently tapping the bottom of the tube. Incubate the tubes at room temperature for 10 minutes or in a water bath or heat block set at 37°C (optional). The reaction requires 10 minutes at room temperature, or approximately 3 minutes at 37°C.
9. Pour into cuvettes for measuring absorbances (if the spectrophotometer is equipped with a flow-through cuvette, aspirate the contents of the test tube directly).
10. Within 60 minutes, read and record the absorbance values for the standard (S) and the unknowns (U) versus the reagent blank (RB) at 500 nm.
11. Calculate the values for controls and the patient specimens (unknowns) using the following equation.

Total Cholesterol Calculation (Manual Method)

$$\text{Total Cholesterol (mg/dL)} = \frac{\text{Abs of unknown (Au)}}{\text{Abs of standard (As)}} \times 200 \text{ (concentration of the standard) (mg/dL)}$$

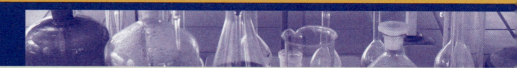

IN THE LAB

HDL Calculation (Manual Method)

$$\text{HDL (mg/dL)} = \frac{\text{Abs of unknown (Au)}}{\text{Abs of standard (As)}} \times 50 \text{ (concentration of the standard) (mg/dL)}$$

12. Discard all supplies used for the procedure in the appropriate containers. A disinfectant should be used to clean the work surfaces and equipment should be cleaned and restored to its former position. Gloves should be discarded appropriately and the hands washed thoroughly in accordance with established policies.

Quality Control

Two levels of control material with known cholesterol levels determined by this procedure should be analyzed each day of testing in a medical laboratory.

Linearity

When performed as directed, the method is linear from 0 to 200 mg/dL.

Reporting of Results

Report your findings from the Total Cholesterol and High-Density Lipoprotein (HDL) procedure in the form supplied by your instructor. Results of total cholesterol and HDL are reported in milligrams per deciliter (mg/dL).

MANUAL CHEMISTRY PROCEDURE #4
AST/GOT (Manual) Chemistry Procedure
Principles

This test is for the quantitative determination of serum aspartate aminotransferase (AST), needed in the diagnosis and treatment of certain types of liver and heart disease. Organ cells deteriorate under certain conditions (e.g., infection, diminished blood flow). The death of these cells releases enzymes that are richer in some organs than others. The physician can rule out certain ailments or suspect others based on this test. Usually, a battery of enzymes tests are run and the results compared for significance.

A working reagent is prepared by reconstituting a substrate upon which the enzyme AST will react. The working reagent is prepared by pouring the contents of a small AST additive (substrate) bottle into a larger AST reagent (coenzyme) bottle. Replace the cap and mix well by gentle inversion (do not shake vigorously). For ease in transferring the working reagent, some kits provide a flip-top cap to replace the screw cap.

The absorbance of freshly prepared working reagent should be at least 1.200 when measured at 340 nm in a spectrophotometer with a 1-cm light path. The reagent

Critical Reminder

The cholesterol procedure, unlike the previous examples, uses a *kinetic reaction* to measure the change in absorbance as a substrate, a product on which an enzyme works specifically (Figure 14-3). This test requires a factor determined from a number of assay conditions on which the reaction is dependent. The previous chemistry procedures were based on an end-point reaction, where a color is produced that correlates in intensity with the concentration of the component being measured. Most product inserts found in the test kits will provide all of the information needed to understand and perform the procedure. Most automated chemistry analyzers use these *kinetic* methods, which measure the change rather than an end-point. This gives a more accurate and rapid analysis than that of the end-point reactions, which must sit for a period of time for the color to develop.

should be combined with reagent grade water or the provided diluent and mixed well before obtaining an initial reading from a spectrophotometer.

Storage of the reagent is possible for up to 10 days when stored at 2°C to 8°C, and for 1 day when stored at 20°C to 25°C (room temperature), providing that the reagent has not expired. The expiry date is provided on the box in which the reagent was received.

The reagent as packaged will be clear and colorless to straw-colored. The additive as packaged will also be clear and colorless. After mixing the two reagents, the working reagent should also be clear and colorless. Discard the working reagent if it is turbid, as this may suggest contamination has occurred.

The preferred specimen is fresh and unhemolyzed serum. The samples should be collected in the usual manner for any other clinical test requiring serum. Separate serum and plasma from red blood cells promptly to minimize hemolysis, although slight hemolysis will not significantly affect results. However, if erythrocytes remain in the sample and become hemolyzed, they contain approximately 10 times more intracellular AST than normal serum. If plasma must be used, the recommended anticoagulants are oxalate, citrate, EDTA, and heparin.

In addition to hemolysis, other interfering substances such as certain drugs (including illicit drugs) may affect AST determinations. Interferences with the AST procedure commonly occur when triglyceride levels exceed 600 mg/dL. Bilirubin values above 14 mg/dL, a common occurrence in jaundiced persons and those with severe liver damage, may also interfere with this method.

Most kits for AST determination are suitable for manual methods as well as semi-automated and automated instruments. The instrument settings are provided through a package insert. The AST procedure is based on a kinetic rate change over a period of time (Figure 14-3).

Equipment and Supplies

1. Gloves, disposable paper towels, and disinfectant or other cleaning solution
2. Report form provided by your instructor
3. Working reagents prepared as directed and monitored for deterioration
4. Spectrophotometer or other analyzer capable of measuring absorbance at 340 nm

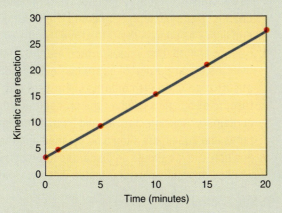

FIGURE 14-3 Kinetic rate reaction predicts the total level of analytes in a short time.
Source: Delmar/Cengage Learning.

IN THE LAB

5. Cuvettes or flow cell (If a thermal cuvette allowing for temperature adjustment is not available, a water bath or heat block set at 37°C will be needed.)
6. Micropipetter with disposable tips
7. Serological pipettes
8. 13 × 100 test tubes and a test tube rack
9. Electronic timing device or clock/watch with second hand (Spectrophotometers with a built-in thermal cuvette will have a built-in timing device.)

Procedure (Manual)

1. Wash hands and don gloves.
2. Assemble necessary equipment and supplies.
3. Zero the spectrophotometer at 340 nm with distilled or deionized water.
4. Place 1.0 mL working reagent (substrate plus diluents) in each prelabeled tube. No standards is required with many of the kinetic reactions. A reagent blank (RB), control (C), and identified sample tubes are needed for each test.
5. Prewarm the reagent at 30°C or 37°C for at least 3 minutes in accordance with manufacturer's instructions.
6. Add 50 µL sample to the 1 mL reagent sample. Mix by vortex or by swirling before incubating at 30°C or 37°C in the water bath or heat block.
7. Incubation of the working reagent is not necessary if a spectrophotometer with a thermal flow-through cuvette is used. However, it is important to ensure that the temperature of the instrument is adjusted to the proper level.
8. After a 120-second delay, record absorbance values every 15 seconds for at least 2 minutes. Determine the absorbance change (Delta change) per minute (Delta A/min) is consistent and linear as seen in the rate curve (Figure 14-3).
9. Record absorbance values, which are the change (Delta A/min) over the linear portion of a rate curve. Uniformity of successive absorbance changes confirms linearity of rate reaction.
10. Discard all supplies used for the procedure in the appropriate containers. A disinfectant should be used to clean the work surfaces and equipment should be cleaned and restored to its former position. Gloves should be discarded appropriately and the hands washed thoroughly in accordance with established policies.

Quality Control

Quality control is important in all departments of a clinical laboratory. Fresh commercial control sera prepared each day may require reconstituting with deionized water or may come as a liquid and is

Critical Reminder

The AST procedure is a kinetic reaction that reacts on a specific substrate. The change in absorbance is measured for a specific period of time depending upon the instrumentation used, and the change in absorbance is measured over a period of time where the reaction proceeds in a linear manner as a smooth progression. The enzyme that is measured is released from liver cells when they are damaged by disease or exposure to toxins and during infectious processes. A factor is determined based on the concentration of substrate in the reagent upon which the enzymes act. The majority of chemistry determinations are performed on automated chemistry analyzers as kinetic methods, which provides for quicker and more specific results. When the enzyme level of a patient's sample is exceedingly elevated, the substrate may be acted upon so quickly that the supply of substrate is completely consumed. Automated instruments used for these types of procedures are programmed to detect such conditions and will prompt the laboratory professional to repeat the procedure using a diluted sample that is then multiplied by the dilution factor to obtain an accurate result.

recommended with each assay batch to monitor procedural para-meters. Use two controls containing normal and abnormal levels of the enzyme if possible. If r esults fall outside the acceptable activity limits, check procedural parameters (i.e., photometer, cuvette, pipettes, tubes, and temperature). If problems persist, call your technical representative. Please note that some control sera may show increases of AST activity if activated with pyridoxyl phosphate.

Reporting of Results

Report your findings from the AST/GOT procedure in the form supplied by your instructor. Activity is expressed in units per liter of specimen (U/L). One unit is defined as the amount of enzyme that catalyzes the conversion of one micromole of substrate per minute under specified assay conditions. Data used in factor calculations are found on the assay sheet provided by the manufacturer. These data are a factor from the manufacturer of the substrate and are derived from the concentration of the sub-strate. The results of the test(s) are calculated by multiplying the absorbance change for one minute by the calculated factor.

AST/GOT Rate Reaction Calculation

U/L = Delta change per minute × Derived Factor = Value of Unknown in IU/L

An example of calculating AST values is shown in Example 14-1.

Example 14-1
AST/GOT Rate Reaction

	0 sec.	15 sec	30 sec	45 sec	60 sec	75 sec	90 sec	105 sec	120 sec
Specimen 1	1.103	1.105	1.110	1.116	1.132	1.148	1.164	1.181	1.199

1. The linear and consistent changes occur from 45 seconds to 105 seconds, for a minute of activity.
2. The delta change in absorption for a minute is 0.065.
3. Results are calculated by multiplying 0.065 by the derived factor (1768).
4. The calculated results in this example = 115 IU/L.

CHEMISTRY PROCEDURE #5
Electrolytes
Principles

Electrolytes may be referred to as a single entity because four of seven components are interrelated, and are balanced between the four basic analytes. The tests for electrolytes refer to positively and negatively charged ions. The positively charged ions, called cations, are sodium, potassium, calcium, and magnesium; sodium (Na+) and potassium (K+) are tested for routinely in a set of electrolytes. Negatively charged ions, called anions, include chloride (Cl$^-$), bicarbonate (HCO^{-3}), and phos-phate; bicarbonate and chloride are the chief electrolytes routinely monitored. Bicar-bonate determinations may be referred to as CO$_2$ (carbon dioxide) as most of the CO$_2$ of the body is found in the bicarbonate molecule . In addition, it is simpler to test for

IN THE LAB

Table 14-1 Normal Values for Serum Electrolytes

Electrolyte	Reference Range mmol/L (mEq/L)
Sodium (Na^+)	135–148
Potassium (K^+)	3.8–5.5
Chloride (Cl^-)	98–108
Bicarbonate (total CO_2)	22–28

*Actual CO_2 as a gas measurement is seldom done currently. A bicarbonate level provides a useful estimate of the CO_2 level in the blood.

bicarbonate than for CO_2, as the later is a gas and testing for it requires a great deal more preparation.

Properly balanced electrolytes are vital for maintaining the narrow range of values necessary for storage of fluids and proper cellular function and excretion (see Table 14-1). Electrolyte imbalances are caused by a variety of medical conditions.

Diabetic comas may occur from electrolyte imbalances (a patient rapidly becomes acidotic, which is a life-threatening condition when the body's fluids fall outside a slightly alkaline range of 7.35 to 7.45). Vomiting, diarrhea, and administration of certain medications may lead to an electrolyte imbalance; such imbalances must be rectified quickly and thus may require accurate laboratory measurements stat (immediately). Imbalances of electrolytes often become life-threatening and affect all organs and systems of the body.

Electrolytes may be measured by small portable instruments at the bedside, providing continual monitoring when necessary. Electrolytes are also included on most routine biomedical panels of chemistry tests used for screening patients and can be performed quickly by automated means. Proper flow of electrolytes between intracellular spaces and extracellular spaces must occur to maintain a balance (Figure 14-4).

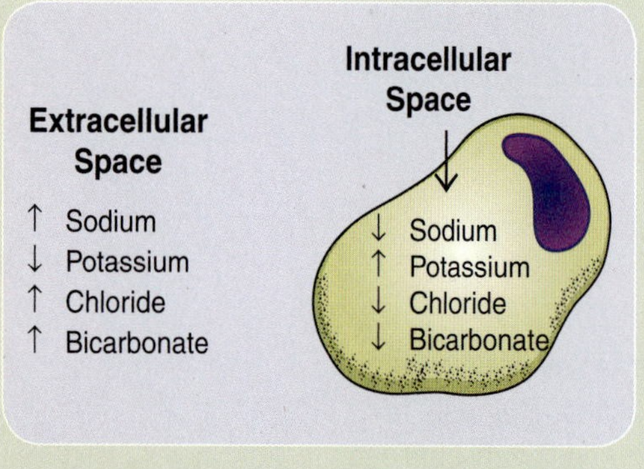

The methodology for measuring electrolytes has advanced greatly over the years. Initially, sodium, potassium and even calcium determinations were performed by flame photometry, where burning of ions emitted light of various wavelengths. Chloride was measured by colorimetry or by the formation of silver chloride when a sample was introduced to a silver wire. Carbon dioxide was measured by manometry or colorimetry. Today, most analyzers use ion-selective electrodes that directly measure these components. A number of instruments are designed to measure either plasma, serum, or whole blood, depending on their operating capacity. Some of these small portable instruments are adapted for use in physician office laboratories and for point-of-care testing in the home or the clinic (Figure 14-5).

Extracellular Space
- ↑ Sodium
- ↓ Potassium
- ↑ Chloride
- ↑ Bicarbonate

Intracellular Space
- ↓ Sodium
- ↑ Potassium
- ↓ Chloride
- ↓ Bicarbonate

FIGURE 14-4 Relative intracellular and extracellular exchanges of concentration.
Source: Delmar/Cengage Learning.

Equipment and Supplies

1. Gloves, disposable paper towels, and disinfectant or other cleaning solution
2. Report form provided by your instructor
3. Non-hemolyzed sample of serum or plasma (not from EDTA anticoagulant as K+ would be artificially increased (Potassium ions (K^+) are greatly elevated in hemolyzed serum or plasma due to the rich supply of intracellular K^+ in RBCs) (note that some instruments require cartridges for testing and quality control)
4. Quality control samples
5. Electrolyte analyzer

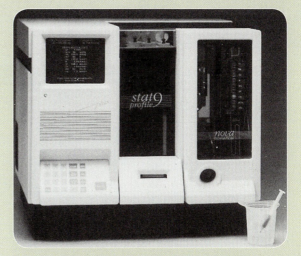

FIGURE 14-5 Nova CCX analyzer that uses ion-selective electrode technology for a variety of analyses. Source: Delmar/Cengage Learning.

Procedure

1. Wash hands and don gloves.
2. Assemble necessary equipment and supplies.
3. Electrolyte procedures do not require specific steps for determining the blood levels of electrolytes, as the procedure for the measurement of electrolytes is almost entirely performed by instruments that require little specimen preparation and little operator expertise and training. The sample is introduced into the instrument, which contains two electrodes. The reference electrode has a known concentration of the ion to be measure. A reference electrode is present for each of the electrolytes to be measured (e.g., sodium [Na^+], potassium [K^+]). The difference between the electrical potential across a membrane in the electrode is proportional to the concentration of the ions (charged atoms). A microprocessor converts the voltage to a digital figure representing the ion concentration of the unknown sample. Each of the electrodes is ion specific and will react only to a particular electrolyte.
4. Procedures for measuring electrolytes in some instruments may differ. The i-Stat analyzer distributed by Abbott Laboratories requires placing the patient's sample into a disposable cartridge with two reservoirs, one for a calibration solution and the other for the sample. Other instruments may use a probe to aspirate the sample into the machine. Some instruments perform a variety of tests other than electrolytes and use various methods to place the sample into the analyzer.
5. Discard all supplies used for the procedure in the appropriate containers. A disinfectant should be used to clean the work surfaces and equipment should be cleaned and restored to its former position. Gloves should be discarded appropriately and the hands washed thoroughly in accordance with established policies.

Reporting of Results

Report your findings from the Electrolytes procedure in the form supplied by your instructor. The four major electrolytes most often tested for are reported as follows:

IN THE LAB

Electrolyte	Normal Values
Potassium (K^+)	3.5–5.0 mEq/L 3.5–5.0 mmol/L (for International Units)
Sodium (Na^+)	135–145 mEq/L 135–145 mmol/L (for International Units)
Chloride (Cl^-)	98–108 mEq/L 98–107 mmol/L (for International Units)
Carbon dioxide (CO_2) (Bicarbonate)	22–29 mEq/L 22–29 mmol/L (for International Units)

mEq/L, milliEquivalents per liter; mmol/L, millimoles/liter

SUMMARY

Tests performed in the chemistry department of a laboratory can reveal a great deal of information regarding a patient's health. Any organ or any system of the body that is not functioning adequately due to a metabolic, carcinogenic, or infectious disease process will yield valuable clues toward providing the medical diagnosis of the patient. A set of chemical determinations will enable the physician to use the results for a diagnosis, even when symptoms and signs may be absent.

Most chemistry panels, which are a set of specialized tests designed to diagnose any number of conditions, are normally performed with large automated systems that may produce hundreds of results per hour with a high degree of accuracy. The chemistry procedures in this chapter should aid the clinical laboratory student in understanding the basic process of measuring samples and reagents. The manual techniques performed in the classroom laboratory prepare the student to understand the functions of large automated systems when performing clinical work within large laboratories.

REVIEW QUESTIONS

1. Describe two basic ways in which clinical chemistry procedures are performed.
2. What is the purpose of a standard?
3. Why is it important to be aware of the quality control values?
4. In your opinion, how would the use of dirty cuvettes (in which the reaction takes place) affect the values obtained?
5. Briefly discuss the technological process from single analyses to the development of multichannel autoanalyzers that perform many tests in a short period.

MICROBIOLOGY

KEY TERMS

Antibiotic therapy
Bacteria
Bacterial incinerator
Crystal violet stain
Decolorizer
Direct method
Fungi, yeasts, and molds

Gene probes
Gram negative
Gram positive
Gram stain
Immunocompromised
Immunosuppressive drug therapy
Indirect method

Iodine stain
Meningitis
Petri dish
Pus
Ringworm
Safranin
Viruses

INTRODUCTION

Throughout history, many theories have been proposed for infections by various organisms that could not be observed, much less understood. Raging fevers and hallucinations were sometimes ascribed to demonic possession or unclean blood, resulting in the letting of blood, which further served to exacerbate any infectious process. Nothing was known of the immune system, although those genetically fortunate enough to survive certain infections then maintained immunity to later contact with the diseases in others. Chance observations of colonies of an unknown growth, found on various products and in liquids, were not thought to be related to any sort of disease process. From outward appearances, they were thought to be mere physical changes in the materials.

The Development of Microbiology

Around 1676, Anton von Leeuwenhoek happened to discover that magnification with the use of a series of lenses produced a view of heretofore unknown teeming colonies of creatures. He described them as vast populations of minute creatures, as he possibly saw some of them moving and assumed they were indeed alive. Von Leeuwenhoek and others of the time apparently attached little significance to this discovery and did not realize the significant impact these images would have on the lives of everyone living. As early as the 1870s, Joseph Lister and others discovered that Petri dishes grew a species of bread mold called *Penicillium* sp. But it was not until 1945 that Alexander Fleming was awarded the Nobel Prize in Medicine for the discovery of penicillin; his original endeavors began in 1928 when he learned that a species of bacteria from the genus *Staphylococcus* were inhibited or killed by this mold.

For most of the early history of microbiology, which chiefly concerned bacteria, organisms were grown on nutrient media after collection from both environmental and body sites. Although viruses are somewhat more difficult to cultivate than bacteria, great strides have been made in identifying them. Protozoa and fungi are more readily seen as microorganisms and in some cases may be identified microscopically. Most procedures for identifying bacterial strains were developed as intensive manual work, but eventually automated systems evolved using the information learned from these manual methods to increase the efficiency and accuracy of microbiology laboratories.

Diagnostic Methodology

In recent years, there has been much development in systems for performing rapid microbiology. New technologies must be approved by government agencies as to their accuracy and validity, so the development of new systems is somewhat cumbersome. Many of the methodologies are extremely expensive, and usually only the larger laboratories are able to justify the cost of the equipment. Therefore, some laboratories do little beyond presumptive identifications of bacteria, then send the specimens to a reference laboratory for further definition. The original method of culturing a specimen and isolating certain colonies from mixed growth may still be required even with some of the new technology. Stains are performed on organisms to determine some of the morphology of the organisms, and these slides are studied microscopically to gain a hint as to the species of organism that has been cultured.

A number of time-consuming manual tests, such as tube and slide tests for certain characteristics of a suspect organism, have now been adapted for quick and efficient processing in automated systems. Originally, samples were inoculated onto Petri dishes with differing nutrient qualities and growth characteristics depending on the constituents of the growth media. These organisms were then stained with a type of stain called Gram stain, which is actually a series of three stains and a decolorizer. Some organisms stain as **Gram negative** or a pink color, while others stain as **Gram positive**, a purple color. Further manual tests are performed to place the organisms onto a flow chart leading toward identification. Fermentation of various sugars and determinations of metabolic end points from the growing organisms further lead to a definitive identification.

After the organisms are fairly well defined, another type of medium is used to grow a pure culture from the isolated colonies on the original **Petri dish**. Antibiotics that are effective toward eliminating the infectious organism are determined based on the body site or type of specimen from which the organism was isolated, as the antibiotic must be able to reach the site of the infection. The organism is finally grown on a special medium where paper discs impregnated with a variety of antibiotics are dropped onto the surface of the inoculated plate. Failure of the bacteria to grow within a certain distance from the edge of the discs indicates sensitivity to the antibiotic, and often the physician then has a choice between several antibiotics. A rather recent phenomenon related to indiscriminate use of antibiotics has been the increasing incidents of culturing organisms that are resistant to almost all and, in some cases, all of the antibiotics available.

Diagnosis and Treatment

To determine if **antibiotic therapy** is appropriate, the organism must be identified and, in many cases, evaluated as to the antibiotic that will be effective against it. Effective antibiotic therapy depends on the site of the infection, as not all antibiotics will reach the tissues or the body site where an infection is present. In addition, depending on the species of bacterial organism present, the antibiotic must be chosen from among a large arsenal to combat the infection. Most importantly, antibiotics are developed for **bacteria**, and not for **viruses**. There are antivirals that chiefly prevent the reproduction of a virus. Antivirals work best if administered before signs and symptoms appear in those with a known viral infection. Other microorganisms that are isolated, identified, and treated through actions of the microbiology department are parasites, of which there are a number that commonly infect people from around the world; **fungi**; **yeasts**; **and molds**.

There are two types of tests for determining the presence of microorganisms that may be infecting a patient. Normally, viral infections are determined by the **indirect method**. Usually, a sample of blood is collected, and the sample is tested for antibodies that the immune system has formed against an infectious agent that has invaded the body. But there is also a direct method for determining some viral infections, which entails growing the viruses on cell cultures, as viruses can only survive by inhabiting living cells. In some procedures, these cells can then be stained or tagged with material that fluoresces and becomes visible microscopically, allowing the determination of the presence of colonies of organisms such as fungi. The **direct method** includes a group of tests requiring the collection of a sample of the body fluids or tissue that may be infected by bacteria. Complicating this method of collection is possible contamination of the sample with organisms normally found on the skin, in the nose and mouth, or in the intestine. Even blood collected for bacteriological agents may be contaminated with skin contaminants and will yield erroneous results. Another method, enzyme-linked immunosorbent assay (ELISA), may detect both antibodies and antigens (the infecting organism itself).

The term *fungi* relates to a group of organisms that also includes yeasts and molds. Molds, yeasts, and fungi have minor differences but may be considered as somewhat related. Molds, unlike certain yeasts and other fungi, seldom pose a problem as infective organisms. Many fungal and yeast infections can be traced to heavy and often unwarranted use of antibiotics that eliminates normally occurring bacteria, called normal flora, that help to ward off invasions of other organisms, including abnormal bacteria and yeasts. Yeasts reproduce via budding, which can easily be seen microscopically. Several species of yeasts and fungi are common causes of infections in humans. The fungal infections most often seen in humans usually cause minor infections of the hair, nails, mucous membranes, and skin. *Candida albicans* often causes systemic infections such as vaginitis and thrush, an oral infection. *Tinea pedis* is another example of a fungus; it causes the common infection called athlete's foot. The fungal infection ringworm is a type of skin infection. Another fungal infection of a serious nature when found in the cerebrospinal fluid is that of *Cryptococcus neoformans*, which may cause meningitis in infants. People with chronic diseases may be immunocompromised, and their primary illnesses can be exacerbated by infections with organisms that are seldom a problem for people who are healthy. A number of fungal infections may be life-threatening and occur due to the same reasons that yeasts may become a problem. Persons with AIDS or taking immunosuppressive drug therapy are at the greatest risk for contracting fungal infections that may result in death.

Safety in the Microbiology Laboratory

It is inherent to the nature of the work in this department that the worker will come in close proximity to a variety of microorganisms. Care should be exercised to avoid becoming a victim by contaminating oneself while handling specimens. For certain virulent organisms, most of the work will be done under a safety hood, where small organisms are filtered from the air by a laminar flow system. Fungal specimens and TB specimens should be tested by using a biological safety cabinet (Figure 15-1). Procedures should be written to include the use of safety equipment and supplies in handling certain specimens. An instrument called a bacterial incinerator (Figure 15-2) is used to routinely remove bacteria from an inoculating needle or loop, where intense heat renders the organisms harmless. The student will be instructed as to the use of this instrument, particularly how to avoid burns, because even the exterior of this instrument becomes heated, and the metal needles and loops that have been treated by heat will remain hot for a period of time after removal from the incinerator. Focusing on exposure control (Table 15-1) and decontaminating work surfaces periodically is essential to preventing infection of workers as well as contamination of samples and equipment.

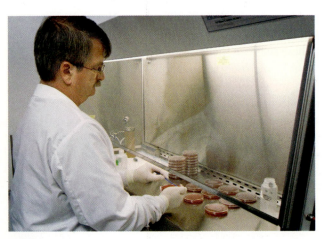

FIGURE 15-1 Biological safety cabinet for working with contagious organisms.
Source: Delmar/Cengage Learning.

RESISTANT STRAINS OF BACTERIA

The overuse or injudicious use of antibiotics when they are not medically indicated has led to the development of strains of bacteria that are resistant to most, if not all, antibiotics.

Therefore, the field of microbiology is growing more important for guiding the proper and effective use of antibiotics. The development of methicillin-resistant *Staphylococcus aureus* (MRSA), a antibiotic-resistant strain of bacteria now found in most hospitals, is a result of heavy use of antibiotics. This organism often causes pneumonia that is difficult to treat.

DEVELOPMENT OF NEW TECHNOLOGY IN MICROBIOLOGY

The term *rapid microbiology* covers methods to confirm more quickly the presence or absence of infectious organisms. Technology now exists that will screen body fluids to determine if any organisms are present before culturing the sample or submitting the specimen to an expensive

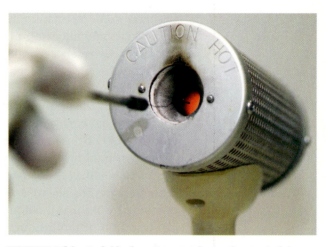

FIGURE 15-2 A bacterial incinerator, a work practice control, is used to avoid aerosols when an inoculating needle is sterilized. **Source: Delmar/Cengage Learning.**

automated process or to a commercial reference laboratory. The original, traditional methods usually require growth of the microorganisms before performing any identification tests, causing a delay in the results. Early identification and treatment are advantageous for the patient, because continued discomfort and in some cases permanent damage may result from delayed treatment. Some early advertisements of rapid methods claim that immediate results will be available, referring to the elimination of or a reduction in the time necessary for the growth phase to produce microorganisms needed for identification testing. The implementation of methodology enabling rapid identification of some common bacterial infections such as the organism that causes strep throat has been slow, in part because of cost and increased labor. This can be attributed to those medical practitioners who prefer to prescribe antibiotics based on clinical symptoms and signs, and then perform testing if the condition is not alleviated. Others believe that the technology will fall to the side of the road, but there are encouraging signs that strides are occurring that will lead to more rapid microbiology results.

Table 15-1 Exposure Control Methods to Protect against Biological Hazards in the Microbiology Laboratory

Hazard	Protective Measures
Blood or blood products	Wear gloves and a buttoned, fluid-resistant laboratory coat
Pathogenic microorganisms	Wear gloves and laboratory coat; use biological safety cabinet
Hazardous aerosols	Place acrylic benchtop shield between worker and tubes when removing stoppers; wear mask, goggles, or face shield when disposing of urine
Contaminated work surfaces	Wipe with 10% chlorine bleach solution (or other surface disinfectant) before and after all procedures and any other appropriate time
Needlesticks	Use self-sheathing needles or quick-release holders; never recap, bend, break, or cut used needles

This may occur based on technology, such as that which identifies bacteria using **gene probes** and fluorescent labeling, that takes less time than traditional methods and is extremely accurate.

Many advances in technology addressing the need for quicker and more accurate identification of microorganisms such as bacteria and viruses have occurred over the past few decades. This technology provides sensitivity panels for prescribing correct antibiotics in a matter of hours rather than days. Traditional methods used since the beginnings of microbiology involve culturing the organism(s) on Petri dishes containing nutritive media and, after growth of visible colonies is accomplished, using biochemical reagents to determine characteristics specific to a particular organism. There are instruments that still use these traditional methods to identify organisms, but another method uses identification of the products of metabolism peculiar to each strain of bacteria. Some of the instruments used frequently in the clinical laboratory are as follows:

Manufacturer	Instrument Name
Becton Dickinson	Phoenix
Biomerieux	ViTek
Dade Behring (Siemens)	MicroScan

An evolving tool uses gene probes to identify genes found in bacteria and viruses. This involves taking a short snippet or fragment of DNA or RNA from a single stranded segment of the double helix arrangement of an entire gene as it naturally occurs. The double helical structure is "unwound" to single strands by chemical means before testing occurs. Because of its specificity toward a particular genetic sequence, this segment can hunt for its complementary strand or fragment amid all of the cellular components that may be encountered in the specimen, which may also contain cellular materials and proteins as well as the infecting organism. The fragment being searched for in the patient specimen is basically a mirror image of the gene probe that is chasing the elusive goal of its identical mate. The fragment will pair with a complementary genetic sequence that has been marked by a chemical or radioactive substance that will bind to a given gene. This marked genetic sequence is then used as a tag to identify or isolate the gene from the microorganism that pairs with the marked genetic structure.

Another technique showing great promise is that of fluorescent labeling. This process is independent of the need to grow the microorganisms. This technique can be used to rapidly detect all viable cells. Including both damaged and fastidious microorganisms that might be difficult to grow in a culture. In addition, there is no need for large numbers of organisms so there is no need for an incubation period.

Technical and financial benefits gained from implementation of some of these methods are significant but they are in reality only useful for those laboratories with a large number of determinations needed on a regular basis. No doubt technology will move in the direction of even more definitive testing, including systems engineered for smaller laboratories and even bedside testing.

N THE LAB

BASIC MICROBIOLOGY PROCEDURES
MANUAL MICROBIOLOGY PROCEDURE #1
Specimen Setup for Isolation and Identification
Principles

Bacterial infections may be contracted from many sources, including food, water, sexual practices, contact with dirty surfaces or equipment, and directly from another human or animal. Coughing and sneezing (which generate droplets and aerosols containing bacteria) onto surfaces and contact between the hands and mucus membranes are convenient routes for passing bacteria and other microorganisms to others.

Typically, bacterial specimens are collected by physicians or nurses and transported to the laboratory. Following collection of a specimen with microbiological organisms, the first step in processing it is to provide an environment (media) on which the organisms will grow to numbers sufficient for identification and other testing, such as antibiotic sensitivity procedures. Many bacteria will not survive extreme heat or cold and should be inoculated on a nutrient media as soon as possible. During collection of the sample, the sterile tube or plated media may be inoculated directly with a bacterial specimen. Unfortunately, it is easy to contaminate a specimen through careless handling. Media that are designed to grow bacteria and fungi are easily contaminated even by the air and the organisms in suspension there.

The source of the culture and the type of organism suspected will dictate the type of media on which the bacterial specimen is placed. Growth of the organisms on the nutrient media is enhanced by conditions close to those encountered in the human body. This is achieved by using an incubator. A sufficient number of organisms must be grown to make possible morphological studies and staining, the first steps in organism identification.

A variety of solid and liquid media are available for meeting the nutritive needs of bacteria and for growing them in numbers that allow for their identification (Figure 15-3). Appropriate media must be chosen for inoculating and streaking plates for isolation of bacterial colonies. Specimens screening is based in part on the site from which organisms were obtained, as certain organisms are more likely to be found in certain anatomic regions of the body.

Safety Alert

The laboratory student or professional must always be aware of and practice personal safety when performing microbiological procedures. Such procedures require the handling of viable organisms as part of the process of accurately identifying and ensuring the growth and survival of those organisms. Some of the equipment used in microbiological procedures is also inherently dangerous, such as the heated incinerator that sterilizes the loops and needles used to inoculate slides and agar plates.

Most laboratory-acquired infections are acquired via the respiratory route when treating patients and handling specimens. To prevent this, it is incumbent upon lab personnel to avoid producing aerosols when incinerating, centrifuging, or otherwise working with samples. A variety of shields and biological safety cabinets are designed to minimize and help prevent the production of aerosols. In addition to respiratory precautions, disinfectants should be used on a continuous basis to prevent the hands from becoming contaminated and then placed near a mucus membrane such as the nose or mouth.

IN THE LAB

Equipment and Supplies

1. Gloves, disposable paper towels, and disinfectant or other cleaning solution
2. Swabs tipped with cotton or synthetic material (to be used to transfer organisms) or reusable or sterile disposable inoculating metal loops and needles
3. Bacterial incinerator if reusable metal loops and needles are being used, OR sterile disposable loops and needles
4. Incubator for enhancing growth of bacteria (set at 36°C–37°C)
5. Agar plates (Petri dishes)
6. Source of organisms such as stock cultures on agar plates or in broth (liquid media) tubes
7. Waterproof sharp marker
8. Disposal containers appropriate for biohazardous waste

Procedure

1. Wash hands and don gloves.
2. Assemble necessary equipment and supplies.
3. If reusable metal loops and needles are being used, turn on incinerator and check that it has reached the optimum level of heat.
4. Select the proper agar plate (Petri dish) and use the marker to label it with appropriate identifying information.
5. Introduce the sterile swab or sterilized or disposable metal loop into the broth tube or pick up an isolated colony of bacteria from an agar plate.
6. Taking care not to touch any other surfaces with the swab or metal loop, lift the lid from a sterile agar plate slightly and inoculate a fourth of the plate by rolling the swab over the surface, taking care not to tear the agar.
7. Replace the lid on the agar plate and dispose of the swab in a biohazard container.
8. Streak the remainder of the agar surface by touching the sterile loop or a needle (this takes skill and a light touch) to the first quadrant and streaking all the way to the opposite side of the second quadrant, repeating the process 7 or 8 times (Figure 15-4). This serves to isolate colonies of bacteria and to allow multiple strains of organisms to be separated.

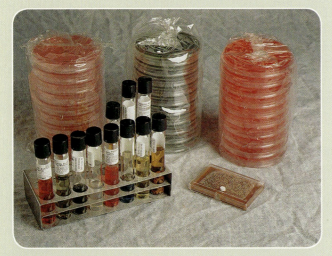

FIGURE 15-3 Different types of nutrient media required for certain bacterial organisms.
Source: Delmar/Cengage Learning.

9. Touch the loop to the second quadrant and streak all the way across the third quadrant, again repeating the process 7 or 8 times

10. Streak the fourth quadrants to produce isolation of bacterial colonies in much the same manner as was done for the second and third quadrants (Figure 15-4). Sterilize the inoculating loop or needle by using the incinerator for several seconds, then place the loop handle into the stand attached to the incinerator. Take care not to contaminate the loop or needle after sterilizing it following use, as the hot metal may burn burn the hands or work surface.

11. Differential biochemical disks aid in identification of certain organisms and are indicated for some cultures. This is done by placing appropriate differentiating discs on the surface of the inoculated agar plate. These discs contain certain chemicals that affect the growth of the bacteria and are based on the source of the culture (throat, etc.) and the suspected species of bacteria. This is done after streaking the media and before incubating the agar plate.

12. Identify the inoculated media on the lid by using a permanent marker capable of withstanding the moist heat of an incubator. The identification information may include a patient's ID number or name.

13. Replace the lid on the inoculated agar plate and place it upside down in an incubator set at 36°C–37°C.

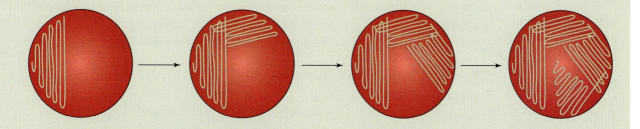

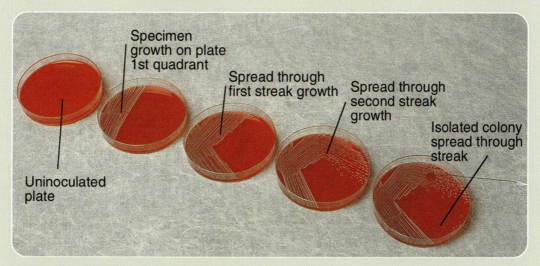

FIGURE 15-4 **Streaking for isolation of bacterial colonies.**
Source: Delmar/Cengage Learning.

IN THE LAB

14. Discard all supplies used for the procedure in the appropriate containers. A disinfectant should be used to clean the work surfaces and equipment should be cleaned and restored to its former position. Gloves should be discarded appropriately and the hands washed thoroughly in accordance with established policies.

15. After 24 hours, examine the agar plate for characteristic bacterial growth. Note that personal safety precautions (wash hands, gloves, clean up) should be followed before and after examining the plate.

Quality Control

Known specimens are cultured and stained on a regular basis to insure conditions are adequate to support the culturing of bacteria.

Reporting of Results

Worksheets are generally kept for each culture initiated. If there is no growth, the plate is reported as "no growth" and is incubated for an additional day. When colony growth is observed, it is important to perform a colony count for some organisms. Samples of colony growth are subcultured (transferred to other agar plates) and the organisms identified and records. More than one organism may be present.. The final report most often takes two days, and should include identification of all organism(s) and if appropriate, an antibiotic sensitivity report indicating the antibiotic to which the organism(s) is/are sensitive.

MANUAL MICROBIOLOGY PROCEDURE #2

Preparation of Smears

Principles

In some cases, exudates (discharge as from a wound) or body fluids such as cerebrospinal fluid (CSF) can be stained directly to gain critical information regarding the type of bacteria that may be present. This is often attempted in cases where a quick presumptive identification is crucial for the patient's health, such as with organisms in CSF. Most slides for staining, however, are obtained from cultures. If mixed cultures of more than one type of bacteria (as observed on an agar plate) are present, separate testing must be done on each type of bacteria. Note that it is not possible to separate the various species of organisms in broth or other liquid mixed cultures. Bacterial smears for staining must be heat fixed prior to initiating the staining process to prevent the organisms from washing off the slide during the staining procedure.

Several methods are employed for preparing smears for staining. The method selected depends upon the type of specimen and type of media, as well as personal preference of the laboratory professional or the skill level of the worker.

Equipment and Supplies

1. Gloves, disposable paper towels, and disinfectant or other cleaning solution
2. Swabs tipped with cotton or synthetic material (to be used to transfer organisms) or reusable or sterile disposable inoculating metal loops and needles.

3. Disposable droppers or Pasteur pipettes
4. Bacterial incinerator or Bunsen burner for heat-fixing slide
5. Source of organisms such as stock cultures on agar plates or in broth (liquid media) tubes
6. Microscope slides (do not need to be sterile but should be free of oil drops, dust, lint, and fingerprints)
7. Forceps to handle slides being heat-fixed
8. Clean tap or deionized water
9. Waterproof sharp marker
10. Disposal containers appropriate for biohazardous waste and sharps container for disposing of slides

Procedure

1. Wash hands and don gloves.
2. Assemble necessary equipment and supplies.
3. Turn on the bacterial incinerator at least 5 minutes before beginning the procedure.
4. Use the marker to identify a clean slide with the specimen number or patient name. Place a drop of clean tap or deionized water onto the center of the slide.
5. Select one of the following methods for preparing smears for straining.
   a. When an agar plate is the source of the organisms, gently touch the tip of a sterile cotton or synthetic fiber swab to a bacterial colony and roll it onto the slide, mixing it in with the drop of water (Figure 15-5Aand 15-5B).
   b. When an agar plate is the source of the organisms, an inoculating needle or loop may be used in lieu of a swab (a needle is easiest for picking from isolated bacterial colonies). Touch the tip of the needle into a single colony of bacteria, then insert the needle tip into the drop of water on the slide and gently roll the needle to remove the organisms from the tip. Spread the mixture to form a smear covering a quarter-sized area. If a loop is used, mix the loop's contents with the water and again spread the mixture over a quarter-sized area.

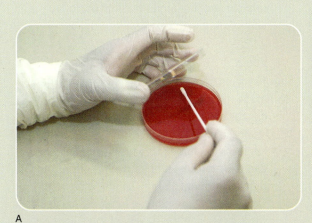
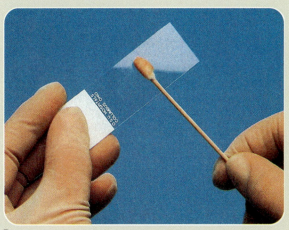

A   B

FIGURE 15-5 Making a smear from a bacterial culture on an agar plate for staining.
Source: Delmar/Cengage Learning.

IN THE LAB

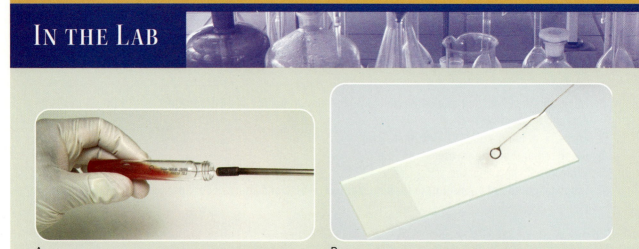

A   B

FIGURE 15-6 Making a smear from a bacterial culture in an inoculated broth or agar slant for staining.
Source: Delmar/Cengage Learning.

c. If using inoculated broth or an agar slant in tubes, a sterilized metal loop or a disposable loop is used to take a loopful of inoculated broth or a small amount of the organisms from the agar slant (Figure 15-6A and 15-6B).

6. Allow the smear to dry (approximately 30 seconds to 1 minute). If excess water is used, the time for drying may be slightly longer).

7. Heat fix the slide by using the forceps to hold the slide near the opening of a bacterial incinerator (Figure 15-7). If a Bunsen burner is available, gently pass the slide through the flame until the slide has become quite hot.

8. Allow the slide to cool to room temperature.

9. The slide is ready for staining.

10. Discard all supplies used for the procedure in the appropriate containers. A disinfectant should be used to clean the work surfaces and equipment should be cleaned and restored to its former position. Gloves should be discarded appropriately and the hands washed thoroughly in accordance with established policies.

Reporting of Results

The slide should be examined for consistency of the mixture. It is possible to have small clumps of bacteria present in the water droplet or the liquid from a broth culture. Excessive numbers of clumps may interfere with distribution of organisms and staining patterns, and require a repeat slide to be made. Smears should be thin enough as to barely be visible. After assessing the quality of the smear for suitability, the slide should then be stained for microscopic examination (see Procedure #3).

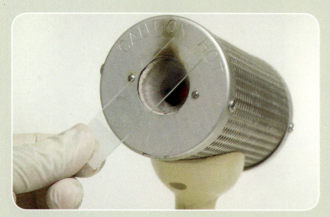

FIGURE 15-7 Heat-fixing bacterial smear to prevent washing from slide during staining.
Source: Delmar/Cengage Learning.

MANUAL MICROBIOLOGY PROCEDURE #3

Performing a Gram Stain

Principles

The most frequently performed stain in the microbiology department is the Gram stain. Staining of bacteria is necessary as it is virtually impossible to see and describe the morphology of the organisms unless they are stained. Bacteria are small and have little natural color for most species, so the Gram stain provides for differentiation as to the shape of the organisms as well as providing further aid in identification by labeling the organisms as either Gram-positive or Gram-negative. Differences in the cell walls of bacteria are based on their chemical constituents, which in turn accounts for the staining difference. Gram-negative cell walls contain more lipids (fats), polysaccharides, and lipoprotein complexes (including amino acids) than do those of the walls of a Gram-positive organism. The cell walls of both Gram-positive and Gram-negative organisms will absorb crystal violet, but Gram negative organisms will lose the crystal violet in the decolorizing step, and will then absorb the safranin, which imparts a pink to orange color to them. The Gram positive organisms will not lose their crystal violet during decolorizing and will appear purple in color.

The four-part Gram-staining procedure is outlined here and provided in detail below. The heat-fixed smear is placed on a staining rack and is flooded with crystal violet (the primary stain). After 30 seconds to a minute, the slide is gently washed under a stream of water and returned to the staining rack. Gram's iodine is then poured over the smear. After 30 seconds to a minute, the slide is again gently washed under a stream of water. The slide is then held at a 30- to 40-degree angle and quickly rinsed with an acetone-alcohol mixture. This will decolorize the organism if it is a Gram-negative species of bacteria. The decolorizing process only takes a few seconds. All color should run from a slide containing predominantly Gram-negative organisms. Finally, a counterstain (safranin) is poured over the slide. Gram-negative organisms absorb and retain the counterstain.

Equipment and Supplies

1. Gloves, disposable paper towels, and disinfectant or other cleaning solution
2. Bibulous paper
3. Bacterial smears (slides) created in Procedure #2 (both Gram positive and Gram negative species) (slides should be cool)
4. Clean tap or deionized water
5. Staining rack on sink and drying rack
6. Gram stain kit containing crystal violet, Gram's iodine, acetone-alcohol decolorizer, safranine
7. Electronic timing device or clock/watch with second hand
8. Disposal containers appropriate for biohazardous waste and sharps container for disposing of slides

Procedure

1. Wash hands and don gloves.
2. Assemble necessary equipment and supplies.

IN THE LAB

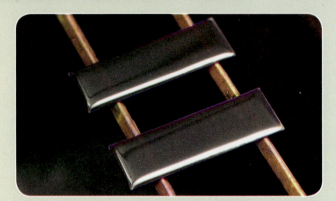

FIGURE 15-8 Slides staining on rack designed for Gram staining. Source: Delmar/Cengage Learning.

3. Place the slide(s) prepared in Procedure #2 on a staining rack positioned over a sink to permit draining of the solutions (Figure 15-8).
4. Flood the slide with crystal violet.
5. After 30 seconds to a minute, gently wash the slide with clean tap or deionized water, using a weak stream of water.
6. Return the slide to the staining rack.
7. Flood the slide with Gram's iodine.
8. After 30 seconds to a minute, again gently wash the slide with clean tap or deionized water, using a weak stream of water.
9. Holding the slide at a 30- to 40-degree angle over the sink, quickly decolorize the slide's contents by flooding the slide briefly (10 seconds) with an acetone-alcohol mixture (do not over-decolorize the slide—only a few seconds are required for this process). All color will run from a slide containing predominantly Gram-negative organisms.
10. Briefly rinse the decolorizer from the slide with a weak stream of clean tap or deionized water, then drain the water from the slide briefly. Return the slide to the staining rack.
11. Flood the slide with a counterstain of safranin.
12. Rinse the slide gently with tap water and place in a vertical position in a slotted rack designed for standing slides on their ends.
13. Gently blot the slide dry with the bibulous paper before examining it under a microscope.
14. Discard all supplies used for the procedure in the appropriate containers. A disinfectant should be used to clean the work surfaces and equipment should be cleaned and restored to its former position. Gloves should be discarded appropriately and the hands washed thoroughly in accordance with established policies.

Reporting of Results

The smear is read microscopically using the oil-immersion objective. Results are reported as either Gram-positive or Gram-negative, and as rods (rod-shaped organisms) or as cocci (spherical in shape). Sometimes rod-shaped organisms that are extremely short are reported as coccobacilli. Some species of cocci occur in pairs and are called diplococci.

SUMMARY

Clinical microbiology is a valuable component of the clinical laboratory, regardless of the lab's size. Although identification of organisms is more sophisticated today, the underlying principles are the same. The microbiologist and the students performing basic microbiological procedures must practice safety for themselves as a primary responsibility. The microbiology student must learn about the basic equipment and supplies required for performing basic procedures, and how to safely store and use these supplies and equipment. A number of media are used for the initial culturing of microorganisms, and each is designed for a specific purpose. Following the inoculation of the appropriate media based on the source of the culture, growth from the media will be stained and evaluated microscopically. Then, certain chemical reactions will be performed to further differentiate the type of organism to be identified. The next step may be that of performing antibiotic sensitivity testing to determine the antimicrobial agent that would be most effective in treating the infection. Equally important as handling samples carefully and avoiding becoming contaminated or contaminating the culture itself by careless handling, the wastes, which are most infectious in nature, require proper handling for disposal.

REVIEW QUESTIONS

1. What is required for bacteria to grow before they can be identified?
2. After growing colonies of bacteria, what is the next step to identifying the organism?
3. What discovery gave a clue that microscopic organisms are present in almost all areas of our lives?
4. What is meant by bacterial susceptibility or sensitivity testing?
5. What is meant by antibiotic-resistant strains of bacteria?

IMMUNOLOGY AND SEROLOGY

KEY TERMS

Acute phase
Agglutination
Convalescent phase
Direct Method
Fomites
Inanimate (nonliving) objects
Indirect Method

Latex reagent
Memory cells
Postzone
Prozone
Qualitative procedure
Quantitative procedure
Rheumatoid arthritis (RA)

Semiquantitative procedure
Serial dilution
Systemic lupus erythematosus (SLE)
Titer
Transfusion
Undiluted

INTRODUCTION

Principle of the Immune Reaction

Most of the organisms and foreign bodies that invade our bodies will elicit an immune response. A number of reactions take place, from reddening and swelling to producing heat and pain. These invasive organisms and other substances such as environmental toxins and chemicals are called *antigens*. Certain white cells of our bodies attempt to combat this invasion; specialized cells try to engulf or eat the antigens (to phagocytize), while others produce antibodies against the antigens. Some of these invasive organisms may be identified by the **direct method** which tests for specific antigens, while other types of antigens may be identified by the **indirect method** where specific antibodies for those antigens are measured.

The terms *immunology* and *serology* are often used interchangeably. Immunology more accurately describes the functions of the immune system, while serology refers to the actual testing of the samples, usually of blood serum. Immunologic laboratory procedures are based primarily on the reactions of specific antibodies to antigens, which may be foreign invaders of the body. Antigens may be transplanted tissue cells, bacteria, viruses, parasites, and even **fomites** or **inanimate (nonliving) objects** such as pollen, chemicals, or toxins that may produce a reaction from the individual who has been invaded by one of these materials. Immunology differs from immunohematology (blood banking; see Chapter 17), which is chiefly related to the deliberate transplantation (**transfusion**) of blood cells and platelets into a recipient, to ensuring that blood is free from organisms such as HIV and hepatitis, and to studying antigens and antibodies associated with blood transfusion and those complications of pregnancy where a mother may produce antibodies against the blood of her fetus. Transplanted blood cells may cause a rapid and serious reaction if they are not compatible with the person receiving the transfusion.

Immunology is based on a study of the components of the immune system and involves a unified attack by the body against dangerous materials that enter or attempt to enter the body. The body engineers specific antibodies against antigens, or foreign invaders, of the body. Once the body has been invaded by a particular antigen, **memory cells** (a type of white cell called leukocytes) will remember the previous invasion, sometimes for the lifetime of the individual. Each subsequent invasion will precipitate a repeat reaction with a rapid buildup of antibodies. This rise in the antibody level will provide the basis for immunological tests. These tests are called *serological tests* because they use serum to perform the laboratory procedures. Sometimes the stage to which a disease has progressed may be determined by the level of antibodies that have been produced against a specific antigen.

Many quick tests that are easy to perform have become available in the past few decades. Many of them are quite simple and have been deemed a "waived" test, not requiring any special training, education, or skills to perform. Tests may be assigned to the waived category under the Clinical Laboratory Improvement Amendments of 1988 (CLIA 88), which provide federal government oversight for laboratory practice. Many of these tests are based on an antibody-antigen reaction.

In some cases, the results for a serological test are reported merely as a positive or negative response, which is called a **qualitative procedure. Semiquantitative procedures** are performed when it is important to determine if the results exceed the normal levels of antibodies that can be expected when no active disease is present. Most serological testing is intended to identify the body's response to attacking foreign invaders. In *autoimmune diseases*, the body produces antibodies against its own tissues or cells. Although no foreign tissue has been transplanted, the tissues may have become altered and are not recognized as normal by the immune system. Testing is performed in the same manner for autoimmune diseases as for responses to bacteria and viruses. A significant number of autoimmune diseases are covered thoroughly in specific courses related to immunology and serology. Examples of autoimmune diseases are **rheumatoid arthritis (RA)** where joint tissue becomes inflamed and therefore altered, and **systemic lupus erythematosus (SLE)**, in which antibodies are formed against the nuclear material of the body's cells.

Quantitative and Semiquantitative Procedures

Quantitative procedures are tests that attempt to quantify the numbers, amounts, or levels of certain constituents of the blood. Some serological procedures are sophisticated enough to qualify as quantitative, but the majority of common serological tests are semiquantitative, in that they measure only the dilutional strength of an antibody level, rather than actual numbers of antibodies. Antibody titers (dilutions of antibodies) are indirect and semiquantitative tests. Because antibodies formed against disease vary widely from individual to individual, a result may be significant or nonsignificant according to the level of antibodies present. Some individuals will not produce an antibody level sufficient to support the diagnosis of a certain disease. Other serological tests are available for determining if white cells themselves are competent for performing their destructive work on foreign invaders. This set of procedures is rarely requested, and is extremely specialized work that is usually beyond the scope of a routine hospital laboratory. Most of these tests are performed in large commercial reference laboratories that perform a sufficient quantity of tests to make it economical to set up the procedure.

Serial dilutions (dilutions of serum) reacted with specific antigens available in commercially prepared laboratory test kits comprise the bulk of serological tests. A titer, which includes dilutions of serum to determine the approximate level of antibodies present, yields valuable data as to the stage of the disease. The acute phase for most organisms infecting the body occurs within hours to days of exposure, depending on previous exposure to a certain organism, which if present may cause a more rapid rise in antibody levels. The convalescent phase comes later when the level of antibodies subsides and the infected person has overcome the disease and is usually free of symptoms of the disease. This information enables the physician to determine whether the patient's immune system has responded adequately or if a chronic, or long-term, disease process is in place.

Critical Reminders
Prozone and Postzone Reactions

Two phenomena—prozone and postzone reactions—can produce false-negative results in common serological reactions called agglutination and precipitation, and the laboratory professional must be alert to these possibilities. There is an optimum proportion of antibody-antigen levels in a sample that yields valid results, but prozone and postzone reactions yield erroneous results. For some procedures, both undiluted and diluted samples are tested for these conditions before a quantitative antibody titer is performed. A prozone reaction occurs when there is an excess of antibodies compared with the amount of antigens present. In undiluted and low-dilution samples, this condition creates a zone with relatively high antibody concentrations where no reaction occurs, yielding a false-negative result. In addition, if low levels of antibody are present, the agglutination may be too weak to observe. A postzone reaction occurs when excess antigen is present, so there is a lack of agglutination or precipitation and a false-negative result is also obtained. In the serial dilution test for antibodies called an antibody titer, a prozone reaction will result in a negative value for the low dilution portions of the test and will become positive at higher dilutions.

METHODOLOGIES EMPLOYED IN IMMUNOLOGY AND SEROLOGY

It is important for the clinical laboratory student to understand that the basic serological test is an indirect test to determine the presence of antibodies against antigens, not to identify the antigen itself. Most tests in serology are of the indirect type, where a known antigen, purchased most often from a commercial provider, is used to test for antibodies against the organism. If antibodies exist against a certain antigen, then it is presumed that the patient is infected or has been exposed and maintains a certain level of antibodies. This system is explained thoroughly in anatomy and physiology classes as well as academic classes for immunology and serology.

Some direct tests are available in a few cases. Antigens present in blood or body fluids and human wastes may be tested for directly, such as parasites in the blood (e.g., malaria) or in the stool of a patient. Some tests in serology and immunology use a system in which radioactive, enzymatic, and other "tags" are attached to an antigen or antibody. These tagged antigens or antibodies are then counted or otherwise detailed for the degree of infection. Other technologically advanced procedures are either available or on the drawing board. This component of the laboratory will most likely offer the most advances for new procedures in the future.

The student will be exposed to only a few basic procedures to begin developing the awareness and skills required to perform most serological tests. Some are rather simple slide tests and others offer results that are semiquantitative, such as dilutions of serum. Many simple slide tests are now available for at-home testing, such as the home pregnancy test, which is actually an antigen-antibody reaction. The tests offered here are only a few of the most basic procedures to help orient the new student to the clinical laboratory, and not to train the student to be technologically competent. That will come later in a comprehensive program for medical laboratory technology.

IN THE LAB

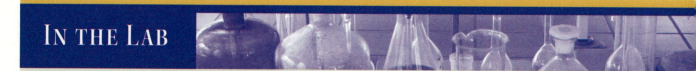

BASIC SEROLOGY PROCEDURES
MANUAL SEROLOGY PROCEDURE #1
Serial Dilution Procedure (Two-Fold Antibody Titer)
Principles

Serial dilutions are used for a number of purposes in a clinical laboratory. Dilutions of serum or plasma are often required for a variety of semi-quantitative and quantitative serological tests. The serial dilution titer is often ordered for certain infectious diseases where dilutions of serum are required for the performance of quantitative tests. The physician may use this procedure to determine if a patient is successfully combating an infection, is in an acute or convalescent state, or has an immunodeficiency. Most often, the dilution will be made of antibodies found in the serum or plasma. In some cases, the dilutions will be made of antigens.

Perhaps the most common serial dilution is the antibody titer. The antibody titer procedure is based on the humoral response of a patient to his or her infective state. In these cases, serial dilutions of the patient's serum to determine a semi-quantitative level of antibodies against a specific antigen may be required. Normal saline, which approximates the amount of sodium chloride found in the plasma, is commonly used as a fluid for diluting the samples. The higher the dilution, the higher is the amount of antibodies or antigens that are being tested for because larger amounts of the diluting fluid are being used. As the dilutional ratio becomes higher, the amount of the original sample becomes smaller and the amount of diluent becomes larger. This concept is sometimes difficult for the beginning laboratory technician or technologist to understand. The following procedure should serve to inform the student of the purpose and theory behind a serial dilution titer.

When a serial dilution is performed on a patient's serum, it is necessary to observe the pattern of positive test results obtained. A phenomenon called a prozone reaction may cause results to be negative in early, less dilute specimens, while increasingly stronger reactions are seen as the dilutions become more dilute. This situation arises when the level of antibodies is extremely elevated and the optimum level of antibody to antigen is exceeded. To find the titer (antibody level) of a certain antibody, clinical laboratory workers prepare serial dilutions of a serum sample, usually in a two-fold dilution pattern, where each subsequent dilution halves the level of antibodies in the diluted serum.

An antibody titer that consists of serial dilutions of serum is a semi-quantitative serological procedure. It is used to determine the stage of infection or the patient's response to a medical condition. In setting up a serial dilution, the patient's sample is diluted the number of times that will yield a significant titer (level of antibodies). Samples are set up by consistently doubling the dilution by a factor of 2 for each tube: 1:2, 1:4, 1:8, etc. (Figure 16-1). This is called a two-fold dilutional titer and is the most common ratio used for antibody titers.

However, dilutions are not always by a factor of 2; sometimes, factors of 10 may be used, such as with dilutions of 1:10, 1:20, etc. This also results in a doubling of the ratio for each successive tube. Sometimes it is necessary to make dilutions for

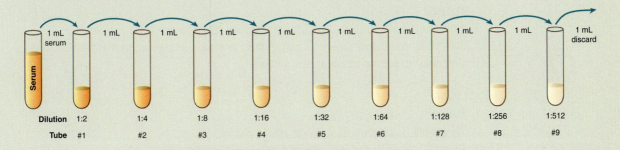

1. Set up 9 tubes, each containing 1 mL of diluent.
2. Transfer 1 mL of patient serum to tube 1.
3. Mix the serum and diluent, and transfer 1 mL of the mixture to tube 2.
4. Repeat the procedure, transferring 1 mL each time after mixing with diluent.
5. Discard 1 mL from the last tube.
6. When dilution series is complete, each of the 9 tubes should contain 1 mL.

FIGURE 16-1 Setting up a two-fold dilution series.
Source: Delmar/Cengage Learning.

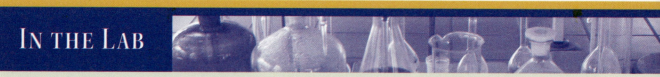

IN THE LAB

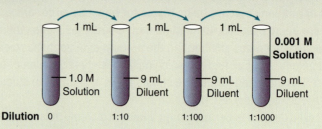

| Dilution | 0 | 1:10 | 1:100 | 1:1000 |

FIGURE 16-2 Making a 10-fold compound dilution.
Source: Delmar/Cengage Learning.

purposes other than for antibody titers, such as a 10-fold dilution. It is sometimes necessary to perform a procedure called a compound dilution, where concentrated reagent or a patient sample requires a larger dilution. For instance, it might be necessary to prepare a 0.0001 M solution from a 1.0 M solution; in such instances, a series of dilutions may be necessary to achieve the low concentration desired. Figure 16-2 depicts how this is accomplished.

Equipment and Supplies

1. Gloves, disposable paper towels, and disinfectant or other cleaning solution
2. Report form for Procedure #1
3. Serological pipettes for measuring diluents
4. Transfer pipettes for diluting specimens
5. At least ten clear test tubes (13 × 100 mm or smaller preferred) and test tube rack
6. Diluent (water or normal saline is commonly used)
7. Waterproof sharp markers
8. Fresh and uncontaminated serum specimen, preferably clear of hemolysis or lipemia
9. Centrifuge with head that will accommodate 13 × 100 mm tubes or smaller
10. Test kit containing antigen corresponding to antibodies being tested for
11. Illuminating lamp with magnifying mirror

Procedure

1. Wash hands and don gloves.
2. Assemble necessary equipment and supplies.
3. Place 10 tubes in a test rack and label as shown below:

Tube #1	1:2	Tube #6	1:64
Tube #2	1:4	Tube #7	1:128
Tube #3	1:8	Tube #8	1:256
Tube #4	1:16	Tube #9	1:512
Tube #5	1:32	Tube #10	Negative Control

4. Place 1.0 mL of the diluent into tubes #1 through #10.
5. Place 1.0 mL of undiluted plasma or serum (solute) into tube #1. This tube now has a total volume of 2.0 mL and a dilution ratio of 1:2.
6. Transfer 1.0 mL from tube #1 into tube #2. Tube #2 now has a total volume of 2.0 mL and a dilution ratio of 1:4.
7. Continue in this manner, transferring 1.0 mL of the preceding diluted specimen through tube #9. Tube #9 will now contain 2.0 mL.
8. Discard 1.0 mL of the diluted specimen from tube #9. Tubes #1 through #9 each now contain 1.0 mL of the diluted specimen.
9. Add the specific antigen for which the antibody titer is being performed to each tube (#1 through #10), and mix the contents.
10. Centrifuge tubes #1 through #10 for 4 minutes.
11. Record the results on the appropriate report form (Procedure # 1 Report Form). Place a (+) in the box indicating a positive reaction. The result will be reflected by the last tube showing a positive reaction (clumping or agglutination). It may be necessary to use an illuminating lamp with magnifying mirror to observe a weak endpoint where very small clumps are present in the last tube to show a positive reaction.

Procedure #1 Report Form: Serial Dilution Procedure (Two-Fold Antibody Titer)

	Tube 1	Tube 2	Tube 3	Tube 4	Tube 5	Tube 6	Tube 7	Tube 8	Tube 9	Tube 10 Control
Dilution	1:2	1:4	1:8	1:16	1:32	1:64	1:128	1:256	1:512	No reaction
Result										

12. Discard all supplies used for the procedure in the appropriate containers. A disinfectant should be used to clean the work surfaces and equipment should be cleaned and restored to its former position. Gloves should be discarded appropriately and the hands washed thoroughly in accordance with established policies.

Reporting of Results

The results for tests such as a quantitative pregnancy test, viral titer, or rheumatoid arthritis test for the rheumatoid factor are expressed in terms of the highest dilution tube in which a reaction can be detected.

MANUAL SEROLOGY PROCEDURE #2

Determining the Presence of C-Reactive Protein in Serum

Principles

C-reactive protein (CRP) is an important diagnostic tool arising from the protein included in acute-phase reactants. CRP is a nonspecific indicator of inflammation and is valuable in screening for chronic diseases such as arteriosclerosis or a buildup of plaque in the vessels of the body, which often predicts the risk for a

IN THE LAB

coronary attack. CRP appears to assist in the binding of complement to damaged cells, foreign organisms, and cells that have invaded the body. This binding enhances phagocytosis or eating by macrophages of opsonin-mediated organisms or cells (those coated with antibodies). The term phagocyte literally means "big eater" and refers to a type of protective cell that develops from a white cell called a monocyte. Phagocytes express a receptor on their cell surfaces for CRP. CRP is also believed to play an important role in innate immunity, as an early defense system against infections. When inflammatory processes are present, CRP levels in a patient may rise to 50,000 times the normal concentration. CRP rises above normal limits usually within 6 hours and peaks at 48 hours following a heart attack or a traumatic injury or infection.

Several procedures for testing for CRP are available from various manufacturers. Testing for CRP is often used in conjunction with other procedures to narrow the possibilities of certain ailments during a diagnosis. Although the procedure was developed in the 1930s, it was seldom used for several decades due to its lack of specificity. However, it has enjoyed increased stature in recent years, as the presence of CRP in the serum or plasma often indicates inflammation of the arteries (arteritis), which may indicate an impending heart attack.

Performing a CRP procedure requires care, including the following precautions:
- All reagents and specimens should be at room temperature before use.
- Avoid contaminating reagents with each other or with test specimens.
- The latex reagent should be gently mixed but not vigorously shaken before use. Dispense contents of the dropper and refill as needed for multiple tests.
- Both positive control and negative controls should be run concurrently with each specimen or batch of specimens. Do not dilute the controls before testing.
- Small amounts of detergent or residue from previous specimens may adversely affect the results, so use only a thoroughly cleaned glass slide. Use only deionized or distilled water to clean the slide and avoid the use of detergents.
- The results must be read at 2 minutes as erroneously false positive results may occur when the time limit is exceeded.

Equipment and Supplies
1. Gloves, disposable paper towels, and disinfectant or other cleaning solution
2. Report form provided by your instructor
3. Kit for measuring CRP, containing latex reagent, positive and negative controls, and a specialized glass slide that makes it easier to see the results (These slides often provide a black background for reading a fine white precipitate.)
4. Test tubes with rack appropriate for the test tube size (size of the test tubes is not important)
5. Deionized water or normal saline for diluting samples to obtain a semi-quantitative result, if required by the test methodology

6. Serological pipettes or semiautomated diluters for making dilutions of samples
7. Mechanical rotator (optional) (The low speed for rotating the slide does not always lend itself to the need for a mechanical rotator and for most kits the slide can be rotated by hand.)
8. Specimen of unhemolyzed serum
9. Electronic timing device or clock/watch with second hand

Procedure

1. Wash hands and don gloves.
2. Assemble necessary equipment and supplies.
3. Specimens are tested from both undiluted and diluted specimens by diluting a specimen to 1:10 with the prepared diluent.
   a. Prepare a 1:10 dilution of specimen by pipetting 0.1 ml specimen into a test tube with 0.9 mL of diluent.
4. Place 1 drop (approximately 50 μL) of undiluted specimen into one of the rings on the slide and 1 drop (approximately 50 μL) of the 1:10 diluted specimen into a second ring.
5. Place 1 drop each of the positive control and 1 drop of the negative control into two additional rings on the slide.
6. Add 1 drop of well-mixed latex reagent to each section.
7. Using a new stirrer (usually provided with the kit) for each ring to avoid carry over from one sample to the next, mix thoroughly and spread the mixture over the entire area.
8. Rock slide evenly and gently by hand 8 to 10 times per minute for 2 minutes.
9. Observe each mixture immediately at 2 minutes for agglutination, which will be visible to the naked eye. Failure to do so may cause erroneous results.
10. Record results of controls and unknown specimens on the appropriate form.
11. Wash slides quickly following completion of the procedure as residue may dry on the slide, then rinse with deionized water.
12. Discard all supplies used for the procedure in the appropriate containers. A disinfectant should be used to clean the work surfaces and equipment should be cleaned and restored to its former position. Gloves should be discarded appropriately and the hands washed thoroughly in accordance with established policies.

Reporting of Results

A number of limitations for the test are observed when interpreting the results of the test. Test results are often confirmed by clinical signs and symptoms as well as correlation with other test results.

1. As in many diagnostic laboratory procedures, results obtained with this test yield data that must be evaluated in light of the total clinical information obtained by the physician.

IN THE LAB

2. Specimens showing gross hemolysis, lipemia, or turbidity should not be used.
3. The strength of agglutination is not indicative of the CRP concentration. Weak reactions may occur with slightly elevated or markedly elevated CRP concentrations.
4. Reaction times longer than 2 minutes may cause erroneous results.
5. The Immunex CRP slide test is classified as moderately complex under CLIA '88 regulations.

Interpretation of a positive test indicating the presence of CRP for a qualitative procedure is as follows:

1. A positive result will show visible agglutination and a negative result will appear smoothly turbid or milky in appearance. A test should be reported as positive if agglutination is found on either the diluted or the undiluted specimen, as the sensitivity of the test kit has been adjusted to avoid a large number of positives for those with normal levels of CRP.
2. When agglutination occurs only in the diluted specimen, it indicates an excess of antibodies in the undiluted specimen. This is called a prozone reaction and indicates that results would increase with additional dilutions of the serum.

Agglutination may occur only in the diluted specimen because of high levels of antibody in the undiluted specimen that are not in proportion to the amount of antigen present.

MANUAL SEROLOGY PROCEDURE #3
Rheumatoid Factor Direct Slide Test (Latex Agglutination)
Principles

A number of methods are available for testing for the rheumatoid factor (RF). RF is similar to an antigen but is actually based on antibodies against the immune globulins, which in themselves are a reaction against the disease. This serological test is therefore slightly different from those that simply test for antibody production against antigens that invade the body (Figure 16-3). The rheumatoid factor (RF) is a high molecular weight protein that is similar to an antibody and can bind to other antibodies. In cases of rheumatoid arthritis (RA), these antibodies bind to IgM antibodies as though they are antigens, producing agglutination. Other factors may yield positive results other than RA. The majority of test kits, such as the one shown for the Rheumatoid Factor (Figure 16-4) reveal agglutination on a special

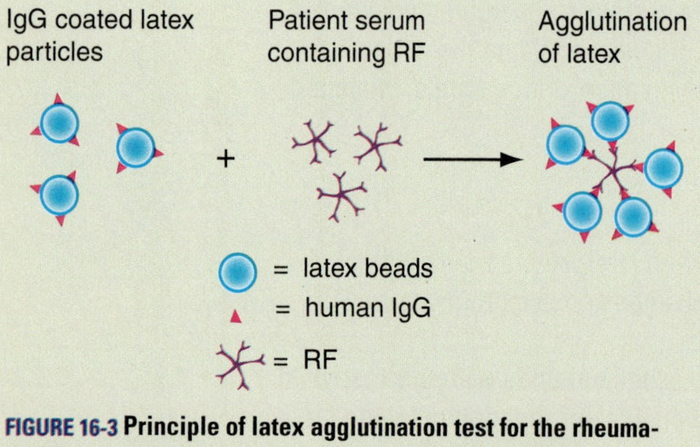

IgG coated latex particles   Patient serum containing RF   Agglutination of latex

= latex beads
= human IgG
= RF

FIGURE 16-3 Principle of latex agglutination test for the rheumatoid factor and other related antigen-antibody reactions. Source: Delmar/Cengage Learning.

slide for positive reactions. Other methods are available that use automated systems such as nephelometers. Nephelometers are similar to spectrophotometers but measure a phenomenon called precipitation rather than agglutination. Some manual tests provide for procedures that include a sophisticated method called enzyme immunoassay.

A number of limitations are associated with this procedure. As with other clinical laboratory procedures, the results obtained with the kits for determining the presence of RF must be evaluated by the physician by cor-relating the clinical picture of symptoms and signs. Those specimens showing gross hemolysis, lipemia, and turbidity should not be used, as these characteristics may indicate deterioration of the sample. The strength of agglutination in the procedure does not indicate the severity of the disease state. Weak reactions are possible with slightly elevated or markedly elevated antinuclear antibody concentrations. The antinuclear antibody test is designed for diagnosis of another autoimmune disease, systemic lupus erythematosus (SLE).

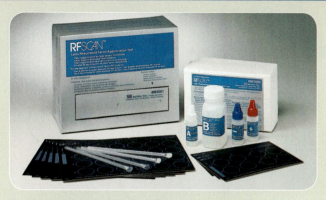

FIGURE 16-4 Rheumatoid factor latex agglutination kit. Source: Delmar/Cengage Learning.

Reaction times of more than 2 minutes may cause erroneous results. The ASI brand of a direct RF slide test is classified as moderately complex under CLIA '88 regulations, indicating that it should be performed by laboratory professionals.

Equipment and Supplies

1. Gloves, disposable paper towels, and disinfectant or other cleaning solution
2. Report form
3. Procedure kit (contains reagent, controls, and diluents)
4. Stirrer pipettes (act as both pipetters and contain a spatula end for stirring).
5. Test tubes (10 × 75 mm, or 13 × 100 mm) for diluting specimens and test tube rack
6. Serological pipettes
7. Volumetric pipette to deliver 0.25 mL
8. Mechanical rotator (optional) (The low speed for rotating the slide does not always lend itself to the need for a mechanical rotator and for most kits the slide can be rotated by hand.)
9. Electronic timing device or clock/watch with second hand

Procedure

1. Wash hands and don gloves.
2. Assemble necessary equipment and supplies.
3. Ensure that all reagents and specimens are at room temperature before use.
4. Exercise care to avoid contamination of reagents with each other or with the test specimens. Reagents contain sodium azide. Do not pipette by mouth!
5. Gently but thoroughly shake the latex reagent before use.

IN THE LAB

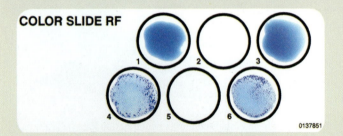

COLOR SLIDE RF

0137851

FIGURE 16-5 Illustration of typical reaction showing both positive and negative reactions.
Source: Delmar/Cengage Learning.

6. Run the positive control and negative control concurrently with each group of specimens tested. Do **not** dilute the controls before testing.

7. Using the stirrer pipettes, deliver one free-falling drop onto a separate circle for each unknown sample to be tested.

8. Place one drop each of the positive control and negative control into two additional rings on the slide.

9. Expel residual reagent in the dropper and refill. Add one drop of well-shaken latex reagent to each section containing sample and controls.

10. Using the flat end of a new stirrer for each ring, mix samples and reagent thoroughly, spreading mixture over entire area.

11. Rock slide evenly and gently by hand 8 to 10 times per minute for 2 minutes.

12. Observe each mixture immediately at the end of two minutes for agglutination (Figure 16-5). Failure to do so may cause erroneous results.

13. Record results of controls and unknown specimens on the appropriate form.

14. Wash slides quickly following completion of the procedure as residue may dry on the slide, then rinse with deionized water.

15. Discard all supplies used for the procedure in the appropriate containers. A disinfectant should be used to clean the work surfaces and equipment should be cleaned and restored to its former position. Gloves should be discarded appropriately and the hands washed thoroughly in accordance with established policies.

Reporting of Results

Typical test results (negative and positive) can be seen in Figure 16-5. Interpretation of results is quite simple. Positive results show visible agglutination and negative results appear uniformly turbid or milky. If either the undiluted or the diluted specimen shows agglutination, the result should be reported as positive. When agglutination occurs only in the diluted specimen, it indicates an excess of antibodies in the undiluted specimen. This is called a prozone reaction and indicates that results would increase with additional dilutions of the serum.

SUMMARY

A patient who has been exposed to or has become infected by a certain virus will form antibodies to combat the invading organism. Tests to determine these diseases may contain antigens that may include the actual organism that is infecting the patient but has been rendered harmless. Testing for a specific reaction between a patient's antibody and an infective organism is called an indirect method because only the antibodies are identified. Testing for the actual antigens (organisms) would be a direct method.

Basic principles of immunology, which may require a serological test using serum, a component of blood, are used to diagnose infectious diseases. In addition, serology is important in diagnosing many other disorders that may cause the formation of antibodies against microorganisms or altered tissues of the body. Knowledge of the immune system from an anatomy and physiology course would be valuable in understanding the concepts of immunology and serology.

This chapter discusses a few tests to orient the learner to the procedures for simple slide-type tests, as well as serial dilution of antibodies present. The value of this procedure is to determine an approximate antibody response to an infective organism. The physician may request an acute and a convalescent test, where two samples are collected 10 days apart. A higher value in the acute sample (the first) would indicate an early process in the disease. If the initial specimen is lower, and the convalescent level of antibodies has leveled off, the patient is recovering from the initial infection.

Treating various types of cancer is a growing segment of advances in immunology. A great deal of research is ongoing in which antibodies against tumor cells would become available. Efforts toward developing antibody treatment against malignant melanoma has gained much attention.

REVIEW QUESTIONS

1. Name at least five entities that may be viewed by the human body as an antigen that might elicit an antibody reaction.
2. Describe the difference between a qualitative and a quantitative test.
3. What is an autoimmune disease?
4. What is meant by a prozone reaction?
5. What is the basic difference between direct and indirect testing?

IMMUNOHEMATOLOGY (BLOOD BANKING)

INTRODUCTION

The original term for **immunohematology** was *blood banking*. Historically, collecting, testing, and storing blood for **transfusion** was extremely labor intensive; to a large extent, it still is. Blood banking is the last area of the laboratory where work is done on a piecemeal basis, with little automation, even though attempts have been and are being made to change this.

Separation of whole blood into its components is a process that entails a significant amount of time for properly, safely, and hygienically preparing products for component **transfusion**. Plasma is separated into platelets, coagulation factors, and volume expanders. White cells are harvested for transfusion into those who are immunocompromised and have low leukocyte counts.

One of the first semi-automated systems in immunohematology was the cell washer. Red blood cells, to be tested for antigens on their surfaces, must be cleaned of extraneous proteins from the plasma that coats the red cells. Cell washers are centrifuges that inject normal saline to maintain the red cell membrane integrity into each tube containing cells to be tested. Cells are centrifuged and the saline is removed from the "button" of red cells that remain following centrifugation. Automation eliminated a large amount of time spent in washing cells and freed technical personnel to perform other procedures while cells were being washed. But this was only the first step in labor-saving automation for immunohematology.

Additional advances have come particularly through the development of automated equipment for performing blood banking procedures such as grouping and typing, as well as for antibody screening and testing for hepatitis B virus (HBV), syphilis, and HIV. In the early 1970s, testing for HBV was entirely manual. The system evolved to use microtiter-based hemagglutination systems, then radioimmune assays and enzyme-linked immunoassays. Automation gradually advanced from plate readers to robotic sample processors, and in the early 1990s to automated microplate processing.

Pressure for automation is in part due to the increased prevalence of blood-borne infectious diseases. In addition to testing for the organism causing syphilis, laboratories in the United States must screen donor blood for the surface antigen of HBV, antibodies to HBV core, hepatitis C virus (HVC), HIV types 1 and 2 (both of which cause AIDS and are clinically the same), and human T-cell lymphotropic virus (HTLV) types I and II. Screening for and quantitating antibodies to cytomegalovirus may be required for certain categories of patients. Discussions have been ongoing as to the necessity of testing all blood components for a number of exotic diseases such as Chagas' disease and the West Nile virus. The need to rapidly identify atypical antibodies from different ethnic groups has spurred the desire for an automated system to perform mass screenings.

Currently available instruments are undergoing modifications to become even more efficient. These instruments are practically all-in-one as to their ability to perform all of the routine procedures for the blood bank relative to the actual testing of the blood, both donor and recipient, for compatibility. The MTS Gel System in widespread use provides convenient identification of blood groups and types with automated and semiautomated systems. Gel grouping and typing are sensitive and specific and can be standardized. Although the costs are higher than for traditional slide and tube methods, it requires fewer man-hours for a higher volume of work. If results are detected by the instrument that do not meet with expected values, the instrument will reject the sample for that particular patient and donor. It is then necessary for the technician or technologist to perform manual tests to confirm the results. Screening tests for diseases are mass-tested on other instruments, and all of these are interfaced with the Laboratory Information System (LIS).

THERAPEUTIC USE OF IMMUNOHEMATOLOGY

Immunohematology is similar to immunology and serology in that in most procedures, antibody and antigen reactions act to form the basis of the bulk of the procedures. The blood bank actually has two major functions assigned to it. Most laboratories maintain a considerable inventory of blood of various groups and types for use in surgery and for trauma where bleeding occurs to an extent that a **transfusion** is needed. Not all hospital blood banks collect their own supply of blood for use within the facility. Those who do collect their own blood are required to first collect, then test the units for certain antigens and sometimes antibodies, and then to store the blood safely until it is used. However, most blood supplies are maintained and blood is shipped regularly to hospital blood banks from large commercial facilities that perform on-site collections around the country, such as the American Red Cross. These facilities also provide a valuable service that is beyond the scope of routine hospital blood banks. They determine rare blood groups and types and provide units of blood for patients who are unable to take the most ordinary groups and types due to **atypical antibodies (alloantibodies)**.

Large commercial blood banks also perform emergency blood drives when disaster strikes and have the staff and capabilities to ship this blood in refrigerated vehicles for long distances to the scene of the disaster. One of the first medical needs for effectively responding to injuries with blood loss is to maintain adequate circulation by using volume expanders. Only blood can be used as a volume expander that is capable of transporting oxygen to all the tissues of the body. Promoting circulation and perfusion of the tissues with oxygen will prevent shock and tissue damage that may lead to death.

Blood banks may also harvest white blood cells for those with immunological problems and platelets for those who are in danger of bleeding due to low platelet counts (platelets contribute to the clotting process). Plasma is extracted from whole blood for use as **volume expanders** in the circulatory system, and in some more advanced procedures, certain **coagulation factors** may be separated from the plasma. There are also large regional storage facilities throughout the United States and the world that are able to store cord blood stem cells for the several decades that they would remain viable, although many hospital blood banks have the capability for washing and glycerinating the cells before shipping them to a storage facility.

Blood supplies are able to be maintained for longer periods than was true a number of years ago, due to improved anticoagulants and nutrients added to the unit to extend the life of the red blood cells (RBC). Although red blood cells have a life span of around 100 to 120 days, the units are only good for approximately 1 month or slightly longer. This is because of the death of a percentage of the RBCs each day leaves components in the unit that would be dangerous to the patient receiving the blood. Under certain conditions, particularly for newborns, Pedi-Paks are used to provide fresh blood for exchange transfusions when a fetus has received antibodies against its own blood type, as occurs with Rh incompatibilities between mother and fetus. Another function of blood banks and some specialty storage centers is that of storing cord blood from newborns and having it available for stem cell transplants when certain disease strike, such as one of the various types of leukemia.

Many technologists and even some medical laboratory technicians find employment in blood banks and become specialists in certain procedures that are highly sophisticated. Testing personnel are also needed in the medical laboratory to test blood for syphilis, hepatitis, and HIV. Most technologists and technicians are used in hospital blood banks. The basic tests performed, even on blood

Table 17-1 Reactions of ABO Groups with Anti-A and Anti-B Sera.

Blood Group	Reactions of Cells With:	
	Anti-A	Anti-B
A	+	0
B	0	+
AB	+	+
0	0	0

+ = agglutination
0 = no agglutination

obtained from commercial blood banks, are the repeat grouping and typing of the cells before storing in the specialized blood bank refrigerator. The temperature must be monitored in the refrigerator, and if the unit malfunctions or is without power, the units of blood must immediately be transferred to other storage or the entire inventory will be lost. Blood that has expired may be separated into certain components and some blood products may be used indefinitely.

A typical blood bank as found in most hospitals chiefly provides a service to determine if a blood donation is compatible with the recipient's immune system (Table 17-1). This procedure, which is actually a combination of several tests, is called a **cross match**. A patient is screened by the medical laboratory worker for atypical antibodies as well as for his blood group (ABO) and his blood type (major type is the **Rh factor**). The identification of ABO blood group and type needed for blood transfusion is also an important component of determining the compatibility of a tissue transplant (Figure 17-1). The RBCs from the donor are tested at room temperature and at body temperature to determine if the recipient (patient) has any antibodies against the cells of the donor. Transfusion of a unit of blood that is incompatible with the donor's immune system makeup would cause problems and might even result in death. As a rare complication, the recipient may have antibodies toward his or her own antigens. The antibodies may either be warm (positive when incubated) or cold (react at room temperature). These **autoantibodies** do not occur normally and may be an indication of the presence of autoimmune hemolytic anemia.

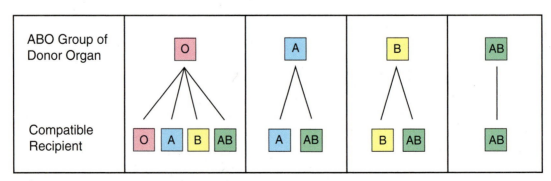

FIGURE 17-1 ABO chart for determining compatibility of tissue in organ transplant.
Source: Delmar/Cengage Learning.

This chapter provides a few routine tests performed in the routine blood banks. The cross match, as mentioned earlier, is a rather long and cumbersome set of tests, so the entire cross match will not be presented here. Medical laboratory students enrolled in immunohematology classes usually learn both theory and practice, and have the opportunity to perform an actual cross match.

SAFETY AND ACCURACY IN IMMUNOHEMATOLOGY

It should now be obvious to the astute clinical laboratory student that there is a relationship between immunology/serology and immunohematology. Both areas work on the premise of antibodies against antigens and require meticulous care in providing accurate and timely results. However, in most routine procedures in blood banking, the basic test are to discover RBC antigens by use of specific antibody solutions obtained from persons with antibodies against various blood groups. Efforts in this department are to obtain a safe supply of blood, test it for communicable diseases, and ensure the patient has no antibodies against the blood of the donor, which would cause a potentially life-threatening reaction. The most atypical antibodies or alloantibodies (those from a donor) often require a specialist in blood banking to determine the offending antibody.

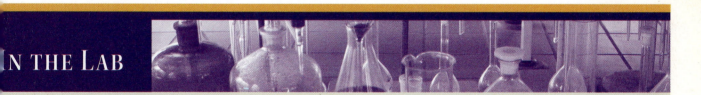

IN THE LAB

BASIC IMMUNOHEMATOLOGY PROCEDURES
MANUAL IMMUNOHEMATOLOGY PROCEDURE #1
Preparation of 2% to 5% Cell Suspensions
Principle

A number of tests require red blood cell (RBC) suspensions and are performed in test tubes. Other tests, such as blood grouping for identifying the ABO group, can be performed either in test tubes or on glass microscope slides.

Red blood cells contain some plasma, which is rich in proteins. Surface proteins may interfere with tests that use antisera against the antigens on the surface of the RBCs. Therefore, the RBCs must be "washed" with normal saline (a salt solution approximately equal to the salt concentration of a person's blood plasma) to enhance reactions in blood bank procedures.

To "wash" RBCs, several drops of RBCs are placed in glass test tubes (12 × 75 mm tubes are preferable). Normal saline from a squeeze bottle is injected into the tube containing the cells. Using a piece of plastic Parafilm, the top of the tube is covered and the tube is then inverted several times to mix the cells and saline. The tube is centrifuged, and the saline is removed, leaving a "button" of RBCs in the bottom. This process is repeated two or three times, according to most blood bank basic

IN THE LAB

procedures. When the saline is again removed, the cells have been cleared of most proteins from the plasma, leaving the cell membranes exposed. In a large hospital's blood bank, specialized centrifuges that automatically wash the RBCs three or four times in quick succession are usually available.

Blood component therapy is most often used to provide RBCs to patients, but may include platelet transfusions, white blood cell transfusions, and coagulation factors found in the plasma of blood, procedures for which washing of the cells may be required. The first step in preparation for any of these procedures, of course, requires determining a blood group (ABO) and type (Rh factors). The donor's blood and the patient's blood are processed to determine if the donor blood is compatible with that of the recipient's blood. These basic steps include a number of procedures where antibodies are tested against the donor's blood to prevent a transfusion reaction. Even if the blood group and types match, there may still be atypical antibodies that may require additional screening of donor blood before suitable matches are found. Proper collection and screening of donor blood also require that a number of procedures be completed to insure the safety of the blood that will be administered to a patient.

Using washed cells, prepare cell suspensions to be used for testing. The following procedures will give practice in preparing the correct concentrations of RBCs for testing

Equipment and Supplies

1. Gloves, disposable paper towels, and disinfectant or other cleaning solution
2. Normal physiological (0.85%) saline (blood bank quality) in squeeze bottle
3. Blood specimen collected in an anticoagulated tube, *OR* RBCs obtained from freshly clotted red cells
4. Commercially prepared screening cell suspensions (used for other blood banking procedures) to act as controls with which cell suspensions may be compared as a standard
5. One disposable 13 × 100 test tube, two disposable 12 × 75 test tubes, and a test tube rack
6. Absorbent pad
7. Pasteur pipettes
8. Applicator sticks if RBCs are to be taken from a clotted specimen
9. Parafilm
10. Waterproof sharp marker for labeling tubes
11. Disposal containers appropriate for biohazardous waste

Procedure

1. Wash hands and don gloves.
2. Assemble necessary equipment and supplies.

3. Fill a 13 × 100 mm test tube with 0.85% normal saline from the squeeze bottle for each blood sample for which a cell suspension is needed. Use this supply of saline as the source of the appropriate drops of saline for the two levels of suspension.

4. Label one of the 12 × 75 mm test tubes as 2% and one as 5%. The two separate concentrations are prepared to ensure an adequate number of red blood cells are available for testing in patients who may be anemic (low RBC count).

5. Using Pasteur or transfer pipettes, prepare 2% and 5% standard RBC suspensions in the labeled tubes as shown below. These suspensions are an approximation and an exact percentage is not critical.

	2% Cell Suspension	5% Cell Suspension
Drops of Saline	98	95
Drops of RBCs	2	5

6. Cover each tube with Parafilm and invert gently to mix.

7. Compare the color intensity in the two prepared suspensions (2 and 5%) with that of the screening cells. Note that one of the two should approximate the color intensity of the commercially prepared screening cells. If the prepared 2% RBC suspension is lighter in color intensity than those of the screening cells, then the 5% RBC suspension should be used for testing. The screening cells are used in blood banking procedures to determine the presence of atypical antibodies in the patient, or to confirm that the blood banking reagents used to test the cells in the prepared suspensions are working correctly.

8. It is important that the technical personnel in a blood bank be able to quickly prepare and approximate cell suspension of 2% and 5% red blood cells. With experience, the blood bank professional can achieve the proper suspension without using prepared standards. The student should practice preparing a 2% and a 5% cell suspension in the 12 × 75 test tubes as follows:

   a. Put 1 drop of the RBCs in each tube.

   b. Using the squeeze bottle, add sufficient saline to achieve a 2% to 5% cell suspension in each of the five tubes.

   c. Compare the color intensity of your suspensions to the standard 2% and 5% suspensions prepared from the table above. They should be roughly the same.

   d. With practice, the student can make approximate 2 or 5% solutions by adding sufficient saline until the color intensity is approximately that of the standard 2 or 5% cell suspensions prepared by counting drops of RBCs and saline.

   e. Repeat the procedure if the standard and the approximate preparations are not close in concentration.

9. Discard all supplies used for the procedure in the appropriate containers. A disinfectant should be used to clean the work surfaces and equipment should be cleaned and restored to its former position. Gloves should be discarded appropriately and the hands washed thoroughly in accordance with established policies.

IN THE LAB

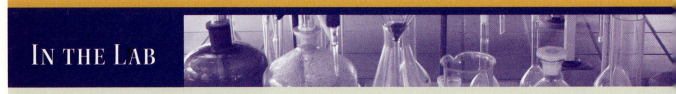

Reporting of Results

When cell suspensions are "too heavy" and excess RBCs are present in the suspension, reactions may be masked by excess antigen based on the number of antibodies in the anti-sera used in a procedure. If a cell suspension is "too light," a reaction may not be strong enough to macroscopically (with the naked eye) observe clumping of RBCs and a microscope may be required.

MANUAL IMMUNOHEMATOLOGY PROCEDURE #2

Direct Blood Grouping by Test Tube Method

Principles

The blood groups are A, B, and O and are referred to as the ABO grouping. Blood typing really has a different meaning, although many call the ABO grouping the blood "type." Human blood contains either A or B antigens, sometimes in combination, or neither A or B antigens, which is then classified as "O" (actually a zero), indicating neither A nor B antigens are present on the surface of the RBCs.

A person who has the A antigen will have antibodies in his plasma or serum against the B antigen. One who has the B antigen will have antibodies against the A antigen. This is true with a few exceptions, as there are blood groups other than A and B. The person with group O blood will have antibodies against both the A and B antigens. Antibodies are used to indicate reverse grouping, and antigens are used as the forward, or direct, grouping.

Performing both a forward grouping and a reverse grouping provides a check for accuracy. There are two major methods for performing blood grouping by the direct method: the slide method and the tube method. Both may be used. Most immunohematology professionals consider the tube method to be more reliable and more sensitive than the slide test. Slide testing is more commonly used for biology students and in some clinical laboratory classrooms, but most blood banks and clinical laboratories rely on tube testing for the ABO group and the Rh type.

Washing the RBCs prior to treating with anti-sera to determine the blood group of the RBCs provides an additional safeguard, as almost all the protein-rich plasma is removed by washing.

A specialized centrifuge called a serofuge is used to speed up the reaction of agglutination or clumping of the RBCs in the tube. It usually requires an approximately 30-second spin to effect a valid result.

Antigens may be found on the surfaces of the RBCs of some patients and results may be extremely weak, or antibodies may be absent or diminished in strength due to the inability of the body's immune system to efficiently produce normal levels of antibodies. The results in these patients may require careful testing and even referral to a specialty reference laboratory where results of testing are in doubt.

The procedure below describes the tube method. In this procedure, the test is for the presence of antigens A and B that may be found on the surfaces of RBCs, depending upon the ABO grouping of the cells.

Equipment and Supplies

1. Gloves, disposable paper towels, and disinfectant or other cleaning solution
2. Report form
3. A 2% to 5% RBC suspension of washed RBCs from the patient being tested, prepared following the steps set out in Procedure #1
4. Waterproof sharp marker
5. Normal physiological (0.85%) saline (blood bank quality) in squeeze bottle
6. Disposable Pasteur pipettes or transfer pipettes
7. Anti-A blood serum
8. Anti-B blood serum
9. Commercially prepared Group A cells (2 – 5% cell suspension)
10. Commercially prepared Group B cells (2 – 5% cell suspension)
11. Disposable 12 × 75 mm test tubes and test tube rack
12. Centrifuge (serofuge) with head that will contain 12 × 75 mm tubes at 2000 rpm
13. Illuminating lamp with magnifying mirror (optional)
14. Disposal containers appropriate for biohazardous waste and sharps container

Procedure

1. Wash hands and don gloves.
2. Assemble necessary equipment and supplies.
3. Prepare a 2% to 5% RBC suspension of washed RBCs from the patient being tested following the steps set out in Procedure #1.
4. Label one 12 × 75 mm tubes "A" and label one "B."
5. Using a Pasteur pipette or transfer pipette, place two drops of the suspension in each tube.
6. Into tube A, put two drops of antisera A, which is prepared from serum from a group B individual.
7. Into tube B, put two drops of antisera B, which is prepared from serum from a group A individual.
8. Tap or gently flick each tube with a finger to mix the cells and antisera.
9. Place both tubes into a centrifuge (called a serofuge in blood banking), and spin for 30 seconds.
10. Gently remove the tubes without shaking and slightly tilt the tubes while observing for clumping, called *agglutination*. An illuminating lamp with magnifying mirror may be used as an optional practice.
11. Record which tube or tubes show agglutination, using the following form. Place a plus sign ("+") for agglutination into the appropriate blank(s) and a minus sign ("−") to indicate no agglutination.

	Tube A	Tube B
Results		

IN THE LAB

12. Discard all supplies used for the procedure in the appropriate containers. A disinfectant should be used to clean the work surfaces and equipment should be cleaned and restored to its former position. Gloves should be discarded appropriately and the hands washed thoroughly in accordance with established policies.

Reporting of Results

Interpret your results for ABO direct blood grouping according to the following criteria.

Agglutination in Tube A = Group A

	Tube A	Tube B
Results	+	−

Agglutination in Tube B = Group B

	Tube A	Tube B
Results	−	+

Agglutination in Tubes A and B = Group AB

	Tube A	Tube B
Results	+	+

No agglutination in Tubes A or B = Group O

	Tube A	Tube B
Results	−	−

MANUAL IMMUNOHEMATOLOGY PROCEDURE #3

Direct Blood or Forward Grouping by Slide Method

Principles

The quality and care practiced by the laboratory professional is critical in the blood bank, as a mistake has an immediate impact upon the patient in many instances. These mistakes can be of misidentification, misinterpretation, or in the performance of the testing. Slide tests, like tube tests for ABO grouping, employ the same technique of introducing antigens on the surfaces of RBCs to anti-sera that contain antibodies that correspond to the antigens for a specific blood group. If the antigen that correlates with the antibody against that particular antigen is not present on the RBCs, no reaction occurs.

The direct grouping performed on a microscope slide is the quickest and easiest method to determine the ABO grouping (Figure 17-2) but is not the choice for most blood banking professionals. The problem with this procedure lies in the possibility of proteins interfering with the reaction, which is avoided in the tube method, as the RBCs that contain the A or B antigen(s) are washed before testing.

Equipment and Supplies

1. Gloves, disposable paper towels, and disinfectant or other cleaning solution
2. Report form
3. EDTA anticoagulated blood sample or a freshly clotted sample
4. Waterproof sharp marker
5. Normal physiological (0.85%) saline (blood bank quality) in squeeze bottle
6. Disposable Pasteur pipettes or transfer pipettes
7. Anti-A blood serum
8. Anti-B blood serum
9. Applicator sticks or plastic stirrers
10. Clean microscope slides or specialized cell typing slides
11. Illuminating lamp with magnifying mirror (optional)
12. Electronic timing device or clock/watch with second hand
13. Disposal containers appropriate for biohazardous waste and sharps container

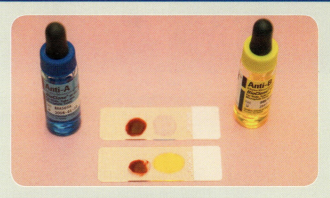

**FIGURE 17-2 ABO slide grouping procedures.
Source: Delmar/Cengage Learning.**

Procedure

1. Wash hands and put on gloves.
2. Assemble equipment and materials.
3. Mark a clean slide into two halves, labeling the left side "A" and the right side "B."
4. Using a Pasteur pipette, transfer pipette, or dropper included with the reagent, place one drop of anti-A serum on the "A" side (do not allow the dropper to touch slide).
5. Using a Pasteur pipette, transfer pipette, or dropper included with the reagent, place one drop of anti-B serum on the "B" side (do not allow the dropper to touch slide).
8. Add one drop of well-mixed blood to each side of the slide using the Pasteur pipette or a pair of applicator sticks (the drop of blood should be no larger than the drop of antiserum).
9. Using a clean applicator stick, mix the blood and antiserum on side A and spread into a smooth round circle about the size of a nickel.
10. Using a clean applicator stick, repeat the procedure on side B.
11. Rock the slide gently for 2 minutes and look for agglutination. An illuminating lamp with magnifying mirror may be used as an optional practice.
12. Record which sides of the slide show agglutination, using the following form. Place a plus sign ("+") for agglutination into the appropriate blank(s) and a minus sign ("−") to indicate no agglutination.

	Side A	Side B
Results		

13. Discard all supplies used for the procedure in the appropriate containers. A disinfectant should be used to clean the work surfaces and equipment

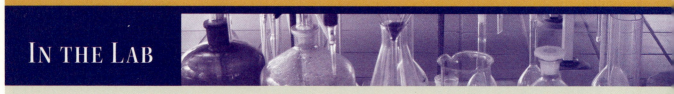

IN THE LAB

should be cleaned and restored to its former position. Gloves should be discarded appropriately and the hands washed thoroughly in accordance with established policies.

Reporting of Results

Interpret your results for ABO direct blood grouping on slides according to the criteria found at the end of Procedure #2, substituting "slide" for "tube."

MANUAL IMMUNOHEMATOLOGY PROCEDURE #4

Indirect (Reverse) Grouping by Tube

Principles

The blood groups A, B, and O normally have antibodies against the blood group the individual does not possess, as described in the direct grouping methodology in Procedure #2. Therefore, in indirect grouping, the test is for the antibodies and not for the antigen. The indirect group method is often used to confirm the forward grouping and should correlate under normal conditions where the patient's immune system is functioning normally. The interpretation for an indirect grouping method is opposite that of the forward grouping. Therefore, antibodies may be used to indicate the reverse grouping, because, for instance, a group A individual would have antibodies against group B RBCs.

This procedure describes the tube method and is sometimes called *back grouping*. This procedure appears to be the easiest for interpretation, because the plasma proteins have been removed by washing the RBCs and will not interfere with the procedure.

Equipment and Supplies

1. Gloves, disposable paper towels, and disinfectant or other cleaning solution
2. Report form
3. A 2% to 5% RBC suspension of washed RBCs from the patient being tested, prepared following the steps set out in Procedure #1
4. Waterproof sharp marker
5. Normal physiological (0.85%) saline (blood bank quality) in squeeze bottle.
6. Disposable Pasteur pipettes or transfer pipettes
7. Commercially prepared Group A cells (2 – 5% cell suspension)
8. Commercially prepared Group B cells (2 – 5% cell suspension)
9. Disposable 12 × 75 mm test tubes and test tube rack
10. Centrifuge (serofuge) with head that will contain 12 × 75 mm tubes at 2000 rpm
11. Illuminating lamp with magnifying mirror (optional)
12. Disposal containers appropriate for biohazardous waste and sharps container

Procedure

1. Wash hands and don gloves.
2. Assemble necessary equipment and supplies.
3. Prepare a 2% to 5% RBC suspension of washed RBCs from the patient being tested following the steps set out in Procedure #1
4. Label one 12 × 75 mm tubes "A" and label one "B."
5. Using a Pasteur pipette or transfer pipette, place two drops of the suspension in each tube.
6. Into tube A, put two drops of commercially prepared Group A cells.
7. Into tube B, put two drops of commercially prepared Group A cells.
8. Tap or gently flick each tube with a finger to mix the cells.
9. Place both tubes into a centrifuge (called a serofuge in blood banking), and spin for 30 seconds.
10. Gently remove the tubes without shaking and slightly tilt the tubes while observing for clumping, called *agglutination.* An illuminating lamp with magnifying mirror may be used as an optional practice.
11. Record which tube or tubes show agglutination, using the following form. Place a plus sign ("+") for agglutination into the appropriate blank(s) and a minus sign ("−") to indicate no agglutination.

	Tube A	Tube B
Results		

12. The strength of an immunohematological reaction is sometimes clinically significant. The reactions are grades as shown in Figure 17-3

Grading of Agglutination

The degree of red cell agglutination observed in any blood bank test procedure is significant and should be recorded. A system of grading is illustrated.

Description	Reaction	Grade
Button is one or two large clumps after being dislodged. Background is clear.		4+ (++++)
Button breaks into a few large clumps. Background is clear.		3+ (+++)
Button breaks into many medium-sized clumps. Background remains clear.		2+ (++)
Button breaks into numerous tiny clumps. Background becomes cloudy.		1+ (+)
A few small, very fine aggregates barely visible to the naked eye.		w+
No visible clumps or agglutinates.		0 (Neg)

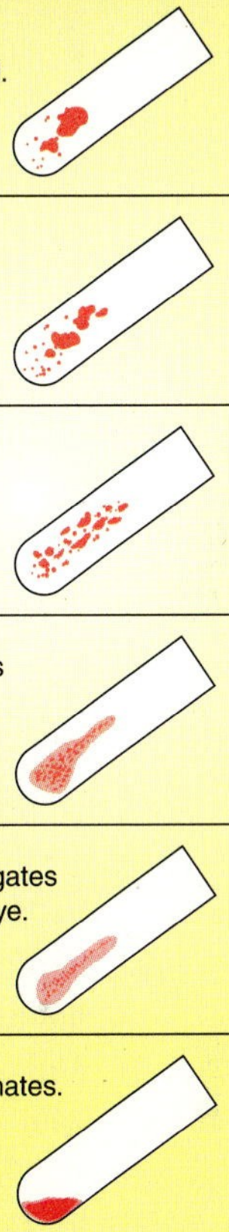

FIGURE 17-3 Illustration of agglutination of varying strengths in ABO tube typing.
Source: Delmar/Cengage Learning.

Reporting of Results

Interpret your results for ABO indirect blood grouping according to the following criteria.

Agglutination in Tube B = Group A

	Tube A	Tube B
Results	−	+

Agglutination in Tube A = Group B

	Tube A	Tube B
Results	+	−

No agglutination in Tubes A and B = Group AB

	Tube A	Tube B
Results	−	−

Agglutination in Tubes A or B = Group O

	Tube A	Tube B
Results	+	+

IN THE LAB

MANUAL IMMUNOHEMATOLOGY PROCEDURE #5
Blood Typing for the Rh Factor, Slide and Tube Method
Principles

The Rh blood system is composed of many antigens, but the first to be discovered was that of the **D antigen**. Normally when screening patients and units of blood for the Rh factor, the only antigen that is initially tested for is the D antigen. Others may be tested for in certain medical conditions, and are pursued following the determination of the presence of the D antigens. RH antigens may occur in a number of combinations, but the "big D" antigen is the one most commonly associated with incompatibilities when preparing units of blood for transfusion, and in certain diseases of the unborn child when the mother is Rh negative. An Rh negative mother may develop antibodies against her baby while it is in the uterus, requiring treatment before and after birth to save the fetus's life.

A "weak" D antigen, often denoted as D^u, is tested for by incubating washed RBCs with anti-D sera and then treating the specimens with a commercial immunoglobulin G (IgG) to detect antibodies bound to the red cells in the initial test procedure for a "normal" D antigen. Several dozen more antigens other than D have been identified in the Rh typing system, but many of them are extremely rare. The most common of these include C (big C), c (little c), E (big E), and e (little e). Individuals who do not have this antigen on their RBCs and who are transfused with blood containing these antigens may develop antibodies against them, which may cause problems in women who have children whose blood contains these antigens.

This procedure provides an initial review of some of the kinds of testing laboratory technical personnel perform. It will cover only the determination of the presence or absence of the D antigen ("big D"). As in the ABO grouping procedure, there are two methods for Rh determination: a tube method and a slide method. Washing of the red cells is not normally done for the slide method, but a newborn's cord blood contains a material that interferes with the normal testing procedure, so washing of the RBCs in this case is necessary. Unlike the ABO grouping, which will occur at room temperature, the test for the Rh factor, when performed as a slide test, requires warming of the slides during the test.

Equipment and Supplies

1. Gloves, disposable paper towels, and disinfectant or other cleaning solution
2. Report form
3. EDTA anti-coagulated blood specimen (for the slide method), and a 2% to 5% RBC suspension of washed RBCs from the patient being tested, prepared following the steps set out in Procedure #1 (for the test tube method)
4. Wax pencil or other permanent marker
5. Normal physiological (0.85%) saline (blood bank quality) in squeeze bottle

6. Disposable Pasteur pipettes or transfer pipettes
7. Anti-D blood serum
8. Rh control (negative control) (available commercially)
9. Positive whole blood Rh control (optional)
10. Clean microscope slides
11. Lighted and heated view box
12. Applicator sticks or plastic stirrers
13. Disposable 12 × 75 mm test tubes and test tube rack
14. Heat block set at 37°C
15. Centrifuge (serofuge) with head that will contain 12 × 75 mm tubes at 2000 rpm
16. Illuminating lamp with magnifying mirror (optional)
17. Disposal containers appropriate for biohazardous waste and sharps container

Procedure—Slide Test for Rh Factor

1. Wash hands and don gloves.
2. Assemble equipment and materials.
3. Mark a clean slide into two halves using a wax pencil, labeling the left side "A" and the right side "control."
4. Place a drop of the EDTA-anticoagulated blood on the test section of the slide and one drop of the negative control on the other section.
5. Place one drop of anti-Rh antisera from a patient who is Rh negative and has developed a high level (titer) of antibodies to the Rh factor (D) on both the test section and the control section of the slide.
6. Place the slides on the warming view box.
7. Mix each side with a clean applicator stick and tilt the slide by rocking the warming view box, ensuring the slide does not move about on the glass surface, by anchoring it with a fingertip.

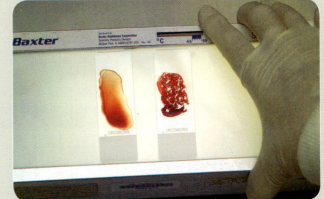

FIGURE 17-4 A heated and lighted viewbox is designed for Rh slide typing, as the test requires heat for reaction. The specimen on the right is positive for "big D" or the Rh factor. Source: Delmar/Cengage Learning.

8. Agglutination of the test drop indicates the presence of the D antigen (Figure 17-4). The control should be negative. If it is not, there is a problem with the test reagents or performance, and the test should be repeated after appropriate modifications.
9. Further interpretation is required with apparently negative results with a modified tube test for confirmation for the weak D (D^u).
10. Discard all supplies used for the procedure in the appropriate containers. A disinfectant should be used to clean the work surfaces and equipment should be cleaned and restored to its former position. Gloves should be discarded appropriately and the hands washed thoroughly in accordance with established policies.

IN THE LAB

Procedure—Tube Test for Rh Factor

1. Wash hands and don gloves.
2. Assemble necessary equipment and supplies.
3. Into a 12 × 75 test tube, place one drop of anti-Rh typing serum.
4. Add one drop of washed RBCs into the tube.
5. Mix cells and antiserum by tapping gently with a finger.
6. Incubate the tube in a 37°C heat block for 5 to 10 minutes.
7. Centrifuge the tube for 1 minute, making sure to balance the tube with a blank tube containing 2 drops of saline or water, or another test if more than one patient is being tested.
8. Observe over a lighted surface such as that of the view box used for the slide test method.
9. Agglutination indicates the presence of the D antigen (Figure 17-4).
10. For interpretation, a negative result requires further testing with a more definitive test, in which a variant of the D antigen may be found as the weak D (D^u).
11. Discard all supplies used for the procedure in the appropriate containers. A disinfectant should be used to clean the work surfaces and equipment should be cleaned and restored to its former position. Gloves should be discarded appropriately and the hands washed thoroughly in accordance with established policies.

Reporting of Results

Interpret your results for the RH procedure according to the following criteria.

Anti-D	Protein Control	Rh Type
+	−	Positive
−	−	Negative
+/−	+	Requires further investigation

SUMMARY

The term *immunohematology* is a combination of *hematology,* or "study of blood," and *immunology*, which comes from the "study of the immune system," although the term "blood banking" is still often heard. Blood component therapy is most often used to provide RBCs, but also includes platelet transfusions, white blood cell transfusions, and coagulation factors found in the plasma of blood.

The first step in preparation for any of these procedures, of course, requires determining a blood group (ABO) and type (Rh factors). The donor's blood and the patient's blood are processed to determine if the donor blood is compatible with that of the recipient's blood. These are basic steps that include a number of procedures where antibodies are tested against the donor's blood to prevent a transfusion reaction. Even if the blood group and types are a match, there may still be atypical antibodies that may require a great deal of screening of donor blood before suitable matches are found.

Proper collection and screening of donor blood also require that a number of procedures be performed. Screening the blood for infectious diseases such as syphilis, HIV, HBV, and other diseases is required before the donor blood is cleared for continued processing and storage in a bank. This chapter provided a number of basic screening tests with which the student should be familiar before entering clinical training sites for a more advanced level of work.

REVIEW QUESTIONS

1. When testing blood donor units for safety, what tests are performed on the units?
2. What is meant by *immunotherapy*?
3. Why do units of blood expire?
4. What is meant by *atypical antibodies*?
5. Why are RBCs washed with normal saline before being tested or used in testing?

STATES AND TERRITORIES WITH LABORATORY PERSONNEL LICENSURE REQUIREMENTS

The following list of states and territories with laboratory personnel licensure and contact information was updated as of January 2009. Consult Web sites for current information regarding application and renewal fees as well as requirements for continuing education. If not otherwise stated, annual renewal is assumed.

California

California Department of Public Health
Laboratory Field Services
Personnel Licensing Section
850 Marina Bay Parkway
Building P, 1st Floor
Richmond, CA 94804
Phone: 510.620.3834
Fax: 510. 620.3697
http://www.cdph.ca.gov/programs/lfs/Pages/default.aspx
Beginning in 2008, Laboratory Field Services (LFS) no longer administers the State-Administered Examination for CLS (generalist) and for the three categories of specialists (limited) licensing (clinical chemist, clinical microbiologist, and clinical toxicologist scientist). Applicants must select one license category as listed on the preceding website. Applicants for specialty (limited) license of chemistry, microbiology, and toxicology can apply to take a California-approved certifying organization exam (ASCP examination for chemistry and microbiology is approved and NRCC examination for toxicology is approved). Applicants for specialty (limited) license of immunohematology and hematology have to take a state administered examination.

Florida

Florida Department of Health
Division of Medical Quality Assurance
Board of Clinical Laboratory Personnel
4052 Bald Cypress Way
Tallahassee, FL 32399-3251
Phone: 850.488.0595
Fax: 850.487.9626
http://www.doh.state.fl.us/mqa
National exams recognized
24 contact hours of continuing education biannually

Georgia

Georgia Department of Human Resources
Office of Regulatory Services
Diagnostic Services Unit
Two Peachtree Street, NW, Suite 33-250
Atlanta, GA 30303-3142
Phone: 404.657.5450
Fax: 404.657.8934
http://ors.dhr.georgia.gov
Facility Licensure Only
Requires CLS/CLT/MT/MLT/MLS/MLT national certification by approved agencies
Education and experience requirements; does not cover POLs or state or federal government laboratories

Hawaii

Hawaii Department of Health
State Laboratories Division
2725 Waimano Home Road
Pearl City, HI 96782
Phone: 808.453.6653
Fax: 808.453.6662
http://dlslab.com/employment/hawaii-license
NCA and ASCP Board of Registry certification exams recognized

Louisiana

Louisiana State Board of Medical Examiners
PO Box 54383 (for Clinical Laboratory Personnel)
New Orleans, LA 70154-4383
Phone: 504.568-6820 (800.296.7549)
Fax: 504.599-0503
http://lsbme.louisiana.gov/ClinicalLaboratoryPersonnel
.htm
National certification exams recognized

Montana

Montana Board of Clinical Laboratory
Science Practitioners
301 South Park Avenue, 4th floor
Helena, MT 59620-0513
Phone: 406.841.2395
Fax: 406.841.2305
http://www.cls.mt.gov
National certification recognized

Nevada

Nevada State Health Division
Bureau of Health Care Quality and Compliance
1550 College Parkway, Suite 158
Carson City, NV 89706
Phone: 775.687.4475
Fax: 775.687.6588
http://www.health.nv.gov/HCQC_
Medical.htm
National certification recognized

New York

New York State Education Department
Office of the Professions
PO Box 22063
Albany, NY 12201
http://www.op.nysed.gov/prof/clt/clp-cltlic.htm
Practice as a clinical laboratory technologist or as a
certified clinical laboratory technician and the use
of the titles "clinical laboratory technologist" or
"certified clinical laboratory technician" in New York
State require licensure, unless otherwise exempt under
the law. Certain educational requirements must be
met in order to achieve this licensure, as specified. A
professional license is the authorization to practice
and use a professional title in New York State and
is valid for life unless it is revoked, annulled, or
suspended by the Board of Regents. Reregistration is
required every three years.

North Dakota

North Dakota Board of Clinical Laboratory Practice
PO Box 4103
Bismark, ND 58502-4103
Phone: 701.530-0199
http://www.ndclinlab.com/
National certification recognized

Puerto Rico

Puerto Rico College of Medical Technologies
Ave. San Patricio F-1
Guaynabo, PR 00968
Phone: 787.792.6400
Fax: 787.792.6627
http://www.ctmpr.com
National certification recognized; must be a member
of the Puerto Rico College of Medical Technologies

Rhode Island

Rhode Island Department of Health
Office of Health Professionals Regulation
3 Capitol Hill, Room 205
Providence, RI 02908
Phone: 401.222.2828
Fax: 401.222.3352
http://www.health.ri.gov/hsr/professions/index.php
National certification recognized

Tennessee

Tennessee Department of Health
Medical Laboratory Board
227 French Landing, Suite 300
Heritage Place MetroCenter
Nashville, TN 37243
Phone: 615.532.3202, 800.778.4123
http://health.state.tn.us/boards/MedLab/
National certification recognized

West Virginia

West Virginia Department of Health &
Human Resources
West Virginia Office of Laboratory Services
167 Eleventh Avenue
South Charleston, WV 25303
Phone: 304.558.3530
Fax: 304.558.2006
http://www.wvdhr.org/labservices/compliance/licensure/
index.cfm
National certification recognized

MEDICAL TERMINOLOGY FOR LABORATORIANS

Word Prefix, Root, Suffix	Definition, Pertaining to
a or an	without, lack of
ab-	away from
ad-	toward
aden/o-	glands
adip/o	fat
adren/o	adrenal gland
albin/o	white
albumin/o	albumin
-algia	pain
amni/o	amnion; fetal sac
andr/o	man
angi/o	vessel (blood)
anis/o	unequal or dissimilar in size
ante-	before
anter/o	front
anti-	against
aort/o	aorta
aque/o	water
-ar	pertaining to
-arche	beginning
arteri/o	artery
arthr/o	joint
articul/o	joint
-ary	pertaining to
-asthenia	lack of strength
ather/o	fatty plaque
-ation	process
atri/o	upper heart chamber
audi/o	hearing

Word Prefix, Root, Suffix	Definition, Pertaining to
aur/o	ear
auto-	self
axill/o	armpit
bi/o	life
bil/i	bile acid
-blast	immature form
blepharo-	eyelid
brady-	slow
bronch/o	bronchial tubes
bucc/o	cheek
burs/o	bursa of joints
calc/o	calcium
-capnia	carbon dioxide
carcin/o	cancerous
cardi/o	heart
carp/o	wrist
caud/o	tail
-cele	hernia
cellul/o	pertaining to cells
-centesis	puncture
cephal/o	head
cerebr/o	brain
cervic/o	cervix (neck, uterus)
cheil/o	lips
chol/e	bile
cholangi/o	bile ducts
cholecyst/o	gallbladder
choledoch/o	common bile duct
chondr/o	cartilage

Word Prefix, Root, Suffix	Definition, Pertaining to
chrom/o	color
-cidal	to kill
cili/o	hair
coagul/o	to clot, or condense
coni/o	dust
constricto/o	narrowing or drawing together
-continence	stop
coron/o	crown
corpor/o	body
crin/o	to secrete
-crine	to secrete
-crit	to separate
cry/o	cold
crypt/o	hidden
cutane/o	epidermis
cyst/o	sac; urinary bladder
cyt/o	cell
dacry/o	teardrops
de-	removal, lack of
di-	two
dia-	through, across
diaphor/e	sweating
dipl/o	double
-dipsia	thirst
dors/o	back
duct/o	to draw out
duoden/o	pertaining to duodenum
dur/o	outermost membrane of brain (dura mater)
-dynai	pain
-dynia	pain
dys-	difficult, painful, poor
e-	out, outside of, without
-eal	pertaining to
ec-	out
-ectasis	dilation stretching, widening
ecto-	outward
-ectomy	excision, removal
-edema	pooling of fluid

Word Prefix, Root, Suffix	Definition, Pertaining to
embol/o	plug, clog
-emesis	vomiting
-emia	pertaining to blood
en-	inward
encephal/o	brain
endo-	within
enter/o	intestine
epi-	above, upon
-er	specialist
erythemat/o	red
eso-	inward
esophag/o	esophagus
-esthesia	sensation, feeling
estr/o	female
eu-	normal, good
exo-	out, outward
extra	out, outside, outward
fasci/o	fascia
fibr/o	fibrous tissue, fibers
flex/o	bending
fluor/o	fluorescent, luminous
-flux	flow
galact/o	milk
gastr/o	stomach
-gen	producing
-genesis	beginning, development
-genic	produced
gingiv/o	pertaining to gums
gli/o	gluelike
glomerul/o	glomeruli of kidneys
gloss/o	tongue
gluc/o	sugar; glucose
glycogen/o	storage of sugar
gonad/o	sex glands
-gram	recording, writing
granul/o	contains granules
-graph	instrument for recording
-graphy	process of recording
-gravida	pregnancy

Word Prefix, Root, Suffix	Definition, Pertaining to
gynec/o	female, woman
hem/o	blood
hemat/o	blood
hemi-	half
hepat/o	liver
herni/o	bulging, hernia
hiat/o	hiatus, opening
hidr/o	sweat
home/o	same
hsit/o	tissue
hydr/o	water
hyper-	abnormal increase, above
hypo-	abnormal decrease, below
hyster/o	uterus
-ia	condition
-iasis	abnormal condition, process
-ic	pertaining to
-ician	specialist, expert
immun/o	immunity
in-	not, no
-ine	pertaining to
infer/o	below, downward
infra-	within
insulin/o	insulin
inter-	between
intra-	within
-ion	process
-ior	pertaining to
is/o	equal
isch/o	holding back
-ism	condition
-ist	specialist
-itis	inflammation
-ium	structure
kal/o	potassium
kerat/o	hard, hornlike
kinesi/o	movement
-kinesis	movement, motion
kyph/o	hunchback

Word Prefix, Root, Suffix	Definition, Pertaining to
labi/o	lips
lacrim/o	tears
lact/o	milk
lapat/o	abdominal wall
laryng/o	voice box (larynx)
lei/o	smooth
leuk/o	white
ligati/o	tie, bind
lingu/o	tongue
lip/o	fatty tissue
-lith/o	stone, calculus
-logist	specialist
-logy	study of
lord/o	sway back
lumb/o	lower back
lymph/o	clear, watery fluid
lymphaden/o	lymph glands, nodes
lymphangio/o	lymph vessels
-malacia	softening
mamm/o	breast
medi/o	mid- or middle
medull/o	inner portion of an organ
-megaly	enlargement
melan/o	black
men/o	menses
mening/o	membrane
meta-	change
-meter	instrument for measuring
metr/o	uterus
-metrist	specialist in measurement of
-metry	to measure
mi/o	contraction
mono-	one
myco-	fungus
mydri/o	to dilate, widen
myel/o	bone marrow, spinal cord
myelin/o	myelin sheath of nerve tract
myos/o	muscle
myring/o	eardrum

Word Prefix, Root, Suffix	Definition, Pertaining to
nas/o	nose
nat/i	birth
natr/o	sodium
necr/o	death
nephr/o	kidney
neur/o	nerve
noct/o	night
norm/o	normal
nulli-	none
o/o	egg
ocul/o	eye
odont/o	teeth
-oid	like another
-ole	small
oligo/o	scanty, inadequate
-oma	tumor
onych/o	nail
oophor/o	ovary
-opia	vision
-opsy	to view
opt/o	sight
opthalm/o	eye
-or	person who performs activity
or/o	mouth
orchid/o	testes
orex/i	appetite
ortho-	straight
-ory	pertaining to
-ose	pertaining to
ov/o	egg
ovari/o	ovary
ox/i	oxygen
ox/o	oxygen
oxy-	quick or sharp
pan-	all
pancreat/o	pancreas
papill/o	nipple-like
-para	give birth
para-	near, beside
-partum	labor, childbirth

Word Prefix, Root, Suffix	Definition, Pertaining to
path/o	disease
-pathy	disease process
-pause	stoppage, cessation
pector/o	chest
ped/o	child
pelv/o/i	pelvis
-penia	decrease, deficiency
-pepsia	digestion
per-	through
peri-	around
perine/o	peritoneum
-pexy	fixation by surgery
phac/o	eye lens
-phagia	swallow or eat
phalang/o	phalanx
phall/o	penis
phamac/o	drug
pharyng/o	pharynx, throat
-phasia	speech
phleb/o	vein
-phobia	unreasonable fear
-phonia	voice
-phoresis	carrying, transmission
phot/o	light
phren/o	diaphragm
physi/o	nature
-physis	to grow
pil/o	hair
pine/o	pineal gland
pituitary/o	pituitary gland
-plakia	patches
-plasia	development, formation
-plastic	pertaining to formation
-plasty	surgical repair
-plegia	paralysis
pleur/a; pleur/o	pleural cavity
-pnea	breathing
pneum/o, pneumat/o, pneumon/o	lungs
-poiesis	production or formation

Word Prefix, Root, Suffix	Definition, Pertaining to
-poietin	hormone with stimulatory effect, e.g., erythropoietin
poikil/o	variation, irregular
polio-	gray
poly-	many
porosis-	porous
post-	after
poster/o	dorsal, back
-prandial	meal
pre-	before
presby-	old age
primi-	first
pro-	before
proct/o	rectum
prostate/o	prostate gland
proxim/o	near, close
pseudo-	false
-ptosis	drooping
-ptysis	spitting
py/o	pus
pyel/o	renal pelvis
pylor/o	distal portion of stomach
quadro-	four
radicul/o	nerve roots
re-	back
ren/o	kidney
reticul/o	connected network
retr/o	backward, behind
rhabd/o	rod-shaped or striated
rhin/o	nose
-rrhage	bursting forth
-rrhagia	bursting forth
-rrhaphy	suture, sew
-rrhea	flow or discharge
-rrhexis	rupture
salping/o	eustachian, fallopian, and uterine tubes
-salpinx	fallopian tube, uterine tube
-sarcoma	malignant tumor of connective tissue

Word Prefix, Root, Suffix	Definition, Pertaining to
-schisis	cleft or splitting
-sclerosis	hardening
scoli/o	curved
-scope	instrument for viewing body cavity
seb/o	sebu (sweat oils)
sect/o	cut
sialanden/o	salivary glands
-sis	condition
somat/o	body
son/o	sound
-spadisa	opening, split or tear
-spasm	involuntary contraction
sperm/o, spermat/o	sperm
spin/o	spine, backbone
spondyl/o	vertebrae
-stasis	standing, stoppage
steat/o	fat
-stenosis	narrowing
stern/o	breastbone
steth/o	chest
-stitial	pertaining to location
-stomy	new surgical opening
-su	condition or thing
sub-	under
super/o	above or toward the head
supinati/o	supination
supra-	above, beyond, excessive
sym-	together, with
synovi/o	synovial membrane (joints)
tachy-	fast
-taxia	coordination, order of
ten/o, tend/o, tendin/o	pertaining to tendons
tenosynovi/o	tendon sheath (covering of tendon)
tens/o, tensi/o	tension, stretch
testicul/o, test/o	testes
tetra-	four
thalam/o	thalamus

Word Prefix, Root, Suffix	Definition, Pertaining to
thel/o	nipple
-therapy	treatment
-thermy	heat
thorac/o	chest, thorax
-thorax	chest
thromb/o	clot
thymo-	thymus gland
thyr/o	thyroid gland
-tic	pertaining to
-tocia, -tocin	labor and childbirth
tom/o	cut
-tome	instrument to cut, book
-tomy	cutting or incision of
ton/o	tension
tonsil/o	tonsils
top/o	place
trabecul/o	meshwork, trabeculae of bone
trache/o	windpipe or trachea
trans-	across
-tripsy	crushing, breaking up
-trophy	nourishment or growth
-tropia	turning
-tropic	stimulating
tub/o	fallopian tube

Word Prefix, Root, Suffix	Definition, Pertaining to
tympan/o	eardrum
-ule	small
ultra-	excess, beyond
-um	structure
ungu/o	nail
ur/o	urinary system
ure/o	end product of waste in urine
urethra/o, ureter/o	ureters
-uria	urine, urination
urin/o	urine
uter/o	uterus
valvul/o	valve
varic/o	dilated, twisted vein
vas/o	vas deferens
ven/o	venous
ventr/o	front
ventricul/o	ventricles of heart
versi/o	turning or tilting
vesic/o	bladder
viscer/o	internal organs
vitre/o	glasslike or gel-like
xer/o	dry
-y	process or condition
zygomat/o	cheekbone

ACCREDITING AGENCIES, PROFESSIONAL SOCIETIES, AND GOVERNMENT AGENCIES

ACCREDITING AGENCIES FOR HEALTHCARE FACILITIES

American Association of Blood Banks (AABB)
8101 Glenbrook Road
Bethesda, MD 20814-2749
301.907.6977
www.aabb.org

College of American Pathologists (CAP)
Clinical Laboratory Accreditation
325 Waukegan Road
Northfield, IL 60093-2750
800.323.4040
www.cap.org

Commission on Office Laboratory Accreditation
(COLA)
9881 Broken Land Parkway, Suite 200
Columbia, MD 21046-1158
800.981.9883
www.cola.org

The Joint Commission
(formerly The Joint Commission on Accreditation of
Healthcare Organizations)
One Renaissance Boulevard
Oakbrook Terrace, IL 60181
630.792.5000
www.jointcommission.org

ACCREDITING AGENCIES FOR EDUCATIONAL FACILITIES

Association of Schools of Allied Health Professionals
1730 M Street, Suite 500
Washington, DC 20036
202.293.4848
www.asahp.org

Commission on Accreditation of Allied Health
Education Programs (CAAHEP)
35 East Wacker Drive, Suite 1970
Chicago, IL 60606-2208
312.553.9355
www.caahep.org

Council for Higher Education Accreditation
One Dupont Circle, NW, Suite 510
Washington, DC 20036-1135
800.981.9883
www.chea.org

National Accrediting Agency for Clinical Laboratory
Sciences (NAACLS)
8410 Bryn Mawr Avenue, Suite 670
Chicago, IL 60631-3415
773.714.8880
www.naacls.org

ACCREDITING AGENCIES FOR LABORATORY AND ASSOCIATED PERSONNEL

American Association of Bioanalysts (AAB)
917 Locust Street, Suite 1100
St. Louis, MO 63101-1413
314.241.1445
www.aab.org

American Association of Medical Assistants (AAMA)
(Waived Tests)
20 N. Wacker Drive, Suite 1575
Chicago, IL 60606-2903
312.899.1500
www.aama-ntl.org

American Medical Association (AMA)
515 N. State Street
Chicago, IL 60610
312.464.5000
www.ama-assn.org

American Medical Technologists (AMT)
710 Higgins Rd.
Park Ridge, IL 60058-5765
847.823.5169
www.amt1.com

American Society for Clinical Pathology (ASCP)
PO Box 12277
Chicago, IL 60612-0277
312.738.1336
www.ascp.org

American Society of Phlebotomy Technicians (ASPT)
1109 2nd Avenue SW
PO Box 1831
Hickory, NC 28602
828.294.0078
www.aspt.org

PROFESSIONAL SOCIETIES FOR LABORATORY PROFESSIONALS

Advance for Medical Laboratory Professionals
2900 Horizon Dr., Box 61556
King of Prussia, PA 19406-0956
laboratorian.advanceweb.com

American Association for Clinical Chemistry
2101 L St. NW, Suite 202
Washington, DC 20037
www.aacc.org

American Society for Clinical Laboratory Science (ASCLS)
6701 Democracy Boulevard, Suite 300
Bethesda, MD 20817-1574
301.657.2768
www.ascls.org

Association for Professionals in Infection Control and Epidemiology (APIC)
1275 K Street NW, Suite 1000
Washington, DC 20005-4006
202.789.1890
www.apic.org

American Society for Microbiology (ASM)
1325 Massachusetts Avenue NW
Washington, DC 20005-4171
202.737.3600
www.asm.org

American Society of Hematology (ASH)
1200 19th Street NW, Suite 300
Washington, DC 20030
202.776.0544
www.hematology.org

Clinical Laboratory Management Association (CLMA)
401 N. Michigan Avenue, Suite 2200
Chicago, IL 60611
Phone: 312.321.5111
www.clma.org

GOVERNMENT AGENCIES WITH AN IMPACT ON CLINICAL LABORATORIES

Centers for Disease Control and Prevention
1600 Clifton Road
Atlanta, GA 30333
800.311.3435
www.cdc.gov

Centers for Medicare and Medicaid Services
7500 Security Boulevard
Baltimore, MD 21244
410.786.3000
www.cms.hhs.gov

NIOSH: The National Institute for Occupational
Safety and Health (NIOSH)
200 Independence Avenue SW, Room 715H
Washington, DC 20201
800.35NIOSH
www.cdc.gov/niosh

Occupational Safety and Health Administration
U.S. Department of Labor
Public Affairs Office, Room 3647
200 Constitution Avenue NW
Washington, DC 20402
202.512.1800
www.osha.gov

U.S. Food and Drug Administration
5600 Fishers Lane
Rockville, MD 20857
888.INFO.FDA
www.fda.gov

GLOSSARY

ABO grouping Landsteiner grouping system for blood groups A, B, AB, and O

Absorbance Measurable amount of light that is not able to pass through a colored solution

Accreditation Nongovernmental, voluntary process in which an agency grants recognition to a facility or institution that meets certain conditions and standards of excellence

Accuracy Measure of how close a derived value is to the true value as verified by other analytical methods

Acetest Test for presence of acetone in urine

Acetoacetic acid Also called diacetic acid; found in urine along with acetone indicating inadequately treated diabetes

Acetone Ketone body found in the blood when fats are metabolized for energy; an organic solvent

Acid (acidity) Having a pH below 7.0

Acid-fast bacilli (AFB) stain Stain used to identify *Mycobacterium tuberculosis* (cause of TB)

Acquired immunodeficiency syndrome (AIDS) Disease of the human immune system characterized cytologically by a reduction in the numbers of CD4-bearing helper T cells

Activated partial thromboplastin time (APPT) Amount of time elapsing between the addition of phospholipids and calcium and the formation of a fibrin clot

Acute phase Early reaction to a disease process with a sharp rise in antibody level

Agglutination Clumping together of materials (such as red blood cells, microorganisms, or particles) in the presence of specific antibodies

Albuminuria Presence of albumin in the urine, resulting from renal impairment

Alkaline (alkalinity) Having a pH above 7.0

American Association for Clinical Chemistry (AACC) Professional organization for registered clinical chemists

American Association for Respiratory Care (AARC) Professional organization for respiratory care professionals

American Board of Pathology Member organization of the American Board of Medical Specialties that certifies pathologists

American Medical Technologists (AMT) Organization providing registry exam for medical laboratory workers and phlebotomists

American Society for Clinical Laboratory Science (ASCLS) Professional forum for medical laboratory professionals; presents professional workshops, supports profession through political action and public awareness campaigns

American Society for Clinical Pathology (ASCP) Provides registry by examination for MLTs, MTs, and phlebotomists

American Society for Microbiology (ASM) International organization for life science professionals in microbiology-related fields

Analyte Constituent of body fluid that is being tested for

Analytical error Error that occurs in the laboratory during testing, either randomly or through equipment malfunction or operator performance

Anatomic (or clinical) pathologist The profession of pathology is divided into two major disciplines: clinical and anatomical. Anatomic pathologists work chiefly with surgical specimens of tissues and organs, and perform postmortem exams. Clinical pathologists work in close collaboration with medical laboratory professionals and referring

445

physicians to insure the accuracy and appropriate utilization of laboratory testing.

Anemia Nomenclature for a number of hematological disorders manifested by low red blood cell counts or by qualitative red blood cell disorders; literal meaning is "without blood"

Antibiotic therapy Administration of antibacterial agents to prevent or minimize infectious processes

Antibody Protein produced by a specialized white blood cell, the B lymphocyte, as a response to an antigen

Anticoagulant Medication used to prevent blood clotting

Anticoagulated specimen Blood specimen collected in a vacuum tube containing chemicals to prevent normal coagulation for when plasma is needed for laboratory testing

Antigen Any substance (usually foreign to the body) that evokes an immune response stimulating the production of an antibody

Antispermatic preparation Spermicide that destroys male reproductive germ cells, as used for contraception

Artery Blood vessels that carry oxygenated blood from the heart to tissues, cells, and organs of the body

Assignment of health care benefits "Assignment of Benefits" is a legally binding agreement between the patient and his or her insurance provider, requesting that reimbursement checks be sent to the physician, clinic, or other medical service provider

Association of Surgical Technologists (AST) Provides accreditation for educational programs of surgical technology

Atypical antibody (alloantibody) Antibody produced by one individual that reacts with an alloantigen of another individual of the same species; antibody other than anti-A, anti-B, or anti-AB; also called isoantibody

Autoanalyzer Automated testing equipment

Autoantibody Produced by the body in an autoimmune reaction to any of its own cells or cell products

Autolet device Spring-loaded device that performs capillary puncture for blood collection

Bacillus Calmette-Guérin (BCG) Vaccine used to provide immunity or protection against

tuberculosis (TB); also used to treat bladder tumors or bladder cancer

Bacteria One-celled microorganism with no organized nucleus and a cell membrane composed of carbohydrates

Bacterial incinerator Instrument that uses extreme heat to kill bacteria on metal devices that are used to collect bacterial colonies from a Petri dish

Basilic vein Large vein on inner side of bicep just above elbow; secondary choice for drawing blood

Basophil Type of white blood cell accounting for less than 1 percent of total white blood cells in the body; essential to mediating nonspecific immune response and producing histamine that dilates blood vessels; stains basic with methylene blue

Beaker Deep, wide-mouthed vessel usually with a lip for pouring; used in the laboratory for measuring and mixing

Beer's Law Describes the linear relationship of the absorption coefficient of light with the concentration of a solution

Beral pipette One-piece, semiquantitative pipette with a built-in suction bulb

Bevel Slanted end of a hypodermic needle

Bilirubin Reddish yellow pigment in bile or blood, derived from hemoglobin of red blood cells; causes jaundice if accumulated in excess

Biohazard Biological agent or condition (such as an infectious or highly contagious organism or an unsecure laboratory procedure) that poses a danger to humans or the environment

Biohazardous material Material contaminated by biological agents

Biological safety cabinet Used to protect the worker who is working with infectious microorganisms

Bloodborne and airborne pathogens Organisms classified as "covered pathogens" for their potential to cause serious disease or death; they include HIV, HBV, and TB; they are given special status in the orientation and training of health care workers

Bone marrow Soft tissue in the cavities of most bones; red marrow produces all blood cells

Breach Breaking of a contract

Break-even point Volume of testing at which it becomes more economical for a medical facility to set up its own testing facility rather than to send tests out to a reference laboratory

Bunsen burner Single-flame gas heating device

Buret pipette Quantitative pipette with a valve to start and stop flow of solution for extremely accurate measurement; used primarily for titration

Calcium ions Factor in blood clotting; released from the bone into the bloodstream

Capillary action Rise or fall of liquid in a small passage or tube; caused by surface tension when a liquid comes in contact with a solid

Capillary pipette Similar to a capillary tube with the exception that a capillary pipette has markings or lines of demarcation indicating an approximate amount

Capillary puncture Procedure where small vessels of the finger, toe, or heel are pricked for small blood samples

Capillary tube Used to contain a small amount of blood that is centrifuged to enable an estimate of whole blood versus plasma for the hematocrit test

Carpel tunnel syndrome Repetitive strain injury that can be caused by long-term manual pipette operation

Causation Causal relationship between conduct and the result derived from that conduct

Caustic Corrosive or burning; destroys body tissue on contact

Celsius International temperature scale on which water freezes at 0°C and boils at 100°C

Centers for Disease Control and Prevention (CDC) Federal agency under the Department of Health and Human Services charged with protecting public health and safety

Centimeter Metric measure of length equaling one-hundredth of a meter

Centrifuge Device that spins samples to separate components based on differences in density

Cephalic vein Superficial vein just beneath the skin of the middle inner part of the bend of the arm (elbow); used for phlebotomy procedures

Cerebrospinal fluid (CSF) Fluid that circulates within the brain's ventricles and spinal column to maintain uniform pressure

Certification Verifies a fact or condition, usually by examination, such as the ability to perform a profession

Chief executive officer (CEO) Top officer in an organization who has the highest decision-making power

Class A The higher standard of volumetric flask as determined by the United States or equivalent; made with a more accurately placed graduation mark and has a unique serial number for traceability. Class B or equivalent containers are used for more qualitative analyses or for educational work

Clinical Laboratory Improvement Amendments of 1967 (CLIA 67) Federal legislation to improve the practice of laboratory medicine

Clinical Laboratory Improvement Amendments of 1988 (CLIA 88) Federal legislation modifying and superseding CLIA 67

Clinical Laboratory Management Association (CLMA) Professional organization for laboratory managers

Clinical laboratory scientist (CLS) Equivalent to a medical technologist (MT)

Clinical laboratory technician (CLT) Equivalent to a medical laboratory technician (MLT); a technical worker in a medical laboratory who is supervised by a CLS (MT)

Clinical pathologist *See* anatomic (or clinical) pathologist

Clinical significance Test result that has relevance to a patient's condition based on a medical professional's judgment regarding that particular patient

Clinically normal people People whose test results are deemed normal because they fall within acceptable standard deviations

Clinitest Test performed by tablet in semiquantitative determination for reducing substances in urine or feces

Clotting time Amount of time that elapses before whole blood forms a clot; a test that measures the amount of time for a fibrin clot to form

Coagulation Change from a liquid to a viscous, thickened state; the clotting process of blood

Coagulation factors Thirteen factors in the blood responsible for the process of blood clotting

Coefficient of variation (CV) Variability of test results expressed in percentage form when the mean value is divided by the standard deviation

College of American Pathologists (CAP) Professional organization supporting M.D. and O.D. pathologists

Colorimetric Term describing clinical chemistry tests in which a color develops that can be measured

Commission on Accreditation of Allied Health Education Programs (CAAHEP) Accrediting organization for allied health education programs

Commission on Colleges (COC) Accrediting organization of the Southern Association of Colleges and Schools

Complete blood count (CBC) Measures white blood cells and red blood cells as well as qualitative characteristics; screens for and monitors a variety of disorders, such as anemia

Continuous quality improvement (CQI) Program that documents improvement in institutional performance over a period of time

Convalescent phase Follows the initial acute phase in a bacterial infection when the antibody level drops as the patient recovers from the infection

Cost center Component of a health care facility, such as a clinical laboratory or pharmacy, which generates revenue for the facility

Crenated Scalloped shaped; used to describe red blood cells in a hypertonic solution

Cross match Process of determining if a recipient of a unit of blood has antibodies against the donor unit

Cryptococcus Spore-forming yeast found in soil and bird droppings that may cause meningitis and other infections in immunosuppressed individuals

Crystal violet stain Stain used to dye bacteria for microscopic evaluation

Cubital vein, medial Vein at the bend of the inner elbow connecting cephalic and basilica veins

Cumulative sum (CUSUM) control chart Data analysis technique for determining if a measurement process has gone out of statistical control

Cuvette Clear container used for measuring spectrophotometric changes in a liquid or a mixture

Cyanmethemoglobin Compound of cyanide and methemoglobin; quantitative measure of its presence in blood identifies various types of anemia

Cytotechnologist Medical technician trained in the identification of cells and cellular abnormalities

Damages Compensation paid to a claimant if he or she is successful in court at proving loss, injury, or harm suffered by another's breach of duty

D antigen Blood grouping antigen that denotes whether an individual is Rh positive or negative

Deciliter Metric measure of volume equaling 0.1 liter or 100 mL

Decolorizer Solution of ethanol and acetone used to remove dye from a stained microbiological specimen

Decontamination Removal of harmful microorganisms or toxic chemicals through physical, chemical, or heating methods

Delta change (Δchange) Any change in value of something being measured

Department of Health and Human Services (HHS) U.S. Federal agency with control over budgets for all human health programs, including the Centers for Disease Control and Prevention and the Food and Drug Administration

Department of Health, Education, and Welfare (HEW) U.S. Former name for the current U.S. Department of Health and Human Services

Dipstick Plastic strip with chemically treated pads that react to various chemical constituents during urinalysis

Director Supervisory head of a laboratory

Direct leukocyte count (DLC) Actual count of white blood cells in a prescribed volume; reported as a percentage

Direct test or method Procedure that directly measures the presence of a virus rather than measuring antibodies formed against the virus

Discrete analysis Analytic process in which test reactions take place in separate compartments; the compartments require cleaning or disposal before subsequent procedures

Doctor of osteopathy (D.O.) Licensed physician who emphasizes treatment of the patient as a whole, rather than focusing on one system or body part

Duty Moral or legal obligation

EDTA Ethylenediaminetetraacetic acid; used as an anticoagulant to preserve morphology of blood cells; the tube for blood collection containing EDTA is lavender

Efficiency Selection of test method that produces the greatest number of correct results; wise use of time and resources

Electrochemistry Testing process that measures chemical reactions that take place in a solution when electric voltage is applied

End-point reaction Procedure in which the reaction between reagent and patient sample is complete and remains stable for a period of time; also called colorimetric reaction

Engineered controls Safety controls that are manufactured, such as sharps disposal containers, self-sheathing needles, and eye-washing facilities

Enzymatic Procedure in which enzymes are used to react with a substrate or as a catalyst

Eosinophil White blood cell with large orange granules; comprises 1% to 3% of all white blood cells; numbers increase in allergic reactions and parasitic infections; releases chemical mediators such as histamines

Equivalency testing Examinations formerly but no longer accepted for credentialing laboratory workers other than formal certification, licensure, or registry

Erlenmeyer flask Graduated flask with a narrow neck and flat bottom

Ethics System of moral principles that governs the conduct of individuals in their personal and professional lives

Exposure Control Committee Sometimes included in the Infection Control Committee; makes policies to prevent exposure to biohazardous and toxic materials

Exposure incident Direct contact with patient blood or body fluids, usually as a result of lack of training, failure to follow proper procedures, or exposure to patient who does not yet show symptoms; incidents must be reported promptly to the supervisor of the department where the incident occurred; if warranted the incident also will be reported to the Infection Control Committee

Extrinsic factor Extrinsic pathway utilizing Factor III; important in the coagulation process following a break in the skin but not present within circulating blood

Factor X Unites intrinsic and extrinsic pathways of blood coagulation; activated factor X activates prothrombin; deficiency may cause a systemic coagulation disorder

Fahrenheit Temperature scale in general use in the United States on which the freezing point of water is 32°F and the boiling point is 212°F

False positive paradox Situation in which the actual incidence of a condition is lower than the statistical false positive rate for that test, making it extremely difficult to identify true positives for very rare conditions

Fecal materials Products remaining from digestion of food in the gastrointestinal system that may contaminate urine specimens

Ferricyanide Compound of iron and cyanide; used to oxidize oxyhemoglobin to methemoglobin as a convenient form used for measuring hemoglobin by spectrophotometer or hemoglobinometer

Fiber fragments Fragments from cloth or paper that may contaminate urine specimens

Financial management Management of costs and revenues to maintain the fiscal viability of a laboratory

Flask Narrow-necked, wide-bottomed vessel used for measuring and mixing in the laboratory

Fluoride Ingredient in anticoagulant that is recommended for glucose determinations when testing will be delayed; not suitable for other determinations

Fomite Inanimate object (such as a dish or article of clothing) that may be contaminated with infectious organisms and serve in their transmission

Food and Drug Administration, U.S. Federal agency responsible for oversight of many health related institutions and practices

F-test Compares the precision of the same method for two different procedures; the standard deviation of the method with the larger variance is divided by the standard deviation of the one showing the smaller variance to show the percentage difference

Fume hood Used to prevent inhalation while working with toxic chemicals

Fungi, yeasts, and molds Related groups in the kingdom of fungi; chlorophyll is not found in this group; may grow as uni- or multicellular organisms; most fungi are not pathogenic and some are normal flora

Gamma globulin Class of blood plasma proteins, most notably including antibodies that help fight infections and disease

Gel technology Imbedding of either antigens or antibodies into a colloidal solution where reactions between antigens and antibodies are often visible; widely used in immunohematology

Gene probe Single-stranded DNA or RNA fragment used to seek out its complementary sequence among a mixture of other singled-stranded fragments

Genetic predisposition Make-up of an individual's genes that causes a statistical increase in certain ailments

Ghost cells Red blood cells whose cellular components have lost their hemoglobin, leaving only the cytoplasmic membrane visible in microscopic examination of urine samples

Giardia lamblia Parasite (protozoan) of the digestive system, identified by its ova (eggs)

Gilson micropipette Pipette operated by piston-driven air displacement that is designed for precise liquid sample measurements

Glassware Refers to laboratory vessels used for measuring and mixing (such as flasks, beakers, graduated cylinders, and pipettes) even when they are made of plasticized materials

Glomerular permeability Capability of the glomeruli of the kidneys to filter and reabsorb liquids and components of the urine

Graduated cylinder Long, cylindrical tube held upright by a stable base that is wider than the vertical stem; marked along its entire length with calibration marks, but not considered as accurate as other volumetric vessels

Gram Metric measure of mass equaling 1/1000 of a kilogram SI (or 0.035 ounce)

Gram negative Bacteria from which color can be washed away when decolorized in the Gram stain procedure; seen as pink on the slide

Gram positive Bacteria from which color cannot be washed away when decolorized; seen as purple on a stained slide

Gram stain Procedure utilizing crystal violet, safranin, eosin, and a decolorizer; the first step in determining the morphology and identification of bacteria

Gravimetric analysis Calibration method for pipettes using a precision analytical balance and the density of water as the constant

Griffin beaker Semiquantitative glassware that is chemically inert and thermally stable; most often used to heat, melt, and mix premeasured substances

Gross lipemia Fats in the blood; plasma from a patient with this condition will be cloudy or even opaque

Hazardous chemical Chemical present in the workplace that is capable of causing harm; OSHA currently regulates exposure to approximately 400 substances

Health Care and Financial Administration (HCFA) Federal agency responsible for funding and supervising health care under Medicare and Medicaid

Health care clearinghouse Maintains medical records for large institutions and other medical care providers by providing financial and administrative transactions

Health care provider May be an organization as well as an individual (also called a health care professional) who delivers appropriate health care services in a systematic way to any individual in need of such services. Typically, health care providers are required to be licensed or certified

Health Insurance Portability and Accountability Act (HIPAA) Federal law that protects privacy rights of patients' health information and medical records; establishes national standards for electronic health care transactions; protects health insurance coverage for workers and their families who change or lose jobs

Health maintenance organization (HMO) System where health care is prepaid with the intention of controlling health costs

Health savings account (HSA) Individual savings account for health care expenses into which funds contributed are not subject to federal income tax at the time of deposit

Hemacytometer Device with microscopic grids designed for use in counting blood cells and platelets from a diluted sample

Hematocrit Represents the percentage of red blood cells in whole blood; valuable in screening for anemias; also called a packed cell volume (PCV)

Hematoma Bruise often accompanied by swelling that is caused by a break in a blood vessel collecting under the skin; often occurs during a venipuncture

Hemoconcentration Higher density of red blood cells due to decrease in the dilutional effect of plasma

Hemoglobin Pigment of red blood cells containing iron; responsible for transporting oxygen to tissues and carbon dioxide to lungs for expulsion

Hemorrhage Uncontrolled loss of blood from body causing loss of oxygenation to tissues; may be fatal if not treated quickly or effectively

Hepatitis B virus (HBV) Causes hepatitis B, an acute inflammation of the liver

Hexane Organic solvent

High-density lipoprotein (HDL) Known as "good" cholesterol for its tendency to carry cholesterol away from the arteries and back to the liver where it is excreted

High efficiency particulate air (HEPA) filter mask Provides protection against airborne infectious diseases, dust, allergens, and nontoxic particles

High-power field (HPF) Microscope magnification level used to count cells

Histotechnologist Laboratory technologist concerned with preparing and processing histological (microscopic) specimens

Human immunodeficiency virus (HIV) Retrovirus that causes acquired immunodeficiency syndrome (AIDS)

Human T-lymphotropic virus 1 and 2 (HLTV-1 and HLTV-2) Human retroviruses that cause T-cell leukemia and T-cell lymphoma; U.S. blood supplies are routinely tested for both

Humors Fluids or semifluids in the body

Hypertonic Having a higher level of dissolved elements in liquid; may relate to body fluids that affect the flow of water between tissues and cells of the body

Hypotonic Dilute liquid containing large amounts of water; often relates to IV fluids, plasma, or urine specimens

Iatrogenic Condition introduced inadvertently by a physician or surgeon or by medical treatment or a diagnostic procedure

Ictotest Tablet method to chemically test for increased level of bilirubin in urine

Illinois Society for Microbiology (ISM) Professional organization supporting medical microbiologists in Illinois

Immunocompromised Having a weakened immune system that is incapable of reacting normally to fight infection

Immunohematology Another name for blood banking; relates to collection, testing, and storage of blood prior to transfusion, and the testing of patients for blood compatibility with units selected for administering

Immunologic hormones Hormones that work to prevent tissue damage during an acute phase reaction

Immunosuppressive drug therapy Drug regimen to inhibit or prevent activity of the immune system, usually to treat autoimmune or inflammatory diseases or to prevent rejection of transplanted organs or tissues

Inanimate (nonliving) object Can act as an antigen to activate immune responses; for example, pollen, chemicals, or toxins

India ink prep Preparation used for determining capsulation of certain organisms when viewed microscopically, most frequently for *Cryptococcus neoformans*

Indirect test or method Diagnoses an infection by testing for antibodies to an antigen rather than by testing for the antigen directly

Infection control Activities directed toward elimination of or prevention of infection; includes work activities as well as immunization

Infection Control Committee Sometimes includes a separate Exposure Control Committee for isolating body fluids and toxic chemicals; makes policies and monitors compliance to prevent spread of infection and to enforce proper storage and removal of wastes

International normalized ratio (INR) System whereby prothrombin times are calculated using the normal control; provides standardization throughout the world where various instruments and reagents are used

International Sensitivity Index Indicates how a particular batch of tissue factor compares to an internationally standardized sample; the ISI is usually between 1.0 and 2.0

International System of Units (SI) Modern standard of the metric system used universally in science; becoming dominant also in international trade and commerce

Intrinsic factor Factors in the coagulation process that are included in the circulating components of blood

Inulin Polysaccharide derived from plants and used in renal function studies

Iodine stain Used to stain starch molecules; useful in performing amylase procedures; skin disinfectant for collecting blood cultures

Ketoacidosis Life-threatening condition in which a patient's blood becomes acid rather than slightly alkaline

Ketones Acetone and diacetic acid bodies found in blood when fats have been metabolized for energy

Kilogram Metric measure of weight equaling 1000 grams; base unit of mass in SI, equal to 1 liter of water

Kilometer Metric measure of length equaling 1000 meters; 1.6 K equals 1 mile

Kinetic reaction Common clinical chemistry method that measures the amount of change occurring in the reagent and sample mixture over a period of time

Laboratory Information System (LIS) Computer system that generates identification labels, interfaces with testing equipment, and transmits test results electronically to other hospital departments or physician's office laboratories

Lancet Sharp device used to puncture skin for collecting small blood samples

Latex reagent Solution containing latex particles that are often used to coat antibody-antigen complexes; enables visual observation of agglutination and precipitation

Lease-purchase Agreement whereby a facility has the use of a piece of equipment as long as the facility purchases consumable supplies and reagents for that equipment

Leeuwenhoek, Anton van Credited with making the first microscope

Leukemia Malignant growth in bone marrow; produces numerous abnormal cells

Leukocyte Any white blood cell

Leukocyte esterase (leukoesterase) Enzyme found in urine specimens when white blood cells have been destroyed

Levey-Jennings charts Graph form of daily quality control records for the laboratory

Licensure Governmental and nonvoluntary method of ensuring competence by a practitioner of a profession

Lifestyle costs Increased costs of health care for those with risky lifestyles, which are passed on to the insured and/or to taxpayers

Light-guided pipetting system Computer-based accessories that use LCD monitors or LED arrays to light source and destination wells in microplates or vials for accurate well-to-well pipetting; text-to-speech features on some systems alert operators to laboratory protocols

Linear Having the characteristic of a straight line; response or output that is directly proportional to the input

Lister, Joseph Developed techniques for aseptically cleaning a surgical suite

Liter Metric measure of volume equaling approximately a quart in the English system of measurement

Low-density lipoprotein (LDL) Known as "bad" cholesterol for its tendency to form plaque in arteries, where blood clots in narrowed arteries could cause stroke or heart attack

Low-power field (LPF) Microscope magnification level used to count certain elements in specimens

Lumen Internal diameter of a needle or tube, or other tubular body cavity such as a blood vessel, intestine, or esophagus

Lymphocyte Type of white blood cell that increases in viral infections; B cells produce antibodies and T lymphocytes recognize invasive antigens

Macroglobulinemia Presence of increased levels of macroglobulins in circulating blood; a plasma cell disorder resembling leukemia that produces copious amounts of immunoglobulin

Macropipettes Pipettes that dispense volumes greater than 1 mL

Macroscopic Visible with the naked eye

Malaria Acute or chronic disease caused by the presence in red blood cells of protozoan parasites of the genus *Plasmodium*; four major strains of the malaria organism are capable of infecting humans, although none are prevalent in North America

Malpighi, Marcello Described renal cells in the 1600s

Mean Average of all values

Median Middle value within a range, with half of the values above and half below

Medical laboratory technician (MLT) Also called a clinical lab technician (CLT)

Medical technologist (MT) Also known as clinical lab scientist (CLS)

Medicare and Medicaid Federal government programs providing health insurance for those over 65 years old, those with low income, or those who meet other special criteria; reimburses medical facilities and physicians at a lower rate than the actual cost of service

Memory cells Lymphocyte other than a B-lymphocyte that maintains memory of past infections and can clone itself rapidly to produce more antibody-forming cells (plasma cells)

Meningitis Inflammation of the meninges, or protective membranes surrounding the brain and spinal cord; severity and treatment vary by cause (viral or bacterial)

Metabolic end-point products Body waste products that can help diagnose genetic disorders

Methemoglobin A form of the oxygen-carrying protein hemoglobin; methemoglobin cannot carry oxygen

Microcapillary reader Instrument used to read percentage of cells in a microhematocrit test

Microliter Metric measure of volume equaling 0.001 mL (1 μL)

Microorganisms Normally one-celled organisms that are microscopic

Micropipettes Pipettes that dispense between 1 μL and 1000 μL (1 mL)

Microscopic Can only be seen though a microscope; extremely small

Mode Most frequently occurring value in a set of data points

Mohr pipette Graduated pipette designed for measuring point to point, so the calibration lines do not extend to the end of the pipette

Molality (m) Weight measure of moles of solute per kilogram of solvent, expressed as mol/kg

Molarity (M) Volume measure of moles of solute per liter of solvent, expressed as mol/L

Molar solution Uses molarity to measure solutes in solution; common form of commercially prepared chemistry reagents for performing clinical chemistry tests

Molecular biology Study and development of cellular physiology; future medical laboratory work may chiefly be done in this realm

Monocyte Largest of the five basic white blood cells; functions in the tissues as a macrophage (eats foreign antigens) when it reaches maturity

Morality System of conduct based on principles or ideals of virtuous human behavior; principles of proper professional conduct concerning the rights and duties of health care professionals, their patients, and their colleagues

Multistix Strip of chemically treated pads that will react colorimetrically when exposed to certain components

Nanotechnology Study and engineering of very small chemical or biological objects that are approximately the size of atoms or small molecules

National Credentialing Agency for Laboratory Personnel (NCA) Formerly a certification organization, now merged with ASCP

National Institute of Standards and Technology (NIST) Federal agency responsible for developing and promoting accurate measurements and standards in many disciplines

Necrotic Dead tissue or cells

Needle gauge Outer diameter of a hypodermic needle; the larger the gauge number, the smaller the needle

Neutrophil Type of granular white blood cell that primarily attacks bacteria

Nitrites Presence in urine indicates infection by certain bacteria

Normal frequency distribution Bell-shaped curve showing the probability distributions of random variables; also called Gaussian or normal distribution

Normality (N) Gram equivalent molecular weight of a solute per liter of solvent

Nosocomial Acquired or occurring in a hospital

Nurse's Creed Standard pledge for graduating nurses; dated to 1893 and adapted from the physician's Oath of Hippocrates; also known as the Nightingale Pledge in honor of Florence Nightingale

Oath of Hippocrates Oath for graduating physicians; named in honor of the Greek physician who was called the Father of Medicine since he first recorded medical experiences for others to review

Other potentially infectious materials (OPIM) All body fluids other than blood that are potentially infectious

Order of draw Established sequence of tubes used for blood collection to avoid contamination by preventing carryover of additives from one tube to another

Ova and parasites Also called O&P or OCP (ova, cysts, and parasites); most often found in fecal specimens; the ova, cysts, or eggs of intestinal parasites are easily identified by their morphology

Oxyhemoglobin Hemoglobin pigment combined with oxygen atoms

Pap smear Papanicolaou test that screens for changes in cervical cells that might indicate infection, abnormality, or cancer

Parameters Acceptable ranges for controls for valid clinical data

Pasteur pipette Semiquantitative pipette, commonly called a dropper, used for transferring small amounts of liquids

Pathologist Physician who interprets and diagnoses the changes caused by disease in tissues and body fluids

Patient's Bill of Rights Formal statement by a medical facility guaranteeing that treatment will meet certain established standards

Percentage Part of a whole expressed in hundredths

Percent solution Amount of solute expressed as parts (by mass or weight) per 100 parts of solution

Personal protective equipment (PPE) Includes goggles, masks, face and eye shields, gowns, and gloves to protect individual workers from contact with patient blood or body fluid

Personnel licensure Government-sanctioned certification of an individual, as opposed to a facility

Petri dish Shallow, cylindrical lidded dish used to culture cells, primarily bacteria

pH Measure of hydrogen ion concentration of a solution; pH of 7 is normal, below is acid and above is alkaline

Physician office laboratory (POL) Testing facility owned and operated by an individual health care provider or group practice

Pipette Narrow tube into which fluid is drawn by suction, many varieties of which are used in the clinical laboratory to transfer extremely small up to sizable amounts of liquid; can be made of glass or plastic, reusable or disposable

Pipette calibration Quality check required periodically to maintain accurate and consistent measurement

Pipette filler Alternative to mouth pipetting for filling pipettes easily

Pipette helper Battery-operated pipette filler designed to be used with disposable pipettes

Pipette tip Used with pipetter for extremely small amounts to provide reproducibility and accuracy with extremely small amounts

Plasma Liquid part of whole blood

Pleural, pericardial, peritoneal, and synovial fluids fluids from body cavities used as specimens for testing

Point-of-care testing (POCT) Laboratory testing that takes place at the patient's bedside

Polycarbonate Plastic used for laboratory materials; transparent thermoplastic characterized by high impact strength and high softening temperature; most volumetric flasks and disposable pipettes with built-in bulbs for aspiration of fluids are composed of polycarbonates

Polycythemia An increase in the proportion of blood volume that is occupied by red blood cells, due to an increase in the mass of red blood cells or a decrease in the volume of plasma

Polyethylene Plastic used for laboratory materials; lightweight thermoplastic resistant to chemicals and moisture and with good insulating properties

Polypropylene Plastic used for laboratory materials

Polystyrene Plastic used for laboratory materials; rigid transparent thermoplastic with good electrical insulating properties, used especially in molded products

Polyvinyl chloride Plastic used for laboratory materials; polymer of vinyl chloride (known as PVC) used especially for electrical insulation, films, and pipes

Population norms Normal ranges that account for ethnic, genetic, and cultural differences, including lifestyle; may vary slightly between geographic locations within the same country

Postanalytical error Error that occurs after testing; usually refers to recording error or data transmission error

Postzone Phenomenon in which agglutination or precipitation does not occur in lower dilution or undiluted samples because of an excess of antigens relative to antibodies, yielding misleading results

PPD (tuberculin) skin test Positive results indicate recent exposure or actual infection with *M. tuberculosis*; medical facilities require testing of workers before direct patient contact

Preanalytical error Error that occurs before testing is performed; often refers to improper sample collection or misidentification of a specimen or patient

Preceptor Working professional who supervises students during workplace training

Precision Reproducibility of results when the conditions of the performance of procedures is the same; not to be confused with accuracy

Predictive value Rate at which a test result would be expected for certain disease states

Preferred provider option (PPO) Developed to encourage the use of assigned physicians and medical facilities as a way to contain costs

Professionalism Competence and skills expected of someone in the career field; cleanliness, proper grooming, and confident manner

Proficiency testing (PT) program Commercial program that laboratories subscribe to; measures accuracy by comparing reported values to those of other facilities doing similar procedures with similar technology

Prothrombin Plasma protein coagulation factor synthesized from vitamin K

Prothrombin time (PT) Used to monitor anticoagulant therapy

Protozoan Unicellular, animal-like organism of the phylum Protozoa that may infect humans who are immunocompromised; several malaria species are examples of protozoans

Prozone Phenomenon in which agglutination or precipitation occurs at higher dilution ranges, but is not visible in lower dilution or undiluted samples because of an excess of antibodies relative to antigens, yielding misleading results

Pus Purulent matter that may gather around the site of an infection, composed chiefly of white blood cells

Qualitative procedure Yields a positive or negative result with no attempt at quantitation

Quality assurance Encompasses all aspects, including personnel and equipment, of performance in a facility; quality control is a vital component of a total quality assurance program

Quality control programs Sets of controls performed along with patient samples to provide for accuracy in the laboratory; results are recorded and compared from day to day; mean averages and population norms are determined in this manner

Quantitative pipette Pipette marked to measure volumes to a significantly accurate level

Quantitative procedure Provides specific numbers, amounts, or levels of analytes

Quantity not sufficient (QNS) Indication on report referring to specimen volume

Random access Type of analytic equipment that is programmable to accept samples out of order

Random error Error that occurs during testing without explanation; often discovered when a single result does not match other clinical data for the same patient

Reference laboratory Laboratory that performs low-volume, very specialized tests beyond the scope or affordability of a typical hospital or medical facility

Registration Process by which a professional association places an individual on a list (registry) of persons possessing minimum competencies in a particular field

Registry List of qualified individuals deemed professionally competent through examination

Reimbursement Payment by insurance plans and government programs to medical facilities and physicians toward the cost of patient services

Reproducibility Also called precision; testing that is run repetitively on the same specimen should yield the same results

Reticulocyte Last immature stage of an erythrocyte (red blood cell)

Retrovirus RNA-containing virus that may be implicated in sarcomas, leukemias, and lymphomas

Rheumatoid arthritis (RA) Chronic, progressive autoimmune disease characterized by inflammation and swelling of joints, muscle weakness, and fatigue

Rh factor/Rh type Genetically determined protein on red blood cells; "Big D" is the major antigen used for positive or negative blood type

Rickettsiae Intracellular parasitic bacterium that is usually tick-borne

Ringworm Common term for a contagious skin infection (tinea) caused by a fungus, *Microsporum* or *Trichophyton*

Risk management Prevention and containment of liability by documenting critical or unusual patient care incidents

Rotor Spinning part of a centrifuge that is powered by a motor

Safety Committee Responsible for monitoring the entire physical plant of a facility for safety issues to protect visitors, patients, and workers; works closely with the Infection Control Committee and/ or Exposure Committee

Safranin Biological stain used to dye blood cells; orange in color

Screening test Sensitive but not completely specific test; used for large groups to identify certain individuals for further definitive testing

Sealing putty Similar to clay and plumber's putty; used for sealing ends of microhematocrit tubes

Semiquantitative pipette Pipette not intended for accurate measurement but for general transfer of liquid from one tube or container to another

Semiquantitative procedure Results do not provide numerical values but are graded relative to normal levels of antibodies when no active disease is present (such as weakly reactive, moderately reactive, etc.)

Sensitivity Proper level incorporated into test procedures to detect clinically significant amounts of analytes to help rule out false positive results

Sequential analysis Tests performed in a prescribed order or in the order they were entered into an analyzer

Serial dilution Sequentially increasing dilutions of serum in a quantitative procedure to measure antibodies or antigens

Serological pipette Quantitative pipette with graduations extending all the way to the tip; can be used to measure point to point or point to top

Serology Study of fluid components of blood, usually for antibodies or antigens

Serum Liquid part of blood that has clotted and has been centrifuged; contains little or no clotting factors or platelets

Severe acute respiratory syndrome (SARS) Illness caused by a single-stranded RNA virus of the genus *Coronavirus*, which is found only in chickens, turkeys, ducks, and migratory fowl; transmitted by respiratory droplets or body fluids

Sharps Sharp objects, such as needles, broken glass tubes, glass slides, and scalpels, that require special care in use and disposal, especially if contaminated with patient blood or other body fluid

Shift Abrupt change from the established mean on a quality control chart; may be positive or negative

Short draws Insufficiently filled sample tubes; results in improper dilution ratio and erroneous test results

SI *See* International System of Units

Significant figures Minimum number of digits required to be meaningful for a particular measurement

Silica Derived from sand, natural material from which laboratory glassware was originally handblown

Sodium nitroferricyanide Used in urinalysis to colorimetrically identify amino acids

Southern Association of Colleges and Schools (SACS) Regional educational accreditation agency for the southern states, recognized by the U.S. Department of Education

Specific gravity Weight of a substance, usually liquid, compared with an equal amount of water

Specificity Measure of the incidence of true negative results; having relevance for a specific disease or will react only with a specific receptor on the surface of a cell

Spectrophotometer Measures the relative intensity of color in a material by comparing with the different wavelengths in the spectrum

Square root Factor of a number that when multiplied by itself equals that number

Standard deviation (SD) Measures the distribution of values around the mean of a data set; an acceptable range for results of quality control materials

Standard Precautions Guidelines recommended by the CDC to reduce risk of the spread of infection in a health care facility; designed primarily to protect patients

Subarachnoid hemorrhage Bleeding in the area between the brain and the thin tissues (arachnoid membrane) that cover the brain

Sulfhemoglobin Compound of hemoglobin and hydrogen sulfide; prevents normal oxygen binding; excess creates a toxic condition

Sulfosalicylic acid (SSA) Reagent used to measure a semiquantitative level of protein in urine

Supernatant Usually clear, lighter overlying material at the top of a tube after centrifugation

Systemic lupus erythematosus (SLE) Chronic, inflammatory autoimmune disorder that may affect skin, joints, kidneys, and other organs; the most common and serious form of lupus

Teflon Synthetic resin used for molding and nonstick coatings; commonly used for laboratory materials

The Joint Commission (TJC) Evaluates and accredits hospital laboratory services and freestanding laboratories; formerly the Joint Commission on Accreditation of Healthcare Organizations (JCAHO)

Thrombocytes Platelets produced in the bone marrow that are involved in forming stable clots, among other functions

Thromboplastin Blood coagulation factor III, found in both blood and tissues

Tissue Committee Hospital committee that reviews tissues removed from surgical procedures to determine if treatment was appropriate

Titer Dilution of a serum containing a specific antibody at which the solution retains the minimum level of activity needed to neutralize or precipitate an antigen

Too numerous to count (TNTC) Notation for when numbers of white blood cells in a biological sample viewed under a microscope exceed 100/HPF

Tort Negligent or intentional civil wrong not arising out of a contract or statute; can include malpractice, negligence, assault and battery (which may also be considered criminal), invasion of privacy, abuse, and defamation of character

Total cholesterol Measures both high-density and low-density lipoproteins

Total solids (TS) meter Measures specific gravity as a screen in urinalysis

Transfer pipette Semiquantitative pipette used for measuring reagents by the number of drops dispensed; bulbs can serve as a reservoir

Transfusion Process of transferring whole blood or blood components from one person (donor) to another (recipient)

Trend When a quality control value consistently increases or decreases from the mean value for six consecutive days

Treponema pallidum Causative organism for syphilis

Trichloroacetic acid (TCA) Reagent used in urinalysis to treat for turbidity

Trichomonas Two species of this genus of flagellated parasitic protozoan cause sexually transmitted infection, mostly in women

t-Test Comparison of standard deviations for two methods for the same procedure should be approximately the same; also called paired "t" test

Tuberculosis (TB) Usually chronic respiratory disease transmitted by the airborne bacterium *M. tuberculosis*; classified as a "covered pathogen"

Tubular reabsorption Process by which solutes (protein and salts) and water are removed from the tubular fluid of the kidney and transported into the blood; called reabsorption because these substances have already been absorbed once (particularly in the intestines)

Turbidity Cloudy appearance of liquid due to precipitant

Tygon Clear, flexible, and extremely chemically resistant plastic commonly used for tubing

Undiluted Full strength, not changed or weakened with the addition of water or any other liquid

Universal Precautions Guidelines recommended by the CDC designed primarily to protect workers with occupational exposure to pathogens in blood or body fluids

Unopette disposable diluting pipette Container with diluents; used to dilute blood in preparation for counting blood cells on hemacytometer

Urinometer Device for determining specific gravity of a liquid by flotation

Urobilinogen Bilirubin that is broken down by bacterial action in the gut

Vein Blood vessel that carries deoxygenated blood from tissues back to heart and lungs

Venipuncture Procedure for collecting blood from a vein

Virus Infective organism that must live intracellularly in order to survive and reproduce

Volume expander Normal saline or plasma administered to maintain adequate blood pressure during or following hemorrhage

Volumetric container Measuring container of various sizes and shapes used in the laboratory

Volumetric pipette Provides extremely accurate measurement of a specific volume of solution; commonly used to make laboratory solutions from a base stock as well as to prepare titrations

Waived test Test that may be performed by noncredentialed laboratory personnel

Warfarin (Coumadin) Anticoagulant medication

Wavelength Distance between beginning and ending of a single wave cycle; used for measuring both end-point and kinetic reactions

Work practice controls Practices rather than devices that the medical worker can use to protect against contamination, such as hand washing

BIBLIOGRAPHY

American Society for Clinical Laboratory Science. (2001). Scope of practice. *ASCLS House of Delegates*, pp. 1–5.

Baer, D. M. (2007, March). Tips from the technical experts: answering your questions. *Medical Laboratory Observer*, 39(3); 48–49.

Beck, S., Briden, M. & Epner, P. (2008). Practice levels and educational needs for clinical laboratory personnel. *Clinical Laboratory Science,* 21(2); 68–77.

Berger, D. (1999). A brief history of medical diagnosis and the birth of the clinical laboratory. *Medical Laboratory Observer* (online). Retrieved October 12, 2009, from http://www.mlo-online.com/history/LabHistory1.pdf.

Centers for Disease Control and Prevention (CDC). (2005). Guidelines for preventing the transmission of Mycobacterium tuberculosis in health-Care settings. *MMWR Recommendations and Reports*, 54(RR17);1–141. Atlanta, GA: Centers for Disease Control and Prevention.

Cosman, T., & Bissell, M. (1991). Ethics and the clinical laboratory. Part II. What has happened to patient confidentiality? *Medical Laboratory Observer*, 23(8), 38–40.

Do, A. N., Ciesielski, C. A., Metler, R. P., Hammett, T. A., Li, J., & Fleming, P. L. (2003, February). Risk of Nosocomial Infection with Occupationally Acquired Human Immunodeficiency Virus (HIV) Infection. National Case Surveillance Data During 20 Years of the HIV Epidemic in the United States. *Infection Control and Hospital Epidemiology.* Atlanta, GA: Centers for Disease Control and Infection. Retrieved from http://www.cdc.gov/ncidod/dhqp/pdf/bbp/2402do.pdf.

Ernst, D. (2008, July). States fail to follow California's lead in certifying phlebotomists. *Medical Laboratory Observer*, 40–42.

Hegner, B., Acello, B. & Caldwell, E. (2008). *Nursing Assistant: A Nursing Process Approach*, 10th ed. Clifton Park, NY: Thomson/Delmar Learning, 2008.

Introducing virtual hospital: University of Iowa Hospitals and Clinics. Schwabauer, M. *Personnel Requirements and Classification.* Retrieved September 24, 2008, from http://medicine.uiowa.edu/cme/clia/module.asp?testID=12.

Massachusetts General Hospital. *History of Pathology at the Massachusetts General Hospital.* Retrieved April 15, 2010 from http://www2.massgeneral.org/pathology/history.htm.

McBride, K. (1978). Task Analysis of Medical Technology Administration and Supervision. *Amer J Med Technol*, 44; 688–695.

National Accrediting Agency for Clinical Laboratory Sciences (NAACLS). (2000). *The laboratory professional of the future. A compilation of data from the September 22, 2000 NAACLS Futures Conference.* Retrieved October 12, 2009 from http://www.naacls.org/news//naacls-news/archives.asp?article_id=742.

National Accrediting Agency for Clinical Laboratory Sciences (NAACLS). (2008). *Differentiate between the CLS/MT and CLT/MLT.* Chicago: NAACLS.

Nurse leads Birmingham, Ala. hospital's war on germs. *Chicago Tribune* (2002, July 22).

Index

Note: Page numbers followed by c, f, and t indicate charts, figures, and tables, respectively.